# Guidelines for Pulmonary Rehabilitation Programs

## FIFTH EDITION

### American Association of Cardiovascular and Pulmonary Rehabilitation

*Promoting Health and Preventing Disease*

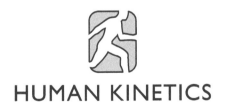

## HUMAN KINETICS

**Library of Congress Cataloging-in-Publication Data**

Names: American Association of Cardiovascular & Pulmonary Rehabilitation, author.

Title: Guidelines for pulmonary rehabilitation programs / AACVPR.

Description: Fifth edition. | Champaign, IL : Human Kinetics, Inc., [2020] | Includes bibliographical references and index.

Identifiers: LCCN 2018052383 (print) | LCCN 2018053038 (ebook) | ISBN 9781492587286 (e-book) | ISBN 9781492550914 (print)

Subjects: | MESH: Lung Diseases, Obstructive—rehabilitation | Needs Assessment | Patient Education as Topic | Rehabilitation—standards | Treatment Outcome | Guideline

Classification: LCC RC776.O3 (ebook) | LCC RC776.O3 (print) | NLM WF 600 | DDC 616.2/403—dc23

LC record available at https://lccn.loc.gov/2018052383

ISBN: 978-1-4925-5091-4 (print)

The web addresses cited in this text were current as of December 2018, unless otherwise noted.

Acquisitions Editor: Amy N. Tocco
Developmental Editor: Melissa J. Zavala
Indexer: Rebecca McCorkle
Permissions Manager: Dalene Reeder
Graphic Designer: Julie L. Denzer
Cover Designer: Keri Evans
Cover Design Associate: Susan Rothermel Allen
Photographs (interior): ©Human Kinetics, unless otherwise noted
Photo Production Manager: Jason Allen
Senior Art Manager: Kelly Hendren
Illustrations: ©Human Kinetics, unless otherwise noted
Production: Westchester Publishing Services
Printer: Seaway Printing

Printed in the United States of America        10   9   8   7   6   5   4

The paper in this book is certified under a sustainable forestry program.

**Human Kinetics**
1607 N. Market Street
Champaign, IL 61820
USA

*United States and International*
Website: **US.HumanKinetics.com**
Email: info@hkusa.com
Phone: 1-800-747-4457

*Canada*
Website: **Canada.HumanKinetics.com**
Email: info@hkcanada.com

E7061

**Tell us what you think!**
Human Kinetics would love to hear what we can do to improve the customer experience. Use this QR code to take our brief survey.

We dedicate these guidelines to all those pulmonary rehabilitation health care providers who, out of dedication and without fanfare, continue to provide this much-needed service.

# Contents

## 4 Collaborative Self-Management and Patient Education . . . . . . . . . . . . . . . . . 55

Gerene Bauldoff, Jane Knipper, and Debbie Koehl

## 5 Psychosocial Assessment and Intervention . . . . . . . . . . . . . . . . . . . 65

Maria Buckley and Kent Eichenauer

## 6 Nutritional Assessment and Intervention . . . . 79

Ellen Aberegg

## 7 Patient-Centered Evidence-Based Outcomes . . . . . . . . . . . . . . . . . . . . 91

Gerene Bauldoff and Eileen Collins

AACVPR Membership Application can be found at www.aacvpr.org. Click on the "Join" button and set up an account to begin your application.

# Preface

Pulmonary rehabilitation is an important intervention for patients with chronic lung disease. It improves patient exercise tolerance and health-related quality of life and reduces limiting symptoms. Pulmonary rehabilitation is comprised of patient-centered exercise training, education, psychosocial and nutritional assessment, and intervention as indicated based on a comprehensive assessment. The goal of pulmonary rehabilitation is to promote and maintain healthy behaviors in patients with chronic lung disease. This edition strives to address the informational needs of those wanting to learn what pulmonary rehabilitation is, those initiating a pulmonary rehabilitation program, and those wishing to update and improve their existing programs to meet AACVPR certification and national quality requirements.

Pulmonary rehabilitation is not a "one size fits all" therapy for the patient with chronic respiratory disease. Instead, it is tailored to the particular problems and needs of the respiratory patient, requiring active collaboration among the patient and an interdisciplinary team of professionals. Often the patient's family or concerned friends are brought into the collaboration process. Pulmonary rehabilitation, as it is currently practiced, is built on an ever-increasing base of scientific evidence, complemented by expert opinion in areas where focused clinical trials are needed. Because of these considerations, practice guidelines continue to be needed for the optimal application of the complex and evolving intervention that is pulmonary rehabilitation. These guidelines are meant to update the *Guidelines for Pulmonary Rehabilitation Programs, Fourth Edition*, published in 2011. Since 2011, the science of pulmonary rehabilitation has advanced considerably, its application has expanded, credentialing of programs has become increasingly important, and reimbursement has changed: thus, the need for new guidelines. This new edition is accompanied by a web resource. The web resource contains links to additional resources, and various forms, tools, and checklists useful for practitioners. The web resource is available at www.HumanKinetics.com/GuidelinesForPulmonaryRehabilition.

The authors involved with this edition are nationally and internationally recognized experts with many years of frontline experience in the delivery of pulmonary rehabilitation. Like pulmonary rehabilitation itself, this has been a collaborative effort, with input from nursing, medicine, respiratory therapy, exercise physiology, physical therapy, psychology, and nutrition.

This endeavor is meant to present the best clinical practice for pulmonary rehabilitation based on current scientific evidence and expert opinion. In this edition, we moved toward more of an evidence-based review in several areas based on the rapid expansion of high-quality scientific evidence since the last edition. We have tried to balance deep evidence-based information with a "nuts and bolts" approach while at the same time referring to important documents such as the American College of Chest Physicians/American Association of Cardiovascular and Pulmonary Rehabilitation (ACCP/AACVPR) Joint Evidence-Based Clinical Guidelines and the American Thoracic Society/European Respiratory Society (ATS/ERS) Statements on Pulmonary Rehabilitation.

## SUGGESTED ADDITIONAL RESOURCES

Those planning to implement a pulmonary rehabilitation program (or add to their existing program) can readily access some important websites, guidelines, and reviews of pulmonary rehabilitation. These complement the guidelines. A listing of some of these documents is given below.

> The American Association of Cardiovascular and Pulmonary Rehabilitation (AACVPR) website: www.aacvpr.org. This provides information on resources, publications, events, the annual meeting, and policy and reimbursement information regarding cardiac and pulmonary rehabilitation.

> The American Thoracic Society website pertaining to pulmonary rehabilitation: www.thoracic.org. Included here is information on the ATS Pulmonary Rehabilitation Assembly, resources for professionals, resources for patients, and access to published ATS statements such as the following:

Holland AE, et al. An official European Respiratory Society/American Thoracic Society technical standard: field walking tests in chronic respiratory disease. *Eur Respir J.* 2014;44:1428-1446.

Rochester CL, et al. An official American Thoracic Society/European Respiratory Society policy statement: enhancing implementation, use, and delivery of pulmonary rehabilitation. *Am J Respir Crit Care Med.* 2015;192(11):1373-1386.

McCarthy B, Casey D, Devane D, Murphy K, Murphy E, Lacasse Y. Pulmonary rehabilitation for chronic obstructive pulmonary disease. *Cochrane DB Syst Rev.* 2015;2:CD003793. This systematic review can be accessed at www.cochranelibrary.com.

Ries AL, et al. Pulmonary rehabilitation: joint ACCP/AACVPR evidence-based clinical guidelines. *Chest.* 2007 131:4S-42S. This is a systematic, evidence-based review of the medical literature on pulmonary rehabilitation, updating a 1997 document. Its summary is reproduced in chapter 1. This paper can be accessed at www.chestjournal .org.

# Acknowledgments

As cochairs of the writing committee of the AACVPR's *Guidelines for Pulmonary Rehabilitation Programs, Fifth Edition*, we would like to individually thank the members of the writing committee for sharing their expertise and passion in creating this book. Our members are nationally and internationally recognized experts in pulmonary rehabilitation. We sought to balance frontline experts with academic experts. This mindful decision resulted in an up-to-date "real world" emphasis regarding how to envision and implement high-quality pulmonary rehabilitation.

The chapter authors were carefully considered for expertise, comprehensive discipline, and geographic representation. The first listed author served as the primary author for the chapter. Except for chapter 1, which Dr. Carlin graciously completed individually, every chapter had multiple experts involved in the writing. All chapters were reviewed by the editors and the AACVPR Document Oversight Committee. Thank you to Richard Josephson, MS, MD, FAACVPR, and Eileen Collins, PhD, RN, FAACVPR, chairs of the committee during the review process.

Since chapter 3, Exercise Assessment and Training, involved such an extensive reenvisioning, this chapter was also sent to pulmonary rehabilitation exercise experts in the United States and Europe for review and input. We want to thank:

- Kim Eppen, PT, PhD, FAACVPR, University of Iowa, Iowa City, United States
- Deniz Inal-Ince, PhD, Haccepette University, Ankara, Turkey
- Daniel Langer, PT, PhD, University of Leuven, Flanders, Belgium

In addition, chapter 5, Psychosocial Assessment and Intervention, underwent significant rewriting and also received additional review and input. We wish to thank:

- Therese Shumaker, MA, RDN, Mayo Clinic, Rochester, Minnesota, United States
- Eva Serber, PhD, Medical University of South Carolina, Charleston, United States
- Megan McMurray, PhD, University of Alabama at Birmingham, United States

As this is the fifth edition of this book, we recognize that this version is built upon the excellent work of the prior editions. We especially want to thank the following fourth edition editors: Rebecca Crouch, PT, DPT, MAACVPR, and Richard ZuWallack, MD, for their expert navigation of this intense process. We also wish to thank the entire fourth edition writing team: Linda Nici, MD; Bonnie Fahy, RN, MS, CNS, FAACVPR; Paula Meek, PhD; Suzanne Lareau, RN, MSN; Carolyn Rochester, MD; Jonathan Raskin, MD, FCCP, FAACVPR; Neil MacIntyre, MD, FAACVPR; Chris Garvey, FNP, MSN, MPA, MAACVPR; Kathleen Steward, PT, DPT; Joseph Norman, PT, PhD, FAACVPR; Gerilynn Connors, BS, RRT, MAACVPR; Lana Hilling, RCP, MAACVPR; and Jane Reardon, RN, MSN, CS, FAACVPR.

*Gerene Bauldoff and Brian Carlin*

## Guidelines for Pulmonary Rehabilitation Programs, Fifth Edition, *Committee Members*

Cochairs: Gerene S. Bauldoff, PhD, RN, MAACVPR, and Brian Carlin, MD, MAACVPR

Ellen Aberegg, LD, MA, RD, FAACVPR

Maria Buckley, PhD, FAACVPR

Eileen Collins, PhD, RN, FAACVPR

Gerilynn Connors, BS, RRT, MAACVPR

Rebecca Crouch, PT, DPT, MS, CCS, MAACVPR

Kent Eichenauer, PsyD, FAACVPR

Chris Garvey, FNP, MSN, MPA, MAACVPR

Anne Gavic, MPA, RCEP, MAACVPR

Jane Knipper, RN, MA, AE-C, MAACVPR

Debbie Koehl, MS, RRT, AE-C

James Lamberti, MD, FCCP

Steven Lichtman, EdD, MAACVPR

Trina Limberg, BS, RRT, MAACVPR

Karen Lui, BSN, MS, MAACVPR

Katherine Menson, DO

Jonathan Raskin, MD, FAACVPR

June Schulz, RRT, FAACVPR

Charlotte Tenebeck, MD

David Verrill, MS, CEP, RCEP, FAACVPR

# Overview of Pulmonary Rehabilitation

## Brian Carlin, MD, MAACVPR
Sleep Medicine and Lung Health Consultants, Pittsburgh, PA

**P**ulmonary rehabilitation is an integral component of comprehensive medical therapy for patients with chronic respiratory disease. Pulmonary rehabilitation provides the greatest improvements in symptoms, exercise capacity, and health-related quality of life of any therapy available for patients with COPD. Pulmonary rehabilitation is now a prominent component for all major guidelines for the treatment of COPD. There is also strong rationale and a growing body of evidence for its use and effectiveness in patients with other respiratory disorders (1).

## DEFINITION

According to the 2013 American Thoracic Society/European Respiratory Society statement on pulmonary rehabilitation, "Pulmonary rehabilitation is a comprehensive intervention based on a thorough patient assessment followed by patient-tailored therapies that include, but are not limited to, exercise training, education, and behavior changes, designed to improve the physical and psychological condition of people with chronic respiratory disease and to promote the long-term adherence to health-enhancing behaviors" (1).

## RATIONALE FOR PULMONARY REHABILITATION

Pulmonary rehabilitation generally provides the greatest benefits of any therapy available for patients with COPD over a wide range of outcome areas, including symptom relief, exercise tolerance, and health-related quality of life. There is an emerging body of evidence indicating it reduces health care utilization and expenditures. These positive effects occur despite the fact that pulmonary rehabilitation does not directly improve lung function such as $FEV_1$. This apparent paradox is explained by the fact that pulmonary rehabilitation identifies, addresses, and treats the systemic problems and comorbid conditions that are common in these patients. Some examples of these other potentially reversible conditions include peripheral muscle dysfunction, the adoption of a sedentary lifestyle, body composition abnormalities, poor self-management skills, anxiety, and depression (1, 2, 3).

# PULMONARY REHABILITATION AND INTEGRATED CARE OF THE RESPIRATORY PATIENT

Patient assessment and goal setting, exercise training, self-management education, psychosocial support, and outcome measurement are conveniently and efficiently packaged as an interdisciplinary pulmonary rehabilitation program. However, pulmonary rehabilitation principles should be integrated into the lifelong management of all people with chronic respiratory disease. The World Health Organization defines integrated care as "a concept bringing together inputs, delivery, management and organization of services related to diagnosis, treatment, care, rehabilitation and health promotion" (4). For years, pulmonary rehabilitation has used an integrated, interdisciplinary approach to the management of chronic respiratory disease. As such, it has been a paradigm for chronic disease management. As we age as a society, the tenets of pulmonary rehabilitation should serve to provide insight and direction as a model for chronic disease management.

Integration of care is an important part of the care of patients with chronic respiratory disease as they often have multiple and important comorbidities, such as cardiovascular disease, osteoporosis, and diabetes. For example, the COPD patient has, on average, 6 to 8 other chronic medical conditions, compared to 1.8 for patients with other chronic illnesses (5). Because of this complexity, single disease-specific guidelines often fall short in meeting the needs of the individual patient and may even have undesirable effects.

The acute exacerbation of chronic respiratory disease can be devastating, with further impairments in lung function, further peripheral muscle dysfunction, further decreases in exercise capacity, decreased activity levels, worsening quality of life, increased health care utilization, and an increased mortality risk. The proper management of the exacerbation requires an integrated care approach, requiring collaboration among health care professionals in the hospital and the community (6). Patients in this setting may be more receptive to "teachable moments," may adopt self-management strategies, and may participate in rehabilitation. The introduction of pulmonary rehabilitation at the time of an acute respiratory exacerbation is important in the integrated care

approach to management, fostering interdisciplinary communication, promoting regular follow-up, and providing a means for seamless transition back to the community (7).

In light of this complexity, the optimal care of the patient with chronic respiratory disease mandates effective collaboration and integration of services within a complex network including the patient, the family, and all health care providers. Optimal care requires integration across settings, across providers, and across time. The motivated and educated patient is a central catalyst to this process. Pulmonary rehabilitation provides the opportunity to both address the complex needs of the individual patient and coordinate the multiple services and interventions to provide effective care.

# HISTORY OF PULMONARY REHABILITATION

The science of pulmonary rehabilitation has an illustrious history, and some important milestones are identified here. However, the ascent of pulmonary rehabilitation to its prominence has resulted from the efforts of countless dedicated professionals, including clinicians and researchers, most of whom have gone unrecognized. Astute clinicians have long believed that a comprehensive care approach to treatment of their patients with chronic respiratory disease is necessary for maximal benefits. This comprehensive approach included breathing techniques, exercise therapy, supplemental oxygen, and bronchial hygiene techniques (8). This, of course, was the prototype of our current pulmonary rehabilitation approach. Thomas Petty, MD, reported in 1974 that COPD patients who participated in comprehensive care at his institution had fewer symptoms and utilized fewer hospital resources than those receiving standard care (9). In 1983, Bebout and colleagues demonstrated a health care utilization benefit from pulmonary rehabilitation (10). Conclusions at this time were based on personal observation, studies with comparator groups, or pre- and post-analyses. The scientific evidence base supporting these conclusions was, therefore, limited. In 1989, Andrew Ries reported on the clinical benefits noted following rehabilitation from the research that was available at the time. This review provided the stage for the development of pulmonary rehabilitation programs throughout the world (11).

Throughout the 1990s, the scientific basis for pulmonary rehabilitation for patients with COPD was further established from a scientific and clinical perspective. In 1991, Richard Casaburi and colleagues reported on the physiological effects of exercise training in 19 patients with COPD (12). Up to this time the prevailing thought was that higher levels of exercise training in COPD patients was impossible because of ventilatory limitation; therefore, meaningful physiological benefits from exercise training could not be achieved. This study demonstrated that exercise training does indeed lead to physiological improvements, and these improvements are dose dependent. In 1996, Maltais and colleagues reported that oxidative capacity in lower-extremity skeletal muscles of patients with COPD was decreased compared to normal subjects (13). In a subsequent study they showed that these oxidative enzymes increased after high-intensity exercise training (14). These studies and subsequent ones demonstrated that COPD does cause biochemical and physiological derangements in exercising muscles and that these derangements can be treated. Decreases in these muscle derangements resulting from pulmonary rehabilitation exercise training led to improvement in physiological function, such as changes in breathing pattern and decreases in dynamic hyperinflation (15). Thus, the effectiveness of pulmonary rehabilitation depends in large part on its improvement in the systemic effects of chronic respiratory disease.

In 1994, Reardon and colleagues showed that a group of patients completing outpatient pulmonary rehabilitation had less exertional dyspnea than a control group who received otherwise standard care (16). A subsequent study by O'Donnell and colleagues demonstrated the physiological changes underlying this improvement in dyspnea (17). In the same year, Goldstein and colleagues demonstrated that pulmonary rehabilitation improves health-related quality of life, further demonstrating that pulmonary rehabilitation leads to improvement in patient-centered outcomes (18).

In 1995, Ries and colleagues reported on 119 COPD patients who were randomized to either eight weeks of comprehensive outpatient pulmonary rehabilitation or eight weeks of education only. Pulmonary rehabilitation resulted in improvements in exercise tolerance, symptoms, and self-efficacy for walking. This was the first randomized controlled study of patients with COPD undergoing rehabilitation and was the basis for the acceptance of pulmonary rehabilitation as a true component of the management of a patient with COPD by the medical community (19).

Between 1998 and 2002, 3,777 patients with emphysema were evaluated and 1,218 were randomized in the National Emphysema Treatment Trial (NETT) (20). This landmark study was designed to evaluate the short-term and long-term risks and benefits of bilateral lung volume reduction surgery (LVRS) to treat severe emphysema, but a key component of the study was that pulmonary rehabilitation was required for all patients entering the study. A subsequent subanalysis from this study showed substantial benefit from pulmonary rehabilitation (21).

In the mid-1990s, a group of rehabilitation professionals reviewed the available evidence regarding the effectiveness of pulmonary rehabilitation and made several "evidence-based" recommendations. Using a true evidence-based review and approach with their methodology, the American College of Chest Physicians (ACCP) and the American Association of Cardiovascular and Pulmonary Rehabilitation published the first evidence-based clinical practice guidelines in the field in 1997 (22). These guidelines summarized the evidence base behind the components and outcomes of pulmonary rehabilitation. An update of these evidence-based guidelines was published 10 years later (2). The summary of these later recommendations and subsequent recommendations from other international societies is provided later in this chapter. The Global Initiative for Chronic Obstructive Lung Disease (GOLD) recommendations published in 2017 clearly state the importance of pulmonary rehabilitation as a key component in the management of patients with COPD (3).

In 2000, Griffiths and colleagues reported on a randomized controlled trial of outpatient pulmonary rehabilitation versus standard care (23). With a sample size of 200, this remains the largest randomized trial of pulmonary rehabilitation. This landmark study corroborated earlier investigations by demonstrating that pulmonary rehabilitation led to improvements in exercise performance and health-related quality of life. Furthermore, it also provided evidence that pulmonary rehabilitation can potentially decrease health care costs. Subsequent nonrandomized multicenter studies in California (24) and the northeastern United States (25) further demonstrated a health resource utilization benefit.

In 2003, Bourbeau and colleagues showed that an outpatient self-management educational program can have substantial benefits for patients with COPD, including a 40% reduction in hospitalizations and a 59% reduction in unscheduled

## Figure 1.1   Evidence-based guidelines

1. A program of exercise training of the muscles of ambulation is recommended as a mandatory component of pulmonary rehabilitation for patients with COPD. *Grade of recommendation: 1A*

2. Pulmonary rehabilitation improves the symptom of dyspnea in patients with COPD. *Grade of recommendation: 1A*

3. Pulmonary rehabilitation improves health-related quality of life in patients with COPD. *Grade of recommendation: 1A*

4. Pulmonary rehabilitation reduces the number of hospital days and other measures of health care utilization in patients with COPD. *Grade of recommendation: 2B*

5. Pulmonary rehabilitation is cost-effective in patients with COPD. *Grade of recommendation: 2C*

6. There is insufficient evidence to determine if pulmonary rehabilitation improves survival in patients with COPD. *No recommendation is provided.*

7. There are psychosocial benefits from comprehensive pulmonary rehabilitation programs in patients with COPD. *Grade of recommendation: 2B*

8. Six to 12 weeks of pulmonary rehabilitation produce benefits in several outcomes that decline gradually over 12 to 18 months. *Grade of recommendation: 1A*

9. Some benefits, such as health-related quality of life, remain above control at 12 to 18 months. *Grade of recommendation: 1C*

10. Longer pulmonary rehabilitation programs (12 weeks) produce greater sustained benefits than shorter programs. *Grade of recommendation: 2C*

11. Maintenance strategies following pulmonary rehabilitation have a modest effect on long-term outcomes. *Grade of recommendation: 2C*

12. Lower-extremity exercise training at higher exercise intensity produces greater physiological benefits than lower-intensity training in patients with COPD. *Grade of recommendation: 1B*

13. Both low- and high-intensity exercise training produce clinical benefits for patients with COPD. *Grade of recommendation: 1A*

14. Addition of a strength training component to a program of pulmonary rehabilitation increases muscle strength and muscle mass. *Grade of recommendation: 1A*

15. Current scientific evidence does not support the routine use of anabolic agents in pulmonary rehabilitation for patients with COPD. *Grade of recommendation: 2C*

physician visits (26). This supported the idea that pulmonary rehabilitation is more than just physical exercise training. The concept of collaborative self-management in chronic disease has grown substantially since this time and is now a core component of all pulmonary rehabilitation programs.

In 2009, the United States Congress passed a bill making pulmonary rehabilitation a Medicare-reimbursed benefit for patients with moderate to severe COPD (27). This law currently serves as the basis for providing pulmonary rehabilitation services for not only the Medicare population but those with other payer backgrounds. These standards will be discussed throughout this text. Subsequent to the passage of this law, a significant amount of ongoing research in the field has been conducted. Now patients with other diseases, including those with pulmonary hypertension, interstitial lung disease, and cystic fibrosis, have been shown to benefit from pulmonary rehabilitation. In addition, the exercise training and educational training as well as the inclusion of self-management skills have become routine parts of the rehabilitation program and are the subject of this text.

Over the next decade, refinements in the provision of pulmonary rehabilitation for patients with COPD were made. This included expansion of the exercise training regimens to include various types of training protocols as well as the use of supplemental equipment (e.g., rollators) for training patients with COPD. Emphasis on self-management skills as well as on the inclusion of patients who

16. Unsupported endurance training of the upper extremities is beneficial in patients with COPD and should be included in pulmonary rehabilitation programs. *Grade of recommendation: 1A*

17. The scientific evidence does not support the routine use of inspiratory muscle training as an essential component of pulmonary rehabilitation. *Grade of recommendation: 1B*

18. Education should be an integral component of pulmonary rehabilitation. Education should include information on collaborative self-management and prevention and treatment of exacerbations. *Grade of recommendation: 1B*

19. There is minimal evidence to support the benefits of psychosocial interventions as a single therapeutic modality. *Grade of recommendation: 2C*

20. Although scientific evidence is lacking, current practice and expert opinion support the inclusion of psychosocial interventions as a component of comprehensive pulmonary rehabilitation programs for patients with COPD. *No recommendation is provided.*

21. Supplemental oxygen should be used during rehabilitative exercise training in patients with severe exercise-induced hypoxemia. *Grade of recommendation: 1C*

22. Administering supplemental oxygen during high-intensity exercise programs in patients without exercise-induced hypoxemia may improve gains in exercise endurance. *Grade of recommendation: 2C*

23. As an adjunct to exercise training in selected patients with severe COPD, noninvasive ventilation produces modest additional improvements in exercise performance. *Grade of recommendation: 2B*

24. There is insufficient evidence to support the routine use of nutritional supplementation in pulmonary rehabilitation of patients with COPD. *No recommendation is provided.*

25. Pulmonary rehabilitation is beneficial for some patients with chronic respiratory diseases other than COPD. *Grade of recommendation: 1B*

26. Although scientific evidence is lacking, current practice and expert opinion suggest that pulmonary rehabilitation for patients with chronic respiratory diseases other than COPD should be modified to include treatment strategies specific to individual diseases and patients in addition to treatment strategies common to both COPD and non-COPD patients. *No recommendation is provided.*

Reprinted by permission from L. Andrew et al., "Joint ACCP/AACVPR Evidence-Based Clinical Practice Guidelines," *Chest* 131 (2004) 7: 4S-42S

have chronic lung disease other than COPD (e.g., interstitial fibrosis, pulmonary hypertension, bronchiectasis, etc.) has been further clarified (1). Over this time, evidence-based guidelines and recommendations have been made by a variety of medical societies throughout the world.

# EVIDENCE-BASED GUIDELINES ON PULMONARY REHABILITATION

The guidelines from the various world societies have been developed over the last decade. They include the most recent literature in the field showing the benefits of pulmonary rehabilitation for patients with symptomatic chronic lung disease. They also include recommendations for outcome assessment. While each guideline used a different methodology for evidence evaluation and recommendations, the overarching results show that pulmonary rehabilitation is an essential component in the overall management for a patient who has symptomatic chronic lung disease. For a detailed review of the methodology used, please refer to the individual guideline publication. The following is a summary of the individual guideline recommendations. In those instances in which a repeat recommendation is made, it is not included in this text.

The American College of Chest Physicians and the American Association of Cardiovascular and

Pulmonary Rehabilitation updated a previous evidence-based guideline in 2007 (2). This is the first set of evidence-based guidelines publications in the field. Their recommendations were categorized as *strong* (grade 1) or *weak* (grade 2). The strength of evidence was determined based on the quality of the data: *high* (grade A, from well-designed randomized clinical trials yielding consistent and directly applicable results or from overwhelming evidence from observational studies), *moderate* (grade B, for the most part randomized clinical trials with limitations that may include methodological flaws or inconsistent results), and *low* (grade C, from other types of observational studies). These guidelines appear in figure 1.1.

Other societies have reviewed and extended these recommended guidelines (appendix E). The British Thoracic Society guidelines include grade D, reflecting *lower level evidence.* The Canadian Thoracic Society addresses some issues not covered by those previously released guidelines (28). In 2015, the American Thoracic Society and European Respiratory Society updated their previous recommendations for pulmonary rehabilitation (1). They noted noteworthy advances in the field.

The most recent guidelines published were by the Australian/New Zealand guideline panel in 2017 (29). Their recommendations included many of the previously noted recommendations from the other groups but extended the recommendations in several areas, particularly with regard to patients with more mild disease and symptomatology, the place of provision of the rehabilitative services to include the home environment, and patients with diseases other than COPD. A summary of the pertinent new recommendations appears in appendix E with the guidelines from the other societies discussed here.

# POSITIONING PULMONARY REHABILITATION WITHIN THE GOLD 2017 GUIDELINES

The current GOLD recommendations (2017) for the management of a patient with COPD include the recommendation for the use of pulmonary rehabilitation as part of the comprehensive treatment of this disease (3). Pulmonary rehabilitation should be considered for COPD patients who have dyspnea or other respiratory symptoms, reduced exercise capacity, restriction in activities, or impaired health status. Pulmonary rehabilitation is considered an option for moderate disease, as symptoms become present on a daily basis. As the symptom burden increases, the need for pulmonary rehabilitation increases.

# CURRENT STATUS OF PULMONARY REHABILITATION

Pulmonary rehabilitation is now firmly established as a standard for the management of COPD patients. In 2009, the United States Congress passed a bill to include pulmonary rehabilitation as a reimbursable service provided under the Medicare law. Benefits in reducing dyspnea, improving exercise tolerance, improvement in health-related quality of life, and reducing health care expenditures have all been shown in a variety of studies over the last three decades for a variety of patients with chronic lung disease (e.g., COPD, interstitial lung disease, pulmonary hypertension), yet challenges remain to the provision of rehabilitation services to those in need.

## Increasing Availability

COPD is the third leading cause of death in the United States. It is known that pulmonary rehabilitation patients with COPD is an essential component of the management of a patient with COPD, yet it is underrecognized and underutilized for those in need. Less than 5% of Medicare patients with COPD have actually been enrolled in a pulmonary rehabilitation program (30, 31). Too few pulmonary rehabilitation programs are currently available to meet this need. Even in areas where pulmonary rehabilitation programs are available, they are underutilized by health care professionals. Many health care providers and patients are unaware of the potential benefits that can be gained following pulmonary rehabilitation as well as whether a program exists in the local community. Increased education of health care professionals and patients on the rationale, indications, and proven benefits should be helpful to address concern that rehabilitation is underutilized. Adequate reimbursement for pulmonary rehabilitation should also help to alleviate the burden.

## Widening Applicability

Widening the applicability of pulmonary rehabilitation should naturally follow the growing evidence base supporting its use in chronic respiratory diseases other than COPD. Widening the applicability should include the use of pulmonary rehabilitation for those patients who have symptoms but who are in a milder stage of the disease, following either an exacerbation or hospitalization, or who are at the end of their lives in collaboration with palliative care. There is a widening applicability for those patients with diseases other than COPD (e.g., interstitial lung disease, pulmonary hypertension, lung cancer) and those with other forms of COPD (e.g., asthma, cystic fibrosis, non-cystic bronchiectasis) (1, 32, 33).

## Maintaining Long-Term Benefits and Promoting Self-Efficacy

The exercise benefits of pulmonary rehabilitation tend to decrease after completion of the formal program. Multiple reasons for this include: poor adherence to exercise and activity prescription, underlying exacerbations, influence of comorbid conditions, and deterioration from the disease itself. The comprehensive multicomponent pulmonary rehabilitation program must address this issue. Potential solutions to this include providing longer pulmonary rehabilitation programs, reintroduction of a modified form of pulmonary rehabilitation after an exacerbation, incorporation of structured exercise and increased activity in the home setting, and promotion of self-management strategies that encourage the patient to be more responsible for his or her health (34).

# SUMMARY

Pulmonary rehabilitation is now recognized as a key component in the management of a patient with chronic lung disease who is symptomatic. Benefits of pulmonary rehabilitation include decrease in dyspnea level, increase in exercise tolerance, improvement of health-related quality of life, and reduction in health care expenditures. With increasing availability and increasing referral of patients with symptomatic chronic lung disease to pulmonary rehabilitation programs, further benefits can be afforded to a larger number of symptomatic patients.

**VISIT THE WEB RESOURCE** ———————————————————
for links to additional resources and various tools, checklists, and forms.

# CHAPTER

# Selecting and Assessing the Pulmonary Rehabilitation Candidate

**Gerilynn Connors, BS, RRT, MAACVPR, FAARC**
Inova Fairfax Medical Campus, Falls Church, VA

**James Lamberti, MD, FCCP**
Inova Fairfax Medical Campus, Falls Church, VA

A comprehensive pulmonary rehabilitation program should be developed for the individual patient with chronic respiratory disease. Health care providers and patients are often unaware of the benefits of pulmonary rehabilitation, and it has been prescribed late in the trajectory of chronic respiratory disease. Patients often present to pulmonary rehabilitation programs with severe impairment and significantly reduced quality of life. It is important for pulmonary rehabilitation specialists to educate the public and medical community about the role of pulmonary rehabilitation across the spectrum of pulmonary disease as well as the importance of prevention and early detection of respiratory disease.

The goal of a comprehensive pulmonary rehabilitation program is selecting the right individual pulmonary rehabilitation program for the right patient. The initial component of a pulmonary rehabilitation program is the interdisciplinary team assessment. The components of pulmonary rehabilitation (e.g., assessment, exercise training, self-management education, psychosocial interventions, and long-term adherence) cannot be appropriately tailored to the individual patient without a thorough initial and ongoing individualized assessment.

A recent definition of pulmonary rehabilitation emphasizes the importance of a thorough assessment: "Pulmonary rehabilitation is a comprehensive intervention based on a thorough patient assessment followed by patient-tailored therapies, which include, but are not limited to, exercise training, education and behavior change, designed to improve the physical and psychological condition of people with chronic respiratory disease and to promote the long-term adherence of health-enhancing behaviors"(1).

## PATIENT SELECTION

Until the past decade, most of the patients referred for pulmonary rehabilitation suffered from COPD. There is an enlarging body of evidence of the clinical usefulness of pulmonary rehabilitation in diseases other than COPD (1) (figure 2.1). Programs should recommend pulmonary rehabilitation for patients who are compromised because of

## Figure 2.1    Conditions appropriate for referral to pulmonary rehabilitation

**Obstructive diseases**

- COPD (including alpha-1 antitrypsin deficiency)
- Persistent asthma
- Diffuse bronchiectasis
- Cystic fibrosis
- Bronchiolitis obliterans

**Restrictive diseases**

- Interstitial lung diseases
- Interstitial fibrosis
- Occupational or environmental lung disease
- Sarcoidosis
- Connective tissue diseases
- Hypersensitivity pneumonitis
- Lymphangiomyomatosis

- ARDS survivors
- Chest wall diseases
- Kyphoscoliosis
- Ankylosing spondylitis
- Posttuberculosis syndrome

**Other conditions**

- Lung cancer
- Pulmonary hypertension
- Before and after thoracic and abdominal surgery
- Before and after lung transplantation
- Before and after lung volume reduction surgery
- Ventilator dependency
- Obesity-related respiratory disease

Definition of abbreviations: ARDS = acute respiratory distress syndrome; COPD = chronic obstructive pulmonary disease.

Reprinted from M.A. Spruit, S.J. Singh, C. Garvey C, et al. "An Official American Thoracic Society/European Respiratory Society Statement: Key Concepts and Advances in Pulmonary Rehabilitation," *The American Journal of Respiratory and Critical Care Medicine*, 188, No. 8 (2013): e13-e64. Copyright © 2013 American Thoracic Society. www.thoracic.org/statements/resources/copd/P=Executive_Summary2013.pdf

their lung disease. It is important that pulmonary rehabilitation staff understand the pathophysiology and clinical presentation of the diverse pulmonary diseases that they may evaluate and treat (2).

## COPD

Patients with COPD often decrease their physical activity because exercise can lead to worsening dyspnea. Pulmonary rehabilitation improves functional exercise capacity and dynamic mechanics of breathing during exercise in patients with COPD. Studies document improvement in health-related quality of life measures such as dyspnea and fatigue (3). In the past, pulmonary rehabilitation has often been reserved for COPD patients with severe airflow obstruction. The Global Initiative for Chronic Obstructive Lung Disease (GOLD) recommends that pulmonary rehabilitation be included in the management of patients with high symptom burden or an increased risk of exacerbations (GOLD groups B, C, and D), without utilizing a spirometry-based $FEV_1$ threshold (4). Centers for Medicare and Medicaid Services (CMS) has approved pulmonary rehabilitation for

patients with moderate to very severe COPD as defined by GOLD spirometry classification ($FEV_1$ postbronchodilator < 80% of predicted and $FEV_1$/FVC ratio < .70). Individual Medicare Administrative Contractors (MACs) may have separate local coverage determinations (LCDs) for pulmonary rehabilitation.

There is often concern from referring providers and pulmonary rehabilitation staff that an individual patient may be "too sick" to undertake pulmonary rehabilitation. A recent study found that one-quarter of patients with COPD referred for pulmonary rehabilitation suffered from frailty. Frailty was defined using the Fried criteria of weight loss, exhaustion, low physical activity, slowness, and weakness (5). Even though frailty was a predictor of noncompletion of a pulmonary rehabilitation program, frail patients demonstrated better outcomes versus non-frail patients in dyspnea, exercise performance, physical activity, and health status (6). Even patients with chronic hypercapnic respiratory failure show benefit from pulmonary rehabilitation (7).

The recent ERS/ATS guideline for the management of COPD exacerbations suggests that patients who are hospitalized with a COPD exacerbation should be considered for initiation of pulmonary rehabilitation within three weeks after hospital discharge. Studies suggest that early pulmonary rehabilitation after hospitalization for an exacerbation reduces subsequent hospital admissions and improves quality of life. However, the ERS/ATS guideline recommends not commencing pulmonary rehabilitation during a hospitalization for a COPD exacerbation (8).

## Pulmonary Diseases Other than COPD

Increased recognition and improved management of pulmonary disease have led to many patients with pulmonary diseases other than COPD being referred for pulmonary rehabilitation. For respiratory diseases other than COPD, pulmonary rehabilitation should be considered for symptomatic patients whose quality of life is impaired by their disease.

Asthma is a common disease, with an estimated adult U.S. prevalence in 2015 of 7.6% (9). Despite optimal pharmacologic therapy, patients with chronic asthma may experience dyspnea, increased work of breathing, and decreased exercise tolerance. A recent meta-analysis reported improved aerobic capacity ($VO_2max$) in asthmatic patients who undertook exercise training (10). A comprehensive pulmonary rehabilitation program can educate patients on important topics such as the recognition and avoidance of asthma triggers, establishment of an asthma action plan, and developing an exercise training program.

Because of advances in disease management, the median predicted survival age for patients with cystic fibrosis (CF) has increased steadily from age 31.3 years in 2002 to age 41.4 in 2015 (11). Higher levels of physical fitness (as measured by aerobic capacity) have been associated with better survival in CF. Aerobic exercise is recommended as an adjunctive therapy for airway clearance and for its additional benefits to overall health (12). A Cochrane review shows improvements in exercise capacity, strength, and quality of life after exercise training, with some evidence of a slower decline in lung function in patients with CF (13). Airway clearance techniques, such as huff cough, vibratory positive expiratory pressure (PEP), autogenic drainage and high frequency chest wall oscillation are important treatments of cystic fibrosis, and training regarding their use and benefits should be included in a pulmonary rehabilitation program for these patients.

Non–cystic fibrosis bronchiectasis is a chronic condition characterized by persistent cough, excessive sputum production, and recurrent respiratory infections. Chronic airflow obstruction may be present and intermittent acute infectious exacerbations can occur. Pulmonary rehabilitation is effective in improving exercise tolerance in patients with bronchiectasis (14). Patients with bronchiectasis may benefit from education on recognition of exacerbations, use of inhaled medications, and airway clearance techniques.

Although the pathophysiology of respiratory limitation in COPD and interstitial lung disease (ILD) is different, the clinical limitations (exercise capacity, dyspnea, muscle dysfunction, and quality of life) are similar. In a large cohort of patients with ILD, pulmonary rehabilitation had a positive impact on functional capacity and quality of life (15). A Cochrane review concluded that pulmonary rehabilitation in patients with ILD is safe and led to improvement in functional exercise capacity, dyspnea, and quality of life (16). The ATS/ERS/JRS/ALAT statement on the diagnosis and management of idiopathic pulmonary fibrosis (IPF) recommended that most patients with IPF should be treated with pulmonary rehabilitation (17). There are few educational resources available for patients with ILD, and a recent study documents the unmet educational needs of this patient group (18). Pulmonary rehabilitation represents a unique opportunity to educate ILD patients regarding their disease and specific approaches to treatment.

In patients with pulmonary hypertension, a meta-analysis concluded that pulmonary rehabilitation results in clinically relevant improvements in exercise capacity without serious adverse events (19). The American College of Cardiology 2013 treatment algorithm of pulmonary arterial hypertension upgraded the recommendation for rehabilitation and exercise training to a Class I with a Level of Evidence A (20). Pulmonary rehabilitation plays an essential role in the management of individuals before and after lung transplantation (21, 22). Pulmonary rehabilitation is recommended prior to lung volume reduction surgery (LVRS) (23). Patients with lung cancer often suffer from exercise intolerance and functional disability, and pulmonary rehabilitation before resectional lung surgery can improve aerobic capacity and 6-minute walk test (6MWT) distance (24).

# Comorbidities

Comorbidities are common in patients with chronic respiratory disease such as COPD and IPF (25, 26). Cardiovascular disease (hypertension, coronary artery disease, congestive heart failure, arrhythmia), metabolic disorders (diabetes mellitus, hyperthyroidism and hypothyroidism, hyperlipidemia), musculoskeletal disorders (orthopedic, osteoporosis, osteoarthritis), behavioral health problems (anxiety, depression, cognitive dysfunction, psychiatric disorders), sleep apnea, swallowing dysfunction, gastroesophageal reflux, advanced liver disease are just a few of the comorbidities that contribute to the symptom burden and functional limitation in patients. Concurrent diseases or conditions may interfere with the pulmonary rehabilitation process and become critical when assessing and outlining a comprehensive pulmonary rehabilitation program for the patient. If possible, the comorbid conditions should be corrected or stabilized prior to program entrance. Any comorbidity that would increase patient risk or interfere substantially with the pulmonary rehabilitation process may be a contraindication. The comorbidity exclusion of a candidate is dependent on the decision of the referring physician and the pulmonary rehabilitation medical director in collaboration with the results of the comprehensive pulmonary rehabilitation assessment.

# Other Considerations in Patient Selection

This section describes considerations in patient selection.

## Smoking

Current cigarette smoking should not be viewed as a contraindication to pulmonary rehabilitation, but rather as an opportunity to assist the individual with smoking cessation. Smoking cessation is an integral component of a comprehensive pulmonary rehabilitation program. Independent of the patient's age, smoking cessation positively affects symptoms, progression of lung function, and mortality in patients with chronic lung disease (27). Assessment of the patient's history of smoking, how often the patient has tried to stop smoking, types of programs and medications used and when the patient was successful in smoking cessation should be determined (28). Current smokers need to determine a quit date and should receive counseling. They should be provided access to a free telephone quit line (800-QUIT NOW) or free smartphone applications (e.g., QuitRight). A recent meta-analysis determined that a combination of behavioral and pharmacologic therapy is effective in assisting smokers with COPD to quit (29). The pulmonary rehabilitation team member should understand the role of nicotine addiction and available pharmacotherapy treatments to provide the patient with the best success, counseling, and support (30).

## Motivation and Adherence

Motivation and adherence of the pulmonary patient should be evaluated during the initial pulmonary rehabilitation assessment. The World Health Organization (WHO) defines adherence in health care as "the extent to which a person's behavior—taking medication, following a diet, and/or executing lifestyle changes, corresponds with agreed recommendations from a health care provider" (31). A prior history of poor adherence should not be a reason for an individual to be excluded from pulmonary rehabilitation. The pulmonary rehabilitation team should strive to understand the factors and underlying issues that may be impacting the individual's compliance. Barriers affecting adherence include socioeconomic, therapy-related, patient-related, condition-related, and the health system or health care team. Education of the referring health care provider and patient of the health benefits of pulmonary rehabilitation will improve adherence. Other adherence-promoting factors include enthusiasm of the referring provider, ease of access to the center, providing the intervention in a more convenient location (such as the home or satellite location), flexibility in program delivery (such as using digital technology for delivery), encouraging self-management, increasing self-confidence, and increasing patient comfort within the program (32).

## Financial Considerations

Insurance authorization and patient out-of-pocket cost should be evaluated prior to starting a comprehensive pulmonary rehabilitation program. Financial burden can impact the patient's participation, motivation, and adherence to treatment. The medical insurance billing codes should be understood by the pulmonary rehabilitation team and are discussed in chapter 9.

## Transportation

Transportation is a socioeconomic factor that can impact a patient's adherence to attend and complete a pulmonary rehabilitation program (33). The time commitment for the patient in traveling to the pulmonary program, the ability of the patient to travel alone, and the patient's restricted mobility limiting access to public transportation should be discussed. A patient using oxygen or with vision problems may have additional issues and possible barriers to driving or commuting to a pulmonary rehabilitation program. Assessment should include the means of transportation by self, family members, and friends or if public transit will be used. The cost of transportation can also impact the overall cost of the program for the patient. Accessible parking and determination if the patient qualifies for a disability parking placard should be covered during the assessment. Travel, transportation, and location of the pulmonary rehabilitation program can be barriers for a patient, and the pulmonary rehabilitation team needs to understand and address these concerns.

# PATIENT ASSESSMENT

This section details all the elements of a patient assessment.

## Interview

The initial assessment should begin with a patient interview (an example is given in appendix A). An in-depth interview with the patient and his family or significant other is necessary to set the stage for the assessment. The importance of the initial interview cannot be overstated. Not only are important data obtained, but the foundations of trust and credibility are established. The interview allows the patient to interact on a personal level with the rehabilitation staff. If the patient did not come in for a tour of the pulmonary rehabilitation program before their initial evaluation, the initial assessment allows the patient to see where the program is located and possibly meet other rehabilitation program participants.

## Medical History

A thorough review of the patient's medical status is essential for the initial assessment. Much of this information can be obtained from patient records

### Figure 2.2   Components of the medical history

- Respiratory history
- Comorbidities (especially coronary artery disease, diabetes, osteoporosis, sleep apnea, orthopedic issues)
- Other medical and surgical history
- Family history of respiratory disease
- Use of medical resources (e.g., hospitalizations, urgent care or emergency room visits, physician visits, exacerbations)
- All current medications including over-the-counter drugs and herbal supplements; includes dose, route, and frequency
- Oxygen: how it is prescribed and how the patient actually utilizes it
- Allergies and drug intolerances
- Smoking history
- Occupational, environmental, and recreational exposures
- Alcohol and other substance abuse history
- Social support

from the referring physician's office or hospital records. The medical history provides information on the severity of respiratory disease, such as symptom burden, exacerbations, medication requirements, supplemental oxygen use, comorbidities, physical limitations, and health resource utilization. The medical history is also important in highlighting comorbid conditions that may have a direct bearing on the patient's health, safety, and response to pulmonary rehabilitation. Components of medical history are included (figure 2.2). For example, unstable angina should be treated and stabilized before pulmonary rehabilitation, and an orthopedic or neurologic disorder may necessitate changes in the frequency, intensity, duration, and mode of exercise.

## Physical Assessment

Physical assessment adds important information to data obtained from the patient's history and from medical record and laboratory review. While a complete physical examination is part of the initial assessment, the aspects of this assessment represent the minimal information that should be obtained.

- Vital signs: blood pressure, pulse, respiratory rate, oxygen saturation, temperature
- Height, weight, BMI
- Breathing pattern
- Use of accessory muscles of respiration
- Chest exam: inspection, palpation, percussion, symmetry, diaphragm position, breath sounds, adventitious sounds (crackles, wheezes, rhonchi), duration of expiratory phase
- Cardiac exam: cardiac rate and rhythm, murmur, gallops, jugular venous distention
- Presence of digital clubbing
- Upper- and lower-extremity evaluation: joint disease, musculoskeletal dysfunction, range of motion, muscle atrophy, edema

## Diagnostic Tests

Diagnostic tests provide essential information to assist in the assessment of the rehabilitation candidate, determine proper billing code use and the development of an individualized treatment plan (ITP). Many of these tests will already be available in the patient's medical record and do not need to be repeated. Additional laboratory tests may also be recommended for selected patients as determined by the initial and ongoing assessments (figure 2.3).

Essential data needed at the initial assessment of the pulmonary rehabilitation candidate includes

- History and physical examination from referring physician to include recent office notes
- Spirometry (postbronchodilator $FEV_1$, FVC, and $FEV_1$/FVC ratio)
- Complete pulmonary function test (spirometry, lung volume, and diffusion capacity) if available

## Symptom Assessment

Information from symptom assessment is often utilized in goal setting, may be used to document outcomes, and may be used by third-party payers to determine the medical necessity for the service. These diagnostic tests and outcome tools help establish a baseline of the patient's current clinical

**Figure 2.3   Diagnostic tests to suggest for selected patients after the pulmonary rehabilitation assessment**

- Complete pulmonary function test (spirometry, lung volumes, diffusing capacity)
- Maximal inspiratory and expiratory pressures
- Cardiopulmonary exercise testing
- Postexercise spirometry
- Sleep study
- Chest x-ray
- Bone densitometry
- Cardiac testing: Holter monitor, echocardiogram, thallium exercise stress test
- Alpha-1 antitrypsin level in patients with COPD
- HbA1c for diabetic patients
- Thyroid panel
- Complete blood count
- Comprehensive metabolic profile

status and are used after program completion to evaluate pre- and post-outcomes.

### *Symptom assessment*

- Dyspnea
- Fatigue
- Frailty and grip strength
- Cough
- Sputum production
- Wheeze
- Hemoptysis
- Edema
- Sleep disorders
- Sinus disease postnasal drainage
- Chest pain
- Gastroesophageal reflux
- Dysphagia
- Extremity pain or weakness
- Feelings of anxiety, panic, fear, isolation
- Depressive symptoms

## Dyspnea

Dyspnea is usually the primary symptom in patients with respiratory disease and must be documented and quantified. Dyspnea is assessed, objectively measured, included in goal setting, and treated throughout the pulmonary rehabilitation program. In the initial patient assessment, its onset, quality, quantity (intensity), frequency, and duration should be documented. It is also useful to identify factors that make this symptom better or worse. One way to clinically assess dyspnea severity is to determine the type of physical activity that typically brings it on, such as carrying laundry up one flight of stairs. It is recommended that an objective measurement tool such as the Modified Medical Research Council Dyspnea Scale (figure 2.4) is utilized.

Dyspnea can also be quantified during exercise training and outcome assessment in pulmonary rehabilitation. Dyspnea during exercise training is commonly rated with a 10-point Borg scale or a visual analog scale. Dyspnea is also included in outcome assessment using instruments such as the Baseline Dyspnea Index (BDI), the UCSD Shortness of Breath Questionnaire (SOBQ), or the dyspnea domain of the Chronic Respiratory Disease Questionnaire (CRQ, or CRDQ). These tools are discussed in chapter 7.

## Fatigue

Fatigue is a common and distressing symptom in patients with chronic respiratory disease, and its importance is often underrecognized and ignored by the pulmonary rehabilitation team. Fatigue impacts the pulmonary patient's quality of life and ability to work, causing financial distress, loss of jobs, anxiety, and depression and can be debilitating. Chronic pulmonary diseases are impacted by fatigue, including COPD (33), idiopathic pulmonary fibrosis, and sarcoidosis (34). The medical community needs to learn how to assess and treat fatigue. Patients with COPD have multiple precipitating and perpetuating factors that lead to fatigue (33) (figure 2.5). Fatigue assessment tools used may vary such as: the Fatigue Severity Scale, the Identity-Consequences Fatigue Scale (ICFS), and the Chronic Respiratory Questionnaire (CRQ). Pulmonary rehabilitation improves fatigue but the exact mechanism is not well understood. Only when we assess fatigue will we gain an understanding of the cause of fatigue, resulting in the pulmonary rehabilitation team being able to determine best treatments for the patient.

## Frailty and Grip Strength

Frailty is a condition characterized by a multisystem decline in functional status that correlates with an increased risk of morbidity and mortality. The most commonly used diagnostic criteria are from the Fried phenotype model: weight loss (> 10 pounds unintentional over the prior year), exhaustion (self-report to questions asked), slowness (15-foot walk time), low activity (patient's physical activity for one week ≤ 270 kcal), and weakness (measured by grip strength) (5). Frailty is an independent predictor of poor outcomes in COPD leading to pulmonary rehabilitation program noncompletion. The frail COPD patient can reverse this syndrome with pulmonary rehabilitation (6). Grip strength assesses weakness in the frailty assessment and is simple to perform and measures overall muscle strength, being a biomarker of the aging process. Grip strength is a predictor of all-cause mortality in middle age and elderly (35). COPD patients with hyperinflation have reduced handgrip strength, which worsens over time (36). Grip strength predicts health-related prognosis

---

### Figure 2.4    Modified Medical Research Council Dyspnea Scale

0    I only get breathless with strenuous exercise.

1    I get short of breath when hurrying on level ground or walking up a slight hill.

2    On level ground, I walk slower than people of the same age because of breathlessness, or have to stop for breath when walking at my own pace.

3    I stop for breath after walking about 100 yards or after a few minutes on level ground.

4    I am too breathless to leave the house or I am breathless when dressing.

Adapted from C.M. Fletcher, "The Clinical Diagnosis of Pulmonary Emphysema - An Experimental Study," *Proceedings of the Royal Society of Medicine* 45 (1952): 577–584.

Patient's environment

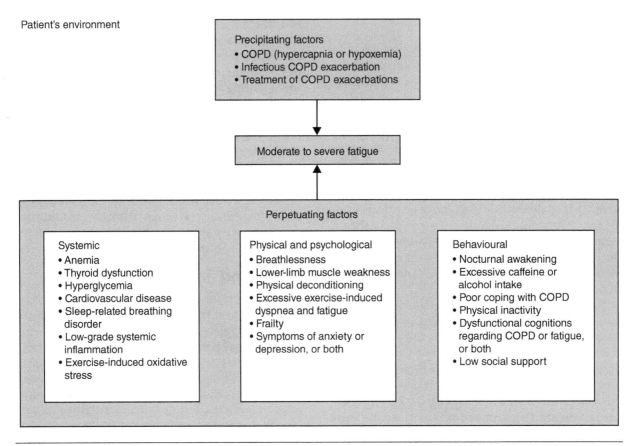

**Figure 2.5** Possible precipitating and perpetuating factors of moderate to severe fatigue in the environment of a patient with COPD.

Reprinted by permission from M.A. Spruit et al. "Fatigue in COPD: An Important Yet Ignored Symptom," *The Lancet Respiratory Medicine* 5, no. 7 (2017): 542–544.

such as functional limitation, functional decline, activities of daily living dependence, and mortality. The maintenance of muscle strength results in improved function, and pulmonary rehabilitation improves physical and musculoskeletal fitness.

### Sleep Disorders

Assessment of sleep-disordered breathing is essential when performing a thorough pulmonary rehabilitation assessment. The assessment should include nocturnal and daytime symptom evaluation and a physical assessment to include BMI, neck circumference, and history of comorbidities such as hypertension. Obstructive sleep apnea is seen in COPD (37) and idiopathic pulmonary fibrosis (38) contributing to worsening morbidity and mortality. Pulmonary rehabilitation should include a sleep disorder assessment; validated tools to use are the Epworth Sleepiness Scale (ESS) and the Pittsburgh Sleep Quality Index Assessment (PSQI).

## Musculoskeletal and Exercise Assessment

The safety of an exercise training program and the appropriateness of the exercise prescription are determined by a thorough initial musculoskeletal assessment (figure 2.6). This assessment includes an evaluation of the patient's ability to exercise, physical limitations, requirements for supplemental oxygen, and need for adaptive equipment. An evaluation of frailty, grip strength, gait, balance, and fall risk should also be included in the assessment. The assessment of physical limitations establishes a baseline of strength, range of motion, posture, functional abilities, and activities. The evaluation should also address orthopedic limitations, any activity restrictions requiring exercise modification, and transferring abilities such as from a chair to a standing position or from the floor to a standing position. See chapter 3 for a detailed description of an exercise assessment. A sample

## Figure 2.6    Information to be obtained in the exercise assessment

- Physical limitations (e.g., strength, range of motion, posture, functional abilities, and activities)
- Fall risk
- Frailty
- Grip strength
- Gait and balance
- Functional assessment
- Orthopedic limitations
- Transferring abilities
- Exercise tolerance
- Exercise hypoxemia, including the need for supplemental oxygen therapy

physical therapy and exercise assessment form can be found in appendix A.

## Pain Assessment

Assessing pain during the initial assessment and during daily sessions throughout the exercise program is also necessary. Considerations include location, duration, intensity, and character. Intensity is usually rated on a 0 to 10 scale or a facial descriptor scale. Assessment also must include factors that aggravate or ameliorate the pain.

## Activities of Daily Living Assessment

Symptoms of respiratory disease such as dyspnea and fatigue often lead to a decreased ability and willingness to perform activities of daily living (ADLs). Patients often do not realize that their activities have been curtailed and often attribute their functional limitations to "getting older." An interview with a significant other frequently adds complementary information to the patient's self-report. ADLs assessment should include which activities have been limited or eliminated because of the disease, its comorbidity, or its therapy. Elimination of an activity often depends on the level of distressing symptoms

it engenders and its importance to the patient. This initial assessment will direct subsequent therapy such as energy conservation techniques, extremity strength and range of motion exercises, proper pacing and breathing techniques, and the need for adaptive equipment. If appropriate, functional task performance and the work environment's demands should be assessed to establish a baseline for planning treatment and measuring outcomes.

ADLs assessment includes distress during, limitations in, or elimination of the following:

- Basic ADLs, such as dressing, bathing, walking, eating
- Household chores
- Leisure activities
- Job-related activities
- Sexual activity

## Nutrition Assessment

Patients with respiratory disease often have significant alterations in nutrition status and body composition. This includes patients who are underweight, those with normal body weight yet depleted muscle mass, and those who are obese. Refer to chapter 6 for initial nutritional assessment.

## Supplemental Oxygen Assessment

Pulmonary rehabilitation professionals need to be familiar with the indications for long-term oxygen therapy as well as the modalities for oxygen storage and delivery (39). Patients will often present to pulmonary rehabilitation having been prescribed supplemental oxygen without an appropriate determination of their specific requirements. One program found that approximately 40% of the patients entering rehabilitation required changes in their oxygen prescriptions during rehabilitation. All changes were to higher flows of oxygen and some to different oxygen devices altogether (40). Pulmonary rehabilitation staff should collaborate with the health care provider and durable medical equipment supplier to select the optimal oxygen delivery system to support adequate oxygenation and lessen the overall impact on the patient's personal freedom and quality of life. The patient should be given a written oxygen prescription and training for oxygen use with daily activities and exercise.

## Education Assessment

Assessing the educational needs of the pulmonary rehabilitation patient begins with a determination of how they understand and manage their disease. The educational assessment provides information needed to formulate the individualized education component of the comprehensive program. The goal of pulmonary rehabilitation education is changing the patient's behaviors to improve outcomes. Education includes collaborative self-management to improve the patient's knowledge of their disease and how best to manage their disease resulting in self-efficacy. The educational focus of pulmonary rehabilitation has transitioned from didactic lectures imparting knowledge to practice and promotion of self-management in collaboration with the health care team. In COPD, assessing if the patient recognizes and understands their disease, what causes an exacerbation, and how to use their inhaled medications are just a few of the important topics. The pulmonary rehabilitation team should understand and assess barriers to learning to include: visual, hearing, cognitive impairment, language barriers, literacy, and cultural diversity. Assessing patient goals should be done during the education assessment, and the goals should be measurable, specific, and realistic. A challenge and goal of pulmonary rehabilitation is to assess and meet the educational needs of pulmonary patients beyond COPD. A study by Morisset (18) looked at the unmet educational needs of patients with interstitial lung disease (ILD) with patients stating areas of concern from dissatisfaction over lack of ILD specific information, lack of emotional support, lack of time for group discussion, and lack of time for patient interaction. Making the pulmonary rehabilitation team aware of the ILD patient's needs can target the education and treatment specific for the ILD patient. The pulmonary rehabilitation program must determine if the educator teaching the patient has the skill and knowledge to be able to tailor the content for the ILD patient and assess if there is adequate psychosocial support and group discussion in the program.

To help with an educational assessment there are validated tools such as the Lung Information Needs Questionnaire (LINQ) and Bristol COPD Knowledge Questionnaire (BCKQ). To assess how a patient understands their lung disease and how to manage their disease resulting in self-efficacy there are reliable tools specific for self-efficacy such as the COPD Self-Efficacy Scale (CSES) and the Pulmo-nary Rehabilitation Adapted Index of Self-Efficacy (PRAISE). See chapter 4 for an extensive description of the educational assessment.

## Psychosocial Assessment

Psychosocial assessment is required by CMS as a condition for coverage of pulmonary rehabilitation. The coverage policy defines a psychosocial assessment as "a written evaluation of an individual's mental and emotional function as it relates to the individual's rehabilitation or respiratory condition and includes: an assessment of those aspects of an individual's family and home situation that affects the individual's rehabilitation treatment and evaluation of the individual's response to and rate of progress under the treatment plan" (41).

Psychosocial assessment should include:

- motivation,
- emotional distress,
- family and home situation,
- substance abuse,
- cognitive impairment,
- interpersonal conflict,
- other psychopathology,
- significant neuropsychological impairment such as memory, attention, and concentration,
- problem-solving impairments during daily activities,
- coping style, and
- sexual dysfunction.

The social history and family component may include:

- the living situation,
- type of home such as single story, number of stairs, and yard,
- family support,
- transportation resources,
- interpreter services needed,
- visual impairment,
- assessment of hearing,
- the patient's interest and activity in family and community activities,
- coping strategies,
- dependence on family and friends,
- stressors,

- relaxation and leisure activities, and
- description of the patient's present mood.

The initial psychosocial assessment should use screening tools to assess symptoms of anxiety, depression, and quality of life. The patient's referring or primary physician should be contacted if significant psychosocial problems are identified. Referral for further evaluation to appropriate professionals such as psychiatrist, psychologist, clinical social worker, or palliative care specialist may be appropriate. Failure to assess and treat the presence of significant psychosocial pathology may result in poor outcomes (42). Refer to chapter 5 for details on psychosocial assessment and intervention.

## Multicomponent Assessment of COPD

A chronic respiratory disease such as COPD affects the entire patient, and no single variable (e.g., $FEV_1$) can capture its extensive effects. Composite disease assessment tools using different aspects of the respiratory disease therefore may be helpful. One such scoring system for COPD is the BODE index, which has four components: body mass index (cachexia is an independent negative risk factor), the level of airway obstruction ($FEV_1$), dyspnea (using a 5-point MRC dyspnea scale), and exercise capacity (6-minute walk distance). The BODE index can range from 0 to 10, with higher scores predicting increasing morbidity (43). The BODE index is a strong predictor of mortality in patients with COPD, and some studies show that it may also be useful as an outcome in pulmonary rehabilitation. The BODE index change after pulmonary rehabilitation provides valuable prognostic information (44).

The assessment of the COPD patient according to the GOLD report should include not only the level of airflow obstruction but also patient's symptoms and exacerbation history (4). GOLD classification of airflow limitation severity in COPD is shown in table 2.1 (4).

Objective measurement of symptoms is important in COPD. A widely used measure of breathlessness is the Modified Medical Research Council Questionnaire (see figure 2.4). Since COPD impacts a patient's quality of life beyond just shortness of breath, GOLD recommends a measure of overall respiratory health status impairment. GOLD suggests using the simple COPD Assessment Test (CAT) (45), instead of a more complex respiratory specific health status questionnaire (e.g., St. George's Respiratory Questionnaire).[4]

COPD exacerbations are defined as an acute worsening of respiratory symptoms that results in additional therapy. The best predictor of having frequent exacerbations (defined as ≥2 exacerbations per year) is a history of prior treated exacerbations (46). A functional definition of exacerbation frequency ("How often have you been prescribed antibiotics or systemic corticosteroids for your lung condition?") is useful during the assessment for pulmonary rehabilitation of a patient with COPD.

GOLD recommends the multicomponent "ABCD assessment tool" (4) (figure 2.7). The number provides information regarding the severity of airflow limitation (spirometry grade 1 to 4) while the letter (groups A to D) refers to the symptom burden and the risk of exacerbation. This multicomponent assessment acknowledges the limitations of spirometry and emphasizes the importance of symptoms and exacerbation risk in prognostication and guiding therapy. For example, a patient with an $FEV_1 < 30\%$, CAT score of 18 and no exacerbations in the past year would be categorized as GOLD Grade 4, Group B.

| Table 2.1 | Classification of Airflow Limitation Severity in COPD (Based on Postbronchodilator $FEV_1$) in Patients with $FEV_1/FVC < 0.70$ | |
|---|---|---|
| GOLD 1 | Mild | $FEV_1 \geq 80\%$ predicted |
| GOLD 2 | Moderate | $50\% \leq FEV_1 < 80\%$ predicted |
| GOLD 3 | Severe | $30\% \leq FEV_1 < 50\%$ predicted |
| GOLD 4 | Very Severe | $FEV_1 < 30\%$ predicted |

Reprinted with permission from Global Initiative for Chronic Obstructive Lung Disease, *"Global Strategy for the Diagnosis, Management and Prevention of COPD."*

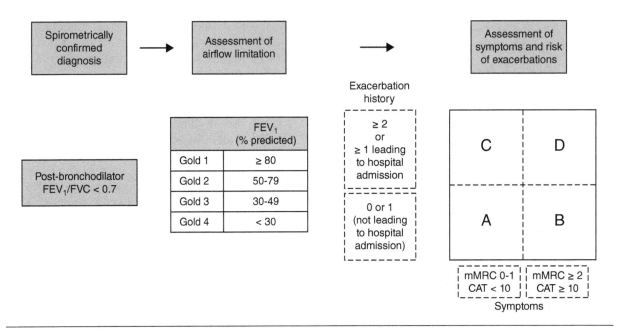

**Figure 2.7**   The ABCD assessment tool.

# Reassessment

Reassessment of the patient during the pulmonary rehabilitation program is necessary to review progress and adjust the program to meet the patient's goals. The outcome tools used to assess the patient, such as quality of life, functional evaluation, anxiety, depression, oxygen use, and airway clearance, are critical in determining a patient's individualized treatment program (ITP) and always part of the reassessment process (see chapter 10). Although a physician referral is necessary for pulmonary rehabilitation, it is also useful to communicate with the patient's health care providers regarding factors that contribute to symptoms, functional limitation and outcomes.

# SUMMARY

Pulmonary rehabilitation is a standard of care for the treatment of patients with chronic lung disease. The pulmonary rehabilitation team should understand patient selection beyond COPD, the pathophysiology, clinical presentation, and comorbidities of the pulmonary patient. Other considerations in patient selection should include smoking, motivation, adherence, financial consideration, and transportation. A thorough pulmonary rehabilitation assessment is the most critical component of a program determining the individual intervention and treatments to improve patient outcomes. The initial patient assessment includes the interview, medical history, physical assessment, diagnostic test, and symptom assessment. The multidisciplinary team assessment should include musculoskeletal and exercise, pain, activities of daily living, nutrition, supplemental oxygen, education, psychosocial, and a multicomponent ABCD assessment of COPD for the patient with COPD. The multidisciplinary team assessment sets the foundation for an individualized and safe comprehensive pulmonary rehabilitation plan of care that includes ongoing assessment, education, therapeutic exercise, psychosocial intervention, and long-term adherence.

**VISIT THE WEB RESOURCE** ─────────────────────────

for links to additional resources and various tools, checklists, and forms.

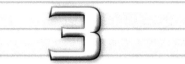

# Exercise Assessment and Training

**Chris Garvey, FNP, MSN, MPA, MAACVPR**
University of California and San Francisco Medical Center

**Rebecca Crouch, PT, DPT, MS, CCS, MAACVPR**
Campbell University and Duke Hospital
Durham, NC

**David Verrill, MS, CEP, RCEP, FAACVPR**
University of North Carolina at Charlotte

Exercise is well established as the cornerstone of pulmonary rehabilitation in persons with chronic lung disease due to its capacity to improve exercise tolerance in people with chronic lung disease (1). Exercise intolerance is multifactorial, resulting from progressive skeletal muscle dysfunction, disabling dyspnea and fatigue, comorbidities, mood disorders, hypoxemia, and in persons with chronic obstructive pulmonary disease (COPD), hyperinflation. Although the majority of evidence for effectiveness of exercise is derived from studies in persons with COPD, growing evidence supports the effectiveness of exercise as part of pulmonary rehabilitation in other lung diseases. The general principles of exercise training in persons with chronic lung disease are the same as for healthy individuals, and are individualized based on history and physical examination, clinical assessment, and objective and subjective findings. To optimize effectiveness, the training load must exceed that normally encountered in daily life to improve fitness and muscle strength (i.e., the training threshold). Exercise levels should

progress throughout pulmonary rehabilitation based on ongoing comprehensive assessment. A key focus of exercise in pulmonary rehabilitation is long-term behavior change to achieve ongoing participation in physical activity and exercise. Several adjuncts have the potential to improve exercise in appropriate patients, including bronchodilation, oxygen, breathing techniques such as pursed-lip breathing, one-leg exercise, and use of rollators (rolling walkers). Critical areas of investigation include technology-supported and home- or community-based exercise (1).

## RATIONALE FOR EXERCISE TRAINING IN CHRONIC LUNG DISEASE

Many factors must be considered when selecting an exercise plan for persons with lung disease. To achieve the greatest benefit from exercise training, the rehabilitation team works closely with the physician to achieve optimization of medical therapy, including appropriate use of medications and oxygen. Successful rehabilitation outcomes depend on effective communication and a coordinated team effort to identify and meet the patient's medical, functional, and psychological needs. The patient and the family are at the center of educational interventions that focus on adaptation and behavior change (see chapter 4).

Exercise training is the cornerstone of pulmonary rehabilitation. Virtually all patients with chronic respiratory disease have strong potential to benefit from exercise training (1, 2). Patients whose physical limitations permit them to exercise at higher intensities can achieve significant improvement in aerobic conditioning, while those with more severe limitations can improve with lower-intensity endurance training (3). While aerobic and resistance upper-body exercise training is essential for all appropriate patients, resistance exercise training has been shown to be essential to improve upper- and lower-body strength and muscle volume, activities of daily living (ADL) performance and health-related quality of life (3–10). The evidence base supporting the functional benefits of both short- and long-term exercise training in COPD is among the strongest in pulmonary medicine (1, 2, 11). While more research is needed on the effect of aerobic and resistance exercise training in patients with other chronic lung diseases, including restrictive and interstitial lung diseases such as pulmonary fibrosis, recent trials have shown positive results (1, 12–15). A warm-up period should be included in each exercise session to provide gradual increases in heart rate (HR), blood pressure, ventilation, and blood flow to the exercising muscles. A cool-down reduces the risk of arrhythmias, orthostatic hypotension, syncopal episodes, and bronchospasm (16, 17).

# MECHANISMS OF EXERCISE INTOLERANCE IN CHRONIC RESPIRATORY DISEASE

Respiratory and nonrespiratory factors, alone or in combination, can significantly decrease the exercise tolerance of persons with chronic lung disease (1, 18–22). Although cardiopulmonary abnormalities are generally considered of fundamental importance, skeletal muscle dysfunction

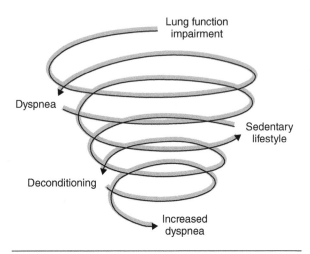

**Figure 3.1**   Dyspnea spiral.

Reprinted by permission from C. Prefaunt, A. Varray, and G. Vallet, "Pathophysiology Basis of Exercise Training in Patients With Chronic Obstructive Lung Disease," *European Respiratory Review* 5, no. 25 (1995): 27–32.

has been increasingly recognized as a key factor that contributes to exercise intolerance (18). Perception of leg effort or discomfort is the main symptom limiting exercise in 40 to 45% of patients with COPD (21). Skeletal muscle dysfunction in COPD is characterized by reductions in muscle mass and strength; atrophy of slow-twitch, oxidative endurance muscle fibers; and reductions in fiber capillarization, oxidative enzyme capacity, and muscle endurance (18). Both resting and exercise muscle metabolism are impaired, with lower exercise tolerance and lactic acidosis occurring at lower exercise workloads compared to healthy persons (18, 21, 23). Systemic inflammation, nutrition impairment, aging, low anabolic hormone levels, corticosteroid-related myopathy, frailty, and hypoxia further contribute to skeletal muscle dysfunction in COPD (23, 24).

Complicating all of these disease effects is physical deconditioning. This is a consequence of patients assuming an increasingly sedentary lifestyle to avoid the unpleasant sensation of dyspnea. Inactivity in turn leads to further deconditioning and increased exertional dyspnea, creating the dyspnea spiral depicted in figure 3.1.

# EXERCISE ASSESSMENT

Prior to exercise assessment, pulmonary rehabilitation providers should carefully review the patient history and physical examination with a focus on disorders that may potentially worsen or become unstable during exercise, including:

- History of cardiovascular disease (coronary artery disease; previous myocardial infarction; chest pain; arrhythmia; new onset, untreated, uncontrolled, or chronic atrial fibrillation with resting rate >110 bpm; ventricular tachycardia; second- or third-degree atrioventricular block; T wave inversion or ST elevation)
- Moderate to severe valve disease
- Symptomatic or new onset heart failure
- Large patent foramen ovale causing shunt physiology

Additional disorders and comorbidities such as significant cognitive, severe psychiatric abnormalities, and intractable pain should be reviewed by the medical director with communication to the referring clinician or specialist to determine the patient's appropriateness as a pulmonary rehabilitation candidate.

Used with permission from University of California San Francisco, C. Garvey and N. Gidwani.

### *Purposes of the Exercise Assessment for Patients with Chronic Lung Disease*

- Quantify exercise capacity before beginning a program (25, 26)
- Evaluate unexplained dyspnea and exercise intolerance (27, 28)
- Observe for abnormal signs and symptoms of exercise intolerance (25–27)
- Establish a baseline for outcome documentation (28)
- Help establish patient-specific goals (29)
- Prognostic evaluation for patient risk stratification (24, 25)
- Drug treatment efficacy evaluation
- Exercise evaluation for research purposes (26)
- Evaluation of patient impairment and disability for insurance purposes and workman's compensation
- Assist in formulating an exercise prescription for exercise training (3, 16, 27, 28)
- Detect exercise-induced hypoxemia and aid with titrating supplemental oxygen therapy (30, 31)
- Evaluate nonpulmonary limitations to exercise (e.g., musculoskeletal problems) (23, 24, 32, 33)
- Help to detect underlying cardiac abnormalities and coronary artery disease (16, 26, 27)

- Help to evaluate status of congestive heart failure (if present)
- Screen for exercise-induced bronchospasm (34)
- Evaluation for heart, lung, or heart/lung transplant (26, 27)

For most respiratory patients *without* known or suspected cardiac problems, exercise testing, even to maximal levels, is relatively safe. Contraindications to exercise testing in this setting are relatively few. Standard lists of absolute and relative contraindications are concerned primarily with patients with known or suspected cardiovascular disease.

General safety considerations when performing exercise testing are as follows (26, 29, 34):

- All test administrators must be trained and competent in performing cardiopulmonary resuscitation.
- Oxygen and emergency equipment should be in close proximity to the testing site.
- If testing is not performed in a hospital environment, adequate emergency procedures must be in place.
- If the patient has been prescribed long-term oxygen therapy, the exercise test should usually be carried out using the prescribed level of oxygen. An exception might be the evaluation of a patient who may no longer need supplemental oxygen. If significant hypoxemia is present during activity, consider titrating the patient during ambulation prior to exercise testing.
- At a minimum, continuous pulse oximetry should be used to measure ($SpO_2$) and HR to monitor the patient's physiological response to exercise.
- Validated dyspnea and exertion scales should be used to measure the patient's perceived shortness of breath and effort during the test (e.g., Borg category-ratio or Borg perceived exertion chart).

# FIELD TESTS (WALKING TESTS)

Field (walking) tests are commonly used for measurement of functional capacity in the pulmonary rehabilitation setting. Advantages include that the tests are functional, generally safe and easy to perform, inexpensive, and do not require extensive or expensive equipment. These tests are easily administered in the majority of pulmonary rehabilitation patients, including those that are debilitated. However, the test does not offer comprehensive physiological monitoring.

# Six-Minute Walk Test

The 6-minute walk test (6MWT) is a widely used outcome measure for pulmonary rehabilitation (34–37). The test is safe, easy to administer, involves the use of minimal technical resources, is well tolerated, and accurately reflects a familiar activity of daily living (walking). The 6MWT measures the maximum distance walked in 6 minutes. To obtain valid and reliable results, it is essential to standardize the test procedure, such as staff, configuration of track, patient instructions and verbal reinforcement during testing, type, use and flow rate of supplemental oxygen, and walking aids (35).

One must consider the energy expenditure changes that occur while performing the 6MWT under certain circumstances, such as while using an assistive walking aid (e.g., rollator) and when a supplemental oxygen source is placed on the walking aid. It has been suggested that there are a reduction of breathlessness and an improvement in the distance walked when using a walking aid or supplemental oxygen (35). One study found as much as a 20 to 25% energy cost savings with the addition of a walking aid that supported supplemental oxygen. These energy savings appear to be most notable in persons with COPD who have lower exercise performance; e.g., 6MWT distance of <300 meters (38). Consequently, if a walking aid is used on the first test, or a required supplemental oxygen source is carried on the walker, the same walking preparation must be used with subsequent testing.

Directions on performing the 6MWT are given below.

## Before the Test

- Standardize the shape of the flat walking course: straight versus continuous circle, oval, or square. If using a corridor, a minimum of 30 meters (98.4 feet) that is free of traffic and obstacles should be used.
- A comfortable ambient temperature and humidity should be maintained for all tests.

- A medical history for the patient has been reviewed and any precautions or contraindications to exercise testing have been taken into account (see absolute and relative contraindications, figures 3.4 and 3.5 later in the chapter).
- Instruct the patient to dress comfortably, wear appropriate footwear, and avoid eating or drinking for at least 2 hours before the test (when possible or appropriate).
- Prescribed inhaled bronchodilator medications should be taken if ordered within 1 hour of testing or when the patient arrives for testing.
- Rest for at least 10 minutes before beginning the test. If two tests are performed on the same day, at least 30 minutes rest should be allowed between tests.
- Record blood pressure BP, HR, $SpO_2$, and dyspnea score while the patient is sitting or standing. Measure HR and $SpO_2$ continuously during the test.
- Describe the walking track to the patient and give the patient standardized instructions (35) (see table 3.1).
- If the patient has not performed a 6MWT in the recent past, two tests should be performed for initial testing due to a significant learning effect. Use the greater of the two test results (35).

## During the Test

The patient should be asked to walk as far as he or she can in 6 minutes. Standardized encouragement and notification of time elapsed should be given at specific intervals according to the European Respiratory Society (ERS)/American Thoracic Society (ATS) 6MWT script (35) (see table 3.1). Rests are allowed and included in the total test time. If the patient stops during the test (once $SpO_2$ is ≥85%), advise the patient every 30 seconds to "please resume walking whenever you feel able" (35).

- The total distance covered is recorded.
- The patient is asked to rate shortness of breath and effort using a validated dyspnea and fatigue scale.
- The patient should walk alone; staff, other patients, or family should not walk with the patient performing the test. If necessary to

## Table 3.1    Script for Standardized Encouragement for 6-Minute Walk Test

| | |
|---|---|
| 1 minute | You are doing well. You have five minutes to go. |
| 2 minutes | Keep up the good work. You have four minutes to go. |
| 3 minutes | You are doing well. You are halfway. |
| 4 minutes | Keep up the good work. You have only two minutes left. |
| 5 minutes | You are doing well. You have only one minute to go. |
| 6 minutes | Please stop where you are. |
| If the patient stops during the test, every 30 seconds (once $SpO_2$ is ≥85%) | Please resume walking whenever you feel able. |

Key: $SpO_2$ = arterial oxygen saturation measured by pulse oximetry

Reproduced with permission of the © ERS 2018: *European Respiratory Journal* Jun 2004, 23 (6) 832–840; DOI: 10.1183/09031936.04.00116004.

have staff close to the patient during the walk for safety, they should walk behind the patient.

- Oxygen flow should be held constant during any test; oxygen titration should not be performed during a measured distance outcome walk test. Subsequent tests should use the same flow rate and modality if possible and safe.
- Staff should not assist the patient in carrying or pulling supplemental oxygen unless the patient cannot safely maneuver oxygen.
- Count laps with a lap counter.
- The patient may use their usual ambulatory assistive device; make note of which device (e.g., single-point cane, rollator walker, standard walker) is used and why.
- Monitor the patient for untoward signs and symptoms, including continuous $SpO_2$ and HR.
- The oximeter should not be held by the patient. Either a finger oximeter or a hand-held oximeter in a pouch should be used.

### Ending the Test

- Once the 6 minutes are completed, the patient is instructed to stop where he or she is.
- Note if the patient exhibits any untoward signs and symptoms.
- Stop the test for:
  - $SpO_2$ desaturation <80%
  - Chest pain

  - Intolerable dyspnea
  - Intolerable leg cramps, signs of intolerance to exercise exertion such as staggering, or unusual diaphoresis
  - Pale or ashen appearance
- Immediately record $SpO_2$, HR, dyspnea, fatigue, and blood pressure while patient is sitting (measurements taken before and after the test should be done with the patient in the same position).
- Record the distance completed in feet or meters, number of rest stops, total time of stops, and final vital signs including the lowest $SpO_2$ level (and oxygen flow rate if used) on a standardized recording form (35, 39).

Figure 3.2 shows a sample evaluation form for use in the 6MWT. The MET level corresponding to the average walking speed can be estimated based on the distance walked in 6 minutes. One MET is the amount of energy required while the body is at rest. This may be useful information for assessing exercise capacity and formulating an initial exercise prescription (see figure 3.3). Other information can be gleaned from the test, including gait analysis, balance, fatigue, and pain assessment.

The 6MWT can be influenced by multiple factors, including motivation, encouragement, learning effect, physical course layout, testing environment, gender, and age. Standardized encouragement must be given. There is a learning effect in performing successive 6MWTs, and distances may increase by 26.3 meters on subsequent tests; therefore, two

**Figure 3.2  Pulmonary rehabilitation 6-minute walk test evaluation form\***

| Parameters | Initial 6-minute walk | | | | Discharge 6-minute walk | | |
| --- | --- | --- | --- | --- | --- | --- | --- |
| | Pre-walk | Walk 1 | MPH | Meters / minute | Walk 1 | MPH | Meters / minute |
| Total distance (m or ft) | _____ | _____ | _____ | _____ | _____ | _____ | _____ |
| # of rests | _____ | _____ | _____ | _____ | _____ | _____ | _____ |
| Time of rest, sec | _____ | _____ | _____ | _____ | _____ | _____ | _____ |
| Validated dyspnea scale | _____ | _____ | _____ | _____ | _____ | _____ | _____ |
| $SpO_2$, % | _____ | _____ | _____ | _____ | _____ | _____ | _____ |
| $F_IO_2$, % | _____ | _____ | _____ | _____ | _____ | _____ | _____ |
| $O_2$, L/min | _____ | _____ | _____ | _____ | _____ | _____ | _____ |
| BP, mmHg | _____ | _____ | _____ | _____ | _____ | _____ | _____ |
| HR, bpm | _____ | _____ | _____ | _____ | _____ | _____ | _____ |
| METs | _____ | _____ | _____ | _____ | _____ | _____ | _____ |
| Patient symptoms (see key) | _____ | _____ | _____ | _____ | _____ | _____ | _____ |
| Walking devices used (see key) | _____ | _____ | _____ | _____ | _____ | _____ | _____ |
| Other comments | _____ | _____ | _____ | _____ | _____ | _____ | _____ |
| Staff initials | _____ | _____ | _____ | _____ | _____ | _____ | _____ |
| Date | _____ | _____ | _____ | _____ | _____ | _____ | _____ |

Key: MPH = miles per hour.

Patient symptoms = chest pain, dizziness, shortness of breath, leg pain, cramps, etc.
Walking devices used = walker (type), cane, etc.
\*Note that two walks are advised if the patient has not recently performed a 6MWT.

Staff signature:_____

---

**Figure 3.3 Calculating MET levels from the 6-minute walk test**

A MET is a metabolic equivalence of a task or a unit for expressing energy expenditure. One MET is the level of energy expenditure (oxygen consumption) at rest at approximately 3.5 ml $O_2$/kg/min (2). Activities can be expressed as requiring a multiple of resting requirements. Formulas are available to estimate energy cost (METs) of various activities, such as walking. MET levels during walking may be calculated by using the following formula (1 ml $O_2$/kg/min of $\dot{V}O_2$ is required for 10 m/min of walking):

$$METs = [baseline\ MET + walk\ MET] / baseline\ MET$$

Example: 100 meters walked in a 6-minute walk

$$METS = [3.5 + (100\ m/6\ min) \times (min/10\ m)] / 3.5 = 1.47$$

An alternative approach (ACSM formula for estimating $\dot{V}O_2$ [METs] for horizontal walking) (16, 37):

$$\dot{V}O_2\ (METs) = [3.5\ ml/kg/min + (0.1 \times \underline{\quad} speed\ (m/min)]/3.5\ ml/kg/min$$

Expressing walking distance as average walking speed in miles per hour (e.g., feet/sec $\times$ 0.68) or 6MWD (feet) $\times$ 10 / 5280 = $\underline{\quad}$ mph

METs can be calculated from speed in mph:

$$METs = [(\underline{\quad}mph)(26.83\ m/min) \times (0.1ml/kg/min) + 3.5\ ml/kg/min]$$

---

walks should be performed during the initial testing, using the furthest distance of the two tests (35-36). If two tests are performed, the recommendation is to wait at least 30 minutes, or up to the next day, to repeat the second test and that the greater of the two values be reported (34-37).

The use of a treadmill for 6MWT is not advised (35, 36, 39). The physical layout of the course may impact walking distance. In the National Emphysema Treatment Trial (NETT), centers that used continuous walking courses, either oval or square, reported longer 6MWT distances than those with straight courses. The difference attributable to the course layout was 110 feet (33.5 meters), or a 10% advantage for continuous courses (40). The difference between straight and continuous courses may be due to the time and effort required for the subject to turn around on a straight course. The preassessments and postassessments in pulmonary rehabilitation, therefore, must use the same course to eliminate this potential variability.

Prediction formulas for the 6MWT distance are available. This information can be used to assess the patient's level of impairment, compared to data from healthy adults (36, 39, 41). If using a prediction formula, the formula should be derived populations similar to the pulmonary rehabilitation program population. The minimal clinically meaningful change or minimum clinically important difference (MCID) in the 6MWT distance has been reported to be a mean of 30 meters (98.4 feet) (35). For those patients who walk a very short distance in their initial 6MWT (<200 meters, or <656 feet), an additional strategy has been suggested to help evaluate improvement which involves calculating the percent (%) change in pre—versus post—pulmonary rehabilitation walk distance (feet or meters) (34).

## Shuttle Walk Tests

There are two types of shuttle walk tests: the incremental and the endurance shuttle walk tests. The ISWT is an incremental, symptom-limited walk test that simulates a symptom-limited cardiopulmonary exercise test (CPET). It measures a symptom-limited walking distance over a marked walking course of 10 meters (33 feet). This distance correlates well with maximal oxygen uptake (42). The ISWT utilizes an audible pacing timer to incrementally increase the pacing frequency (table 3.2). The subject walks according to the pacing timer frequency until they are too breathless to continue or cannot keep pace with the external pacing signal. Like the 6MWT, the primary test result of the ISWT is the total distance walked. As with the 6MWT, the ISWT should be performed twice prior to an intervention, with the best result

## Table 3.2   Example of Layout and Pacing Algorithm for Shuttle Walk Distance Test

| Level | Speed m/s | Number of shuttles per level | Distance ambulated at the end of each level (m) |
|---|---|---|---|
| 1 | 0.50 | 3 | 30 |
| 2 | 0.67 | 4 | 70 |
| 3 | 0.84 | 5 | 120 |
| 4 | 1.01 | 6 | 180 |
| 5 | 1.18 | 7 | 250 |
| 6 | 1.35 | 8 | 330 |
| 7 | 1.52 | 9 | 420 |
| 8 | 1.69 | 10 | 520 |
| 9 | 1.86 | 11 | 630 |
| 10 | 2.03 | 12 | 750 |
| 11 | 2.20 | 13 | 880 |
| 12 | 2.37 | 14 | 1020 |

Reprinted by permission S.J. Singh et al., "Development of a Shuttle Walking Test of Disability in Patients With Chronic Airways Obstruction," *Thorax* 47 (1992): 1019–1024.

recorded (41). The patient should rest for 30 minutes between tests. Directions for performing the ISWT are given below.

The endurance shuttle test (ESWT) is a standardized, externally controlled, constant-paced walking test for the assessment of endurance capacity. The ISWT is initially performed to determine exercise capacity, and then a paced walk speed corresponding to 85% of walking speed on the ISWT is used to determine the walking speed for the ESWT (42, 43). The ESWT is a field test equivalent of the constant workload test. The primary outcome of the ISWT is distance, measured to the nearest 10 meters, whereas the primary outcome of the ESWT is time, consistent with other endurance tests (35–37).

Since exercise endurance improves more than peak oxygen concentration (peak $\dot{V}O_2$) after pulmonary rehabilitation exercise training, the ESWT is more responsive to pulmonary rehabilitation than the ISWT (28, 35–36). For the ISWT, a change of distance of 47.5 meters has been described as associated with feeling "slightly better," while a change of 78.7 meters has been associated with feeling "better"; therefore, the MCID for the ISWT

distance in COPD is 47.5 meters (35). Preliminary data suggests the MID for the ESWT is in the region of 180 seconds (35).

### Before the Test

- A medical history for the patient has been reviewed and any precautions or contraindications to exercise testing have been taken into account.

- Instruct the patient to dress comfortably, wear appropriate footwear, and avoid eating or drinking for at least 2 hours before the test (when possible or appropriate).

- Prescribed inhaled bronchodilator medications should be taken if ordered within 1 hour of testing or when the patient arrives for testing.

- Two cones are set 9 meters apart. The distance walked around the cones is 10 meters.

- The patient should rest for at least 15 minutes before beginning the test.

- Record blood pressure, HR, $SpO_2$, and dyspnea score while the patient is sitting or standing.

### During the Test

- Standardized instructions should be used via an audio recording.
- No encouragement should be given throughout the test.
- Record each shuttle that is completed on the recording sheet.
- The subject is asked to rate dyspnea and effort using a validated scale.
- The patient should walk alone; staff, other patients, or family should not walk with the patient performing the test.
- Do not assist the patient in carrying or pulling his/her supplemental oxygen.
- The patient may use an ambulatory assistive device; make note of which device (e.g., single-point cane, rollator, standard walker) is used and why.
- A comfortable ambient temperature and humidity should be maintained for all tests.
- Monitor the patient for untoward signs and symptoms.
- Stop the test for:
  - Chest pain suspicious of angina.
  - Evolving mental confusion or lack of coordination.
  - Evolving light-headedness.
  - Intolerable dyspnea.
  - Leg cramps or extreme leg muscle fatigue.
  - Persistent $SpO_2 \leq 85\%$.
  - Any other clinically warranted reason.

### Ending the Test

- The patient is more than 0.5 meter (1.6 feet) away from the cone when the beep sounds (allow one lap to catch up).
- The patient determines that he or she is too breathless to continue.
- For the endurance shuttle walk test (ESWT): The patient reaches 85% of predicted maximum HR.
- The patient exhibits any untoward signs and symptoms.
- Immediately record $SpO_2$, HR, and dyspnea rating while the patient is sitting or standing (measurements taken before and after the test should be done with the patient in the same position).

- Two minutes later, record $SpO_2$ and HR to assess the recovery rate.
- Record the total number of shuttles completed.
- Record the reason for terminating the test.

Adapted from C. Garvey, *AACVPR Pulmonary Rehabilitation Outcome Toolkit*, https://www.aacvpr.org/Member-Center/Pulmonary-Rehab-Outcomes-Resource-Guide 2017.

Proponents argue that, when compared to a self-paced 6MWT, the shuttle tests are less influenced by motivation or pacing, correlate better with exercise capacity in patients with chronic lung disease, and may be a more sensitive indicator of functional change with rehabilitation or other therapies (35). Performance on the ISWT relates strongly to direct measures of peak $\dot{V}O_2$, allowing the prediction of peak $\dot{V}O_2$ (41). During the ISWT, the cardiorespiratory response to exercise (peak $\dot{V}O_2$) develops in an incremental fashion similar to formal CPET, thus making this a simple test requiring less technical expertise and equipment (35, 42). Furthermore, the ISWT is easier to administer, is less expensive, and incorporates an activity that patients perform on a daily basis (i.e., walking).

# GRADED EXERCISE TEST AND CARDIOPULMONARY EXERCISE TESTS

Clinical exercise testing, often described as a graded exercise test (GXT), may additionally include expired gas or metabolic analysis. It is then often described as a cardiopulmonary exercise test (CPET) and provides important clinical information for the pulmonary rehabilitation practitioner. The rationale for performing the GXT is patient-specific (see "Purposes of the Exercise Assessment for Patients with Chronic Lung Disease"). Exercise limitations during the GXT or CPET may be due to various causes. Ventilatory requirements during graded exercise are often higher than expected in patients with chronic lung disease due to the increased work of breathing, increased dead space ventilation, earlier onset of lactic acidosis, respiratory muscle dysfunction, impaired gas exchange (hypoxia), increased ventilatory demand due to deconditioning, and peripheral muscle dysfunction (e.g., lower limb dysfunction) (1).

Maximal exercise tolerance is typically measured with a GXT performed on either a treadmill or stationary cycle ergometer in the laboratory

(1, 16, 25, 26). In most clinical circumstances, cycle ergometry using an electronically braked ergometer is the preferred mode of exercise. However, a treadmill may be an acceptable alternative depending upon the purpose of the test. Arm ergometry may be substituted for those patients who are unable to perform lower-extremity exercises, although arm ergometer tests traditionally produce a lower $\dot{V}O_{2peak}$ (16, 25, 44). The GXT can be performed with either a ramped test or incremental increases in exercise load (e.g., 15 to 25 watts/minute on a cycle or arm ergometer) using a variety of established protocols until the patient reaches a symptom-limited maximal level of exertion. Physiologic responses to graded exercise that are commonly evaluated during the GXT include HR, ECG, blood pressure (BP), $SpO_2$, arterial blood analysis via arterial line on selected pulmonary patients, and ratings of perceived exertion and dyspnea. Symptoms of dyspnea can be rated by using the Borg category-ratio (CR10) dyspnea scale or a visual analog scale (VAS). With the addition of expired gas analysis for CPET, it is possible to evaluate parameters such as $\dot{V}O_2$, carbon dioxide production, and ventilatory threshold. Figure 3.4 provides a few of the parameters that can be assessed and analyzed during the CPET (27, 44). The addition of arterial blood gas analysis allows for the most accurate assessment of arterial oxygenation (e.g., alveolar–arterial oxygen gradient, oxygen partial pressure, $PaO_2$), carbon dioxide ($CO_2$) levels, dead space/tidal volume ratio ($V_D/V_T$), and acid-base balance measurements. CPET provides the most robust method for exercise evaluation in chronic lung disease, but due to its complexity and expense, widespread use may be limited in many pulmonary rehabilitation programs.

## Contraindications for Graded Exercise Testing

For most respiratory patients without known or suspected cardiac problems, exercise testing to even maximal levels is relatively safe. Regular 12-lead electrocardiographic graded exercise test (GXT), incremental maximal exercise testing (IMET), and cardiopulmonary exercise testing (CPET) in the medically supervised setting have been shown to be very safe when performed by physicians or specially trained health professionals (45).

---

**Figure 3.4    Common metabolic parameters assessed with cardiopulmonary exercise testing**

- $\dot{V}O_2$ (mL/kg/min and L/min)
- % predicted peak $\dot{V}O_2$
- Peak $\dot{V}O_2$ uptake (mL/kg/min)
- First and second ventilatory thresholds (VT, mL/kg/min)
- Workload at the first and second VT
- % predicted VT
- Heart rate (HR) and heart rate reserve (HRR)
- Ventilatory reserve (VR)
- Respiratory exchange ratio (RER)
- Oxygen pulse (mL $O_2$/kg/beat)
- Minute or pulmonary ventilation ($V_E$)
- Tidal volume (TV)
- Respiratory rate (f, breaths/minute)
- $V_E/VCO_2$ and $V_E/O_2$ (ventilatory equivalents) slopes, presented as ventilation/volume of expired carbon dioxide or oxygen
- Fraction of inspired oxygen ($F_IO_2$)
- Fraction of expired carbon dioxide ($F_ECO_2$)
- Partial pressure of end-tidal carbon dioxide ($P_{ET}CO_2$)
- Exercise oscillatory ventilation
- Circulatory power (CircPw, mmHg/mL/kg/min)
- End-tidal $PCO_2$ and $PaO_2$ (e.g., from arterial blood gas measurements)
- Physiologic dead space-to-tidal volume ratio ($V_D/V_T$)
- $P_{ET}O_2$

---

Common contraindications and precautions for CPET and GXT have been presented by the American Thoracic Society (ATS) and American College of Chest Physicians (ACCP) (26), as well as the American Heart Association (AHA) and American College of Sports Medicine (ACSM) (16, 44). While these two sets of guidelines are quite similar, there are subtle differences that the pulmonary

## Figure 3.5 ATS/ACCP absolute and relative contraindications for cardiopulmonary exercise testing including ISWT

**Absolute**

- Acute myocardial infarction (3–5 days)
- Unstable angina
- Uncontrolled arrhythmias causing symptoms or hemodynamic compromise
- Syncope
- Active endocarditis
- Acute myocarditis or pericarditis
- Symptomatic severe aortic stenosis
- Uncontrolled heart failure
- Acute pulmonary embolus or pulmonary infarction
- Thrombosis of lower extremities suspected dissecting aneurysm
- Uncontrolled asthma
- Pulmonary edema
- Room air desaturation at rest ≤85%*
- Respiratory failure

- Acute noncardiopulmonary disorder that may affect exercise performance or be aggravated by exercise (i.e., infection, renal failure, thyrotoxicosis)
- Mental impairment leading to inability to cooperate

**Relative**

- Left main coronary stenosis or its equivalent
- Moderate stenotic valvular heart disease
- Severe untreated arterial hypertension at rest (>200 mmHg systolic, >120 mmHg diastolic)
- Tachyarrhythmias or bradyarrhythmias
- High-degree atrioventricular block
- Hypertrophic cardiomyopathy
- Significant pulmonary hypertension
- Advanced or complicated pregnancy
- Electrolyte abnormalities
- Orthopedic impairment that compromises exercise performance

*Exercise patient with supplemental $O_2$.

Reprinted from American Thoracic Society/American College of Chest Physicians. ATS/ACCP Statement on Cardiopulmonary Exercise Testing," *American Journal of Respiratory Critical Care Medicine* 167 (2003); 211–277.

rehabilitation practitioner needs to consider. Figures 3.5 and 3.6 present common precautions and contraindications to consider prior to performing symptom- or sign-limited submaximal and maximal GXT or CPET for patients with chronic pulmonary disease.

It should be noted that in patients with primary pulmonary arterial hypertension (PAH) and moderate to severe pulmonary hypertension (PH), pulmonary artery pressure often increases with exercise and there is an increased risk of sudden death. Although caution is advised when testing patients with PAH, CPET can be performed safely in both pediatric and adult populations when prescribed by a clinician with expertise in care of PH patients (46, 47, 48). It is ultimately up to the patient's pulmonologist or clinic supervising physician to determine which patients with PH are suitable for CPET. More research is required to ascertain the risks and benefits of testing those with severe PAH and moderate to severe PH in the clinical setting.

It is also vitally important to terminate the GXT or CPET at the appropriate endpoints. Figures 3.7 and 3.8 present common criteria for terminating the symptom- or sign-limited maximal graded exercise test. Two sets of criteria are presented—those from the ATS/ACCP (26) and those from the AHA, American College of Cardiology (ACC) and ACSM (16, 25, 44). The second set of criteria is divided into both absolute and relative indications for exercise test termination.

It is vitally important that all applicable safety precautions are set in place prior to any form of exercise testing. General safety considerations for cardiopulmonary exercise testing are presented in figure 3.9 (29, 49).

In pulmonary patients, two other assessments should also be considered during the GXT. First,

## Figure 3.6　AHA and ACSM absolute and relative contraindications to symptom-limited graded exercise testing

### Absolute

- Acute myocardial infarction within 2 days
- Ongoing unstable angina
- Uncontrolled cardiac arrhythmia with hemodynamic compromise
- Active endocarditis
- Symptomatic severe aortic stenosis
- Decompensated heart failure
- Acute pulmonary embolism, pulmonary infarction or deep vein thrombosis
- Acute myocarditis or pericarditis
- Acute aortic dissection
- Physical disability that precludes safe and adequate exercise testing

### Relative

- Known obstructive left main coronary artery stenosis
- Moderate to severe aortic stenosis with uncertain relationship to symptoms
- Tachyarrhythmia with uncontrolled ventricular rates
- Acquired advanced or complete heart block
- Recent stroke or transient ischemic attack
- Mental impairment with limited ability to cooperate
- Resting hypertension with systolic >200 mmHg or diastolic >110 mmHg
- Uncorrected medical complications, such as significant anemia, important electrolyte imbalance, and hypothyroidism

Reprinted with permission from the American College of Sports Medicine, *ACSM's Guidelines for Exercise Testing and Prescription*, 10th ed. (Philadelphia: Wolters Kluwer-Lippincott Williams & Wilkins, 2018), 118.

## Figure 3.7　ATS/ACCP indications for exercise test termination

- Chest pain suggestive of ischemia
- Ischemic ECG changes
- Complex ectopy
- Second- or third-degree heart block
- Fall in systolic pressure of 20 mmHg from the highest value during the test
- Hypertension (250 mmHg systolic; 120 mmHg diastolic)
- Severe desaturation: $SpO_2 \leq 80\%$ when accompanied by symptoms and signs of severe hypoxemia
- Sudden pallor
- Loss of coordination
- Mental confusion
- Dizziness or faintness
- Signs of respiratory failure
- Definition of abbreviations: ECG = electrocardiogram; $SpO_2$ = arterial oxygen saturation measured by pulse oximetry

Adapted from. American Thoracic Society/American College of Chest Physicians. "ATS/ACCP Statement on Cardiopulmonary Exercise Testing," *American Journal of Respiratory Critical Care Medicine* 167 (2003): 211–277.

up to 30 minutes postexercise (33). Commonly used criteria to define specific limitations during exercise testing are given in figure 3.10 (29).

# FUNCTIONAL PERFORMANCE ASSESSMENT

In addition to formal exercise testing, patients should be assessed by questioning and physical assessment regarding functional performance status. This should include evaluation of respiratory muscle function, breathing mechanics, and thoracic mobility (e.g., diaphragmatic excursion, accessory breathing patterns, and rib cage flexibility). Equally important is the evaluation of balance, fall risk, and any orthopedic or musculoskeletal limitations; for example, the patient's gait

dynamic hyperinflation can develop with increasing ventilation; this can be assessed periodically with maximal flow-volume loops and measurements of inspiratory capacity (3). Second, exercise-induced bronchospasm can be assessed by spirometry for

## Figure 3.8 AHA/ACC/ACSM indications for terminating a symptom-limited maximal exercise test

**Absolute**

- ST elevation (>10 mm) in leads without preexisting Q waves because of prior MI (other than aVR, aVL, or $V_1$)
- Drop in systolic blood pressure of >10 mmHg, despite an increase in workload, when accompanied by other evidence of ischemia
- Moderate to severe angina
- Central nervous symptoms (e.g., ataxia, dizziness, or near syncope)
- Signs of poor perfusion (cyanosis or pallor)
- Sustained ventricular tachycardia or other arrhythmia, including second- or third-degree atrioventricular block that interferes with normal maintenance of cardiac output during exercise
- Technical difficulties monitoring the ECG or systolic blood pressure
- The subject's request to stop

**Relative**

- Marked ST displacement (horizontal or downsloping of >2 mm, measured 60 to 80 ms after the J point in a patient with suspected ischemia)
- Drop in systolic blood pressure >10 mmHg (persistently below baseline) despite an increase in workload, in the absence of other evidence of ischemia
- Increasing chest pain
- Fatigue, shortness of breath, wheezing, leg cramps, or claudication
- Arrhythmias other than sustained ventricular tachycardia, including multifocal ectopy, ventricular triplets, supraventricular tachycardia, and bradyarrhythmia that have the potential to become more complex to interfere with hemodynamic stability
- Exaggerated hypertensive response (systolic blood pressure >250 mmHg or diastolic blood pressure >115 mmHg)
- Development of bundle-branch block that cannot be distinguished from ventricular tachycardia
- $SpO_2 \leq 80\%$

Key: ECG = electrocardiogram; MI = myocardial infarction; $SpO_2$ = arterial oxygen saturation measured by pulse oximetry

Reprinted with permission. Modified from: Fletcher GF, Balady G, Froelicher VF, Hartley LH, Haskell WL, Pollock ML. Exercise standards: a statement for healthcare professionals from the American Heart Association Writing Group: special report. *Circulation* 1995; 91:580–615. ©1995 American Heart Association, Inc.

should be evaluated for abnormalities that may require individualized alterations to the exercise plan and ambulatory assistive devices. Figure 3.11 outlines some of the important considerations in this assessment (23).

Musculoskeletal problems are especially prominent in the pulmonary rehabilitation population. (1, 17, 18, 21). It is important to make a thorough assessment of the patient's baseline levels of strength, range of motion, posture, orthopedic limitations, and simple ADL (e.g., lying to standing, dressing, climbing steps).

# EXERCISE PRESCRIPTION

Exercise prescription requires understanding the principles of exercise training, exercise mode, frequency, and duration. Additionally, exercise progression is an important concept used in prescribing exercise.

## Principles of Exercise Training

Many factors must be considered when selecting an optimal exercise plan for persons with respiratory disease. To gain the most benefit from exercise training, it is imperative that the rehabilitation team work closely with the physician to achieve optimization of medical therapy, including the use of oxygen for treatment of hypoxemia. Successful rehabilitation outcomes depend on communication and a coordinated effort of the team to identify and meet the patient's medical and functional needs.

Exercise training in pulmonary rehabilitation should encompass upper- and lower-extremity

---

### Figure 3.9   General safety considerations when performing exercise testing for pulmonary patients (29, 49)

- All test administrators must be trained in cardiopulmonary resuscitation and demonstrate competency in use of exercise prescription in chronic lung disease.
- Oxygen and emergency equipment should be in close proximity to the testing site.
- If testing is not performed in a hospital environment, adequate emergency procedures and equipment must be in place.
- If the patient is using long-term ambulatory oxygen therapy, the exercise test should usually be carried out using the prescribed level of oxygen. An exception might be the evaluation of a patient who may no longer need supplemental oxygen.
- At a minimum, pulse oximetry should be used to measure HR and $SpO_2$ to monitor the patient's physiological response to exercise. Dyspnea and established exertion scales should be used to measure the patient's perceived effort and shortness of breath and effort during the test.

---

### Figure 3.10   Criteria for determining limitations during a symptom-limited graded exercise test

**Ventilatory Limits**

- Maximal exercise $V_E$/MVV >80%
- Rising $P_aCO_2$
- Rising $V_D/V_T$
- Development of dynamic hyperinflation
- Development of exercise-induced bronchospasm

**Gas Exchange Limits**

- Falling $SaO_2$ or $SpO_2$

**Cardiovascular Limits**

- Exercise HR >80% age-predicted maximal HR
- Falling blood pressure
- Serious dysrhythmia
- Cardiac symptoms (e.g., chest pain)
- Hypertensive or hypotensive response
- Deconditioning

**Other Limits**

- Orthopedic
- Peripheral vascular
- Musculoskeletal
- Metabolic
- Motivational or psychological

---

endurance training, strength training, and possibly respiratory muscle training. Frequency, intensity, time (duration), type (mode), volume, pattern, and progression of exercise should be included in each patient's initial treatment plan (ITP) as part of the exercise prescription. These components should be based upon the patient's disease severity, degree of conditioning, functional evaluation, and initial exercise testing data.

## The FITT Principles of Aerobic Exercise Prescription for Pulmonary Patients

The ACSM (16) developed the FITT (Frequency, Intensity, Time, Type, Volume, Pattern, and Progression) technique from evidence-based guidelines for exercise prescription in both apparently healthy and some diseased populations. For patients with chronic lung disease, evidence supports aerobic exercise recommendations for those with COPD (1, 2, 16, 50–52) (table 3.3).

Specific evidence-based exercise training guidelines for patients with asthma are not currently available. However, exercise training is normally well tolerated in asthmatics who are successfully managed with proper pharmacotherapy (53). Position statements on exercise in those with asthma (54) and systematic reviews of this topic (54) support the ACSM FITT principles for exercise for asthmatics (16, 55) (table 3.4).

## Figure 3.11   Functional Status Assessment Considerations

- Muscle strength and endurance
- Joint range of motion limitations
- Postural abnormalities (e.g., kyphosis, scoliosis, rounded or elevated shoulders)
- Oxygen equipment (e.g., type, weight and mobility of device)
- Subjective endurance and work tolerance
- Prior level of function
- Dyspnea
- Level of understanding of fitness and exercise
- Fear of exertion
- Ability to pace activities and energy conservation
- Balance abnormalities, gait instability, or increased risk of falling
- Pain levels and locations
- Ability to perform household chores (e.g., vacuuming, laundry, cooking)
- Ability to groom oneself (e.g., showering, dressing)
- Ability to move around home (e.g., climb stairs, walk to bathroom)

## Exercise Type (Mode)

It is most beneficial to direct exercise training to those muscles involved in functional daily living. This typically includes training the muscles of both the upper and lower extremities to improve cardiovascular endurance, muscular strength and endurance, and range of motion. Exercise training of the lower extremities often results in dramatic increases in exercise tolerance of patients with COPD (1–3, 52, 60–65, 67, 79–81) and other respiratory diseases (12–15, 82). Exercises that improve neuromotor abilities, such as balance and coordination to decrease fall risk, are equally important with the pulmonary population (23, 29, 74, 83–85). This topic is explored further later in this chapter.

The mode of exercise will vary by the available equipment and space available at the pulmonary rehabilitation facility. Indoor track or treadmill walking is a common mode of lower-body exercise training for most pulmonary rehabilitation programs and may be the most beneficial type of exercise, as walking requires total body movement. For those who can walk, it is recommended to be included in their pulmonary rehabilitation exercise training program and can help contribute to overall functional gains for most people (training specificity). Other aerobic exercise modalities include cycle ergometers (both upright and recumbent), arm ergometers, rowing machines, step machines, recumbent cross-training devices, seated and upright elliptical trainers and use of one-legged training (see table 3.5). Water exercise is ideal for those with arthritic or musculoskeletal abnormalities due to the lack of stress on the joints and overall body conditioning. Nordic walking is another promising option for walking in persons with chronic lung disease (1).

## Frequency and Duration

In general, the frequency and duration of medically supervised pulmonary rehabilitation exercise may vary from three to five times per week (1–3, 16, 34, 63, 64), 20 to 90 minutes per session (2, 16, 34, 68), and extend over a period of 8 to 12 weeks (1–3, 52, 65–69). Eight to 12 weeks of pulmonary rehabilitation produces benefits in several outcome areas that eventually decline over 12 to 24 months (52, 69). While there remains no general consensus of opinion on the optimal duration of pulmonary rehabilitation, the duration should be adequate to provide maximal individualized benefits without becoming burdensome. Although research has shown inconsistent findings of the overall benefits of long-term pulmonary rehabilitation maintenance programs of up to 3 years in duration (69–75), longer duration programs (e.g., beyond 12 weeks) may produce greater sustained benefits than shorter-term programs (52, 69–70, 75–79). Longer programs are thought to produce greater gains and maintenance of benefits, with a minimum of 8 weeks recommended to achieve a substantial effect (1, 79–83). The optimal duration for the individual would normally be the longest duration that is possible and practical given programs longer than 12 weeks have been associated with greater long-term benefits versus shorter programs (1, 52, 75, 76, 79).

Importantly, the beneficial effects in symptoms and 6MWT distance achieved with long-term pulmonary rehabilitation training have been shown to vanish after 24 weeks of follow-up (68). Thus,

## Table 3.3    ACSM FITT Aerobic Recommendations for Those with COPD

| FITT | Aerobic |
|---|---|
| Frequency | At least 3–5 days/week |
| Intensity | Moderate to vigorous intensity (i.e., 50%-80% peak work rate or 4–6 on the Borg CR10 Scale or 12–14 RPE scale) |
| Time | 20–60 minutes/day at moderate to high intensities as tolerated; if the 20–60 minute durations are not achievable, accumulate ≥20 minutes of exercise interspersed with intermittent exercise rest periods of lower-intensity work or rest |
| Type | Common aerobic modes, including walking (free or treadmill), stationary cycling, and upper-body ergometry |

Key: CR = category-ratio, RPE = rating of perceived exercise

Data from ACSM (2018).

## Table 3.4    ACSM FITT Aerobic Recommendations for Those with Asthma

| FITT | Aerobic |
|---|---|
| Frequency | 3–5 days/week |
| Intensity | Begin with moderate intensity (i.e., 40%-59% of HRR or $\dot{V}O_2R$); if well tolerated, progress to 60%-70% of HRR or $\dot{V}O_2R$ after 1 month. |
| Time | Progressively increase to at least 30–40 minutes/day |
| Type | Aerobic activities using large muscle groups such as walking, running, cycling, swimming, or pool exercises |

HRR: Heart rate reserve; $\dot{V}O_2R$: Volume of oxygen consumption reserve.

Data from ACSM (2018).

there may be an optimal duration of training for the pulmonary rehabilitation participant to "peak" in many physiologic parameters, and further research should lend insight into this optimal threshold of training.

If program constraints will not allow for supervised exercise at least 3 days per week, two supervised and one or more unsupervised sessions per week, in the home, with specific guidelines and instruction, may be an alternative option (1, 2, 16). If the patient is very debilitated, the duration of the initial exercise sessions can be shorter with more frequent rest breaks; however, the ultimate goal is to achieve fewer or no rest breaks and at least 30 minutes of endurance exercise within the first few weeks of rehabilitation.

Exercise training of the arms is very beneficial in patients with chronic lung disease, although most of the evidence comes from patients with COPD (78, 86, 87). Patients with moderate to severe COPD,

especially those with mechanical disadvantage of the diaphragm due to hyperinflation, have difficulty performing ADLs that involve use of the upper extremities (87). Arm elevation is associated with high metabolic and ventilatory demand, and activities involving the arms can lead to irregular or dyssynchronous breathing (86). This happens because some arm muscles are also accessory muscles of inspiration. Benefits of upper-extremity training in COPD include improved arm muscle endurance and strength, reduced metabolic demand associated with arm exercise, and increased sense of well-being. In general, benefits of upper-extremity training are task specific. Because of its benefits, upper-extremity training is recommended in conjunction with lower-extremity training as a routine component of pulmonary rehabilitation (1, 2, 52, 83–89).

Arm ergometry exercise is well tolerated by most pulmonary patients and is particularly beneficial for those who can only walk short distances, who

## Table 3.5 Upper- and Lower-Body Modalities Used for Cardiovascular Conditioning in Pulmonary Rehabilitation

| Modality | Upper Body (UB), Lower Body (LB) or Combined (C) |
|---|---|
| Indoor track or ground walking (patient may walk with or without a rollator or walker) | LB |
| Treadmill | LB |
| Stationary upright cycle ergometer | LB |
| Upright dual action stationary cycle, one-legged training | C |
| Recumbent cycle | LB |
| Pool for water exercise/swimming | C |
| Stepping machine or steps with handrails | LB |
| Stationary arm ergometer | UB |
| Stationary rower | C |
| Modified aerobic activities (e.g., dance, Tai Chi, calisthenics) | C |
| Elliptical trainer (with or without arm cranking) | LB or C |
| Recumbent dual action stepping ergometer (e.g., NuStep™) | C |
| Wall or machine pulleys | UB |
| Seated aerobic activities (e.g., arm lifting, leg lifts) with or without hand or ankle weights | C |

are obese, who have neuromuscular or orthopedic diseases, or who are wheelchair bound.

Caution should be taken with certain exercises in select patients, including those with osteoporosis (known or suspected due to oral steroid therapy) who may have decreased bone density and have an increased risk of vertebral compression fractures. These precautions include avoiding excess spinal flexion and rotation (90). Postoperative thoracic surgery patients (e.g., lung transplant) are generally restricted from upper-body exercise for 6 to 8 weeks postoperative to allow for internal and external incisional healing. Clearance for upper-body exercises is usually based on approval from the thoracic surgeon or transplant team (23).

## Intensity of Exercise

The most challenging aspect of developing the exercise prescription for the pulmonary patient is estimation of the proper exercise intensity (16, 57, 81). The rehabilitation team must be prudent in ensuring that the exercise intensity is not too intense to provoke adverse physiologic reactions, yet is sufficient enough to promote a training effect. Individualized initial and ongoing assessments of subjective and objective findings are used to carefully advance intensity of exercise, often following incremental advancement of time. Supervised exercise training coupled with use of dyspnea control techniques works to enhance coping with fear and discomfort associated with breathlessness that often limits exercise capacity; therefore, most types of exercise that the patient enjoys or is willing to do can be beneficial. When developing the exercise prescription, the rehabilitation team must incorporate the patient's individual activity goals into the training plan. For example, if the patient wants to be able to walk the dog for 30 minutes each day at a relatively slow but steady pace without rest stops, the intensity of training should, in part, be designed to help accomplish that goal.

As previously noted, both low- and high-intensity exercise training may be used to improve patient exercise tolerance. Principles of basic exercise training suggest that the intensity of exercise should be related to degree of disability, disease state, exercise test results (e.g., 6MWT, CPET, GXT, ISWT), time, workload, physiologic responses observed during exercise, and other factors. Please refer to tables 3.3, 3.4, and 3.5 for exercise intensity recommendations for patients with COPD and asthma, respectively.

## High-Intensity Exercise Training

Aerobic endurance training for those with chronic lung disease may be performed at low, moderate and even high intensities (3, 55-59). High-intensity training of 60 to 80% of peak work rate may be undertaken to gain maximal physiological improvements in aerobic fitness. These improvements include increased $\dot{V}O_2$max, delayed anaerobic threshold, decreased HR for any given work rate, increased oxidative enzyme capacity, biochemical cellular changes, and capillarization of muscle (3, 55-58). These physiologic changes can result in a lower ventilatory requirement for a given exercise task as well as a more efficient pattern of breathing, with reduced dead space ventilation due to increased tidal volume and decreased respiratory rate. High-intensity training has been associated with substantial gains in exercise endurance (3).

Not all patients can tolerate sustained high-intensity exercise at the outset of training. Those patients working at their maximal tolerated exercise level will achieve gains over time (55, 57). Interval training, alternating periods of high and low intensity (or rest), has been shown to be an effective training option for persons who cannot sustain extended continuous periods of higher-intensity exercise (55, 56, 59).

Traditional physiologic changes associated with aerobic fitness from high-intensity training are not required to improve exercise tolerance and function in many patients with chronic lung disease. This is important because unpleasant dyspnea and leg fatigue associated with high-intensity exercise may interfere with its incorporation into the patient's daily lives, which affects overall exercise adherence. Moreover, it has not been proven conclusively that high-intensity exercise, with achievement of physiological gains in aerobic fitness, leads to greater improvement in day-to-day functional activity. Thus, lower-intensity aerobic exercise training can lead to significant improvements in exercise endurance, even in the absence of measured gains in aerobic fitness (60-62).

Exercise prescription using METs and MET minutes (see table 3.6) is commonly employed in pulmonary rehabilitation, using a predetermined MET range level for exercise intensity determined from a test of functional capacity. If the results from a CPET are available, one can prescribe exercise using the $\dot{V}O_2$ reserve technique from peak $\dot{V}O_2$ values (16). Peak functional capacity can also be estimated from common metabolic equations employed using GXT and 6MWT results. The rehabilitation team may also choose to have the patient perform any of the following to help gauge exercise intensity:

- Work up to a selected level on a perceived exertion scale or dyspnea level (e.g., 4 to 6 on the Borg CR10 Scale or 12 to 14 on a 6 to 20 RPE scale) (16, 91-93).

- Utilize a numeric rating scale (NRS) (94) or VAS (95-96) (see figure 3.12) to quantify perceived exercise intensity.

Any of these techniques can help guide the pulmonary rehabilitation practitioner in the development of the intensity component of the exercise prescription. Further information on the use of these scales may be found within the selected references.

Another guide for prescribing exercise intensity is using an exercise target HR range (e.g., heart rate reserve or Karvonen method) determined from an initial or follow-up exercise test, or from observations of the patient's HR responses during exercise sessions (16). However, target HR range is not always applicable during exercise training sessions in pulmonary rehabilitation programs due to a myriad of factors that can influence resting and exercise HR responses of the patient with chronic lung disease such as medications, resting dyspnea and deconditioning. Nevertheless, it is prudent to be aware of the patient's HR responses at rest and during exercise. Many pulmonary rehabilitation programs use intermittent "quick-check" HR monitoring during exercise from ECG, HR taken from pulse oximeter readings, and, if available, HR monitored via telemetry to a base station during exercise training. Any uncertainty regarding accuracy of HR based on oximetry reading should be correlated with checking radial or apical HR.

## Table 3.6 Methods for Determining Exercise Intensity for Pulmonary Rehabilitation Participants

| Method | Description |
|---|---|
| Heart rate reserve (HRR) (16) | Target Heart Rate (THR) = $[(HR_{max} - HR_{rest}) \times \%$ intensity$] + HR_{rest}$ |
| $\dot{V}O_2$ reserve ($\dot{V}O_2R$) (16) | Target $\dot{V}O_2 = [(\dot{V}O_{2max} - \dot{V}O_{2rest}) \times \%$ intensity$] + \dot{V}O_{2rest}$<br><br>Note: $\dot{V}O_2R$ may be determined from CPET results or estimated $\dot{V}O_2$ from established metabolic equations from GXT results, 6-minute walk tests, or other measurement of peak functional capacity. |
| Visual analog scale (VAS) (157, 158) | The VAS can be presented in a number of ways, including scales with a middle point, graduations, or numbers (numerical rating scales); meter-shaped scales (curvilinear analogue scales); "box-scales" consisting of circles equidistant from each other; and scales with descriptive terms at intervals along a line (e.g., Likert scale). |
| Numeric rating scale (NRS) (92, 93) | Unidimensional numeric rating scale (0–10) that measures the general severity or perceived intensity of subjective symptoms or dyspnea at a given point in time. |
| Borg CR10 Scale modified for dyspnea (16, 90, 91) | Level of perceived dyspnea measured on a 0–10 scale, with 0 being "no breathlessness at all" and 10 being "maximal." |
| % of METS (16) | 1 MET (metabolic equivalent) = 3.5 mlO$_2$/kg/min. If the subject's actual or measured $\dot{V}O_{2peak}$ was 19.7, their peak MET level is 5.6 METS (19.7 ml O$_2$/kg/min. / 3.5) (103). If you use ACSM recommended aerobic exercise intensity levels for asthmatics (40 to 59% $\dot{V}O_2R$), the MET exercise intensity range = 2.2 to 3.3 METS (.40 × 19.7 to .59 × 19.7). |
| MET minutes (16) | A MET minute is a unit used in exercise prescription to quantify energy expenditure by factoring in the time spent exercising. Example: You want your patient to exercise at 60% of their functional capacity (6.7 METS) for 30 minutes, 4 days/week. 4 METS × 30 min. = 120 MET minutes/day. 120 × 4 days/week = 480 MET minutes/week (weekly exercise prescription at a 4 MET level). |
| Kilocalories (kcal) from METS (16) | Example: 65 kg patient<br><br>1 MET = 1 kcal/kg × hour; 5 METS = 5.05 kcal/kg × hour (65 kg subject)<br><br>5.05 kcal/kg × hour × 65 kg = 5.47 kcal/min<br><br>60 min/hour<br><br>You would like your patient to burn ~150 kcal during their exercise session, so they would exercise ~27 minutes. |

Key: ACSM = American College of Sports Medicine; CPET = cardiopulmonary exercise test; GXT = graded exercise test; $\dot{V}O_2$ = oxygen uptake

Data from ACSM (2018); Biskobing (2002); Borg (1982).

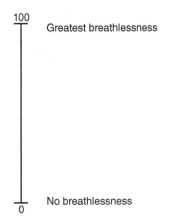

100 — Greatest breathlessness

0 — No breathlessness

**Figure 3.12**   Visual Analog Scale

## Oxyhemoglobin Monitoring During Exercise Training

In exercising patients with chronic lung disease, it is very important to evaluate and monitor $SpO_2$ to determine the need for supplemental oxygen. In particular, the arterial oxygen levels of patients with chronic lung disease change with exercise in an unpredictable fashion and cannot be reliably predicted by any measurement made at rest (97). In general, oxyhemoglobin saturation should be maintained at or above 88% during exercise (16, 29, 98-99). Cutaneous oximetry from finger or hand-held pulse oximeters provide an estimate arterial oxygen saturation ($SaO_2$) with general reliability of $SpO_2$ during walking, including 6MWT, with mean differences of 1 to 2% (35, 36). Measurements of $SpO_2$ are generally reliable when an accurate pulse signal is observed. Change in $SpO_2$ may be more variable in patients with interstitial lung disease, including idiopathic pulmonary fibrosis and systemic sclerosis, such as scleroderma (35). Use of alternative probe sites, including forehead, earlobe, or alternate fingers, may be considered if improved SpO2 accuracy is achieved. Supplemental oxygen therapy should be always readily available in the rehabilitation setting for those patients with hypoxemia during exercise.

Interestingly, some studies indicate that supplemental oxygen allows for higher levels of exercise training in COPD patients who do *not* have significant desaturation or are nonhypoxemic (2, 100-101), including those who participate in high-intensity training (72), while other studies do not have the same findings (102). The mechanisms underlying this potential benefit are unclear, but might involve decreased dyspnea from decreased carotid body stimulation, allowing for a slower respiratory rate and longer expiratory time, thereby decreasing dynamic hyperinflation. Reduced pulmonary vascular resistance may also be important. It is premature to recommend oxygen supplementation for nonhypoxemic pulmonary rehabilitation participants at this time until further research has been conducted.

Previously unrecognized exercise-induced oxygen desaturation should be documented and promptly reported to the patient's physician to facilitate a home oxygen prescription. Pulse delivery of oxygen via electronic demand device may not provide adequate $SpO_2$ for those patients during activity. Instead, continuous flow delivery of oxygen may be required, particularly in the patient with fibrotic lung disease. Patients should ultimately be tested during the maximal intensity level exercise they may undertake when at home, using the type of portable oxygen system that they use outside the program. The adequacy of the patient's oxygen system and flow rate recommendations during activity and exercise should be reported to the patient's physician. Patients requiring oxygen should be encouraged to obtain an oximeter and trained in ongoing monitoring of $SpO_2$ and oxygen in collaboration with the prescribing clinician.

In obstructive lung disease, it is also important to optimize bronchodilation and other pharmacological therapy before and during exercise training. This includes assuring not only that maintenance bronchodilators are taken, but also that short-acting bronchodilators are taken (when indicated) before initiating exercise (1, 2). Optimization of respiratory status allows for exercise training at higher intensities in patients with dyspnea limitation. Short-acting bronchodilators should also be part of any emergency kit in the exercise area.

# VOLUME, PATTERN, AND PROGRESSION OF EXERCISE TRAINING

Currently the optimal volume (total amount of exercise during each session), pattern (sequence of exercise on various modalities, including rest periods), and progression of exercise training (providing an adequate training effect) remain unknown and require further investigation. A collaborative, multidisciplinary approach is typically used to develop the optimal volume, pattern, and progression of exercise based upon patient-specific characteristics. Gradual increases of exercise workload and intensity should be incorporated over time to provide the optimal training effect for the patient. This will vary by the severity and type of lung disease, the physical capabilities of the patient, age, gender, mobility, and many other factors. With further research, evidence-based guidelines may be developed with regard to these three very important parameters.

# RESISTANCE EXERCISE TESTING

Chronic pulmonary disease not only damages the lungs but contributes to overall skeletal muscle dysfunction as well (16, 21, 52, 91). It has been well established that patients with COPD have diminished peripheral and overall muscular strength (22, 103–106). This decrease in strength is accompanied by a reduction in muscle cross-sectional area (105), muscle mass (1, 2, 52, 103) and mobility (103). Peripheral muscle atrophy and weakness combined with weak chest and thoracic muscles along with reduced muscle capillarization contribute to decreased energy expenditure, decreased resting metabolic rate, and a more sedentary lifestyle. Many pulmonary rehabilitation participants present not only with significantly reduced strength, but osteopenia and osteoporosis as well from the detrimental effects of sedentary living, chronic hypoxemia, malnutrition, and prolonged use of corticosteroid therapy. These combined effects may result in overall muscle weakness, increased risk of falls, and permanent injury or disability. Resistive exercise training can help the patient.

Recent investigations have shown that resistive exercise training is beneficial in patients with COPD by increasing QOL (52), upper- and lower-body strength (1, 2, 4, 5, 8, 11, 52), and muscle size or mass (5, 52). For these and other benefits, resistive exercise training has now become an integral component of most pulmonary rehabilitation programs. Unfortunately, the effects of resistance training on disease outcomes are not well understood and few evidence-based resistive exercise recommendations currently exist in the literature for those with chronic lung disease. Most research has traditionally been performed on patients with COPD. The effects of resistive exercise training have not been well researched in patients with restrictive lung disease, pulmonary hypertension, cystic fibrosis, and other chronic lung conditions. Published evidence-based guidelines also vary somewhat with respect to resistance exercise prescription in pulmonary patients (95). Other confounding factors for developing evidence-based guidelines include a variation across studies of the number of repetitions performed, amount of weight lifted, rest interval duration between devices, total volume of work performed, pulmonary medications taken that may affect physiologic responses, upper-body versus lower-body exercise protocols, and the patient population, which oftentimes includes men only.

Therefore, the pulmonary rehabilitation practitioner who performs resistive exercise testing and training should rely on individual patient characteristics and published recommendations as well as their own knowledge of exercise prescription techniques. This is especially important for other clinical pulmonary populations until further research studies have been performed and consistent evidence-based guidelines established.

Resistance exercise testing and training serve many important purposes in today's pulmonary rehabilitation program, including:

- To let the patient know how they compare to those in their age and gender group,
- To let the patient know how much they are improving or regressing throughout pulmonary rehabilitation,
- To help determine the patient's ability to perform basic ADLs (e.g., dressing, picking up items, housework, squatting),
- To measure individual success in resistive exercise with validated normative data,
- To boost confidence and self-efficacy,
- To help assess posture, balance, and mobility issues and to prescribe posture and balance exercises,
- For documentation of preresistive and postresistive testing results for documentation of patient improvements in muscular strength and endurance for outcomes assessment, and
- To assess and determine the individual needs of the patient with respect to their unique overall muscular weaknesses.

Prior to resistance training, the patient should be evaluated for any joint or musculoskeletal abnormalities or discomfort. The standard for determining muscular strength in pulmonary populations in most research studies has traditionally been the one repetition maximum test (1-RM) (7, 16, 103, 107–109). This test involves having the patient perform an adequate warm-up and then lifting as much weight as they can for one maximal repetition with correct form and without straining. Protocols for determining the 1-RM threshold vary by the investigation. Some investigators utilize 3-RM, 5-RM, and even 10-RM preliminary testing to determine the final 1-RM threshold. While 1-RM testing has been shown to be safe in both male and female pulmonary rehabilitation participants (7, 104), machine weight exercise oftentimes may not be prescribed until later in the program (if at all), depending upon the patient. Various techniques to determine the initial resistive training workload exist. These techniques include performing a "modified" RM (e.g., 3-RM to 8-RM), where the pulmonary rehabilitation practitioner progressively increases the workload to determine the maximal amount of weight that can be lifted up to eight times with proper form and physiologic responses, and then prescribing a percent of this workload for exercise prescription. Another technique involves a gradual "titration" of weight over time. With this technique, the practitioner initially has the patient perform 10 repetitions comfortably on a piece of upper- or lower-body weight equipment and with lighter weights. The patient then progresses to 15 repetitions per session, increasing the weight load incrementally based on dyspnea or rating of perceived exercise by 1 to 2 pounds gradually over time. Finally, a validated rating of perceived exertion scale or a VAS may be used to rate resistive exercise intensity, starting with low resistance and low numerical ratings and progressively increasing to higher resistance and higher ratings over time. Patients should be reassessed prior to any increase in resistance training intensity or duration.

An inexpensive and effective "resistive circuit" may be developed if space is available. An example of this type of resistive circuit training could include the following stations:

- Dumbbell lifts (chair and dumbbells of varying weights required)
- Bands or tubes (chair and elastic bands or tubes of various tensions required)
- Medicine ball toss station (chair and medicine balls of various weights required)
- Hand-grip squeeze station (tennis balls, squeeze balls, or handgrip devices required)
- Leg-lift station with ankle weights or weighted shopping bags (chair and ankle weights or cloth shopping bags with full cans or stones required)
- Stair-step station (adjustable step or set of steps required)
- Station where the patient can perform multiple resistive exercises using their body weight such as standing leg lifts, arm circles, chair raises, squats, or repetitive sit to stand (stable chair required)

Thus, with some creativity, an excellent, relatively inexpensive resistive training circuit can be developed for both the upper and lower body to incorporate the resistive component into pulmonary rehabilitation sessions.

## Types of Resistance Modalities

Resistive exercise training can be performed using a number of inexpensive modalities in pulmonary rehabilitation. Patients in the pulmonary rehabilitation setting may be introduced to resistive exercise early in the program with elastic bands or tubes of varying strengths, hand weights, ankle weights, dumbbells, or may use their own body weight with or without chairs (e.g., leg lifts, seated leg extensions, squats, sit to stand, chair presses with both arms). Modalities such as these may be incorporated into warm-up/cool-down activities, used during a specific time period during the pulmonary rehabilitation session in a circuit station format (as described previously), or performed one-on-one with the patient and a pulmonary rehabilitation practitioner. Weight machines and pulley devices using heavier resistance may be used for the participant once they have acclimated to aerobic exercise training and have been cleared by their referring clinician for heavier workloads (108). There are currently no evidence-based recommendations on the time frame for the pulmonary rehabilitation participant to begin heavier resistive training after program entry. Thus, each patient must be evaluated individually with respect to resistive workload, taking into consideration their type and severity of lung disease, existing comorbidities (e.g., cardiovascular status), musculoskeletal limitations, and degree of frailty.

## Rate of Progression

The rate of progression is a very important component of the resistive exercise prescription and

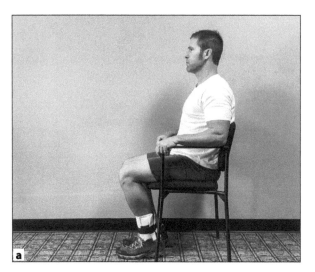
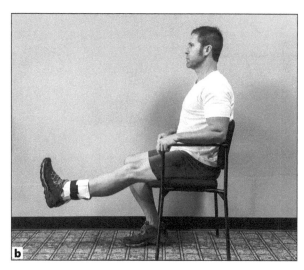

Seated knee extension. *(a)* Sit in chair with back supported. Ankle weight strapped around ankle. Start with knees bent to approximately 90 degrees, feet resting on floor. *(b)* Straighten one knee and dorsiflex ankle ("toes pointing toward nose"). Pause, then return to start position. Repeat. Perform this exercise on both legs. Considerations: For taller individuals, use higher chair surface or rolled-up towel behind knee. For those with knee pain, work within a pain-free range of motion. Purpose of exercise: strengthen quadriceps/thigh muscles.

Photos courtesy of Kim Eppen.

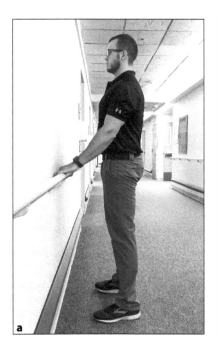
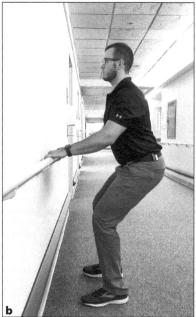
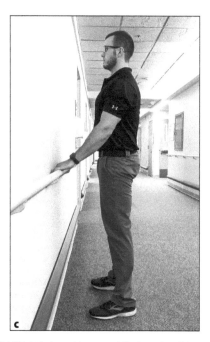

Partial squat or knee bend. *(a)* Stand up straight while holding on to a firm surface. *(b)* Slightly bend knees while keeping hips back (body weight more on heels, not balls of feet). *(c)* Return to standing position. Repeat. Purpose of exercise: leg strengthening. This is a good option to start with for people who can't perform full sit-to-stand exercise.

Photos courtesy of Kim Eppen.

should be individualized to the patient based upon risk stratification criteria stated previously. The most important part of rate of progression is utilization of the overload principle. Upper- and lower-body musculature must be stressed in a gradual, progressive manner over time for the patient to gain the most benefits from resistive training (1, 109). The principle of overload involves increasing the exercise dosage over time to maximize gains in muscular strength and endurance.

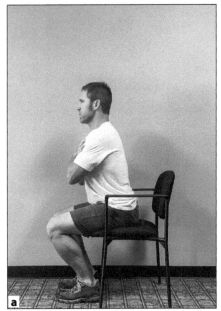
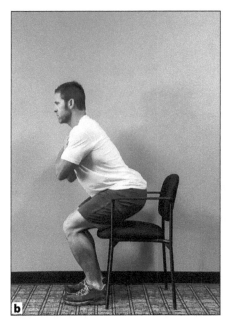
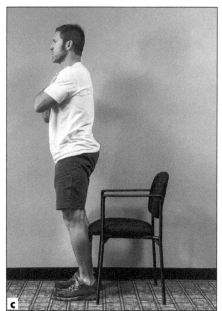
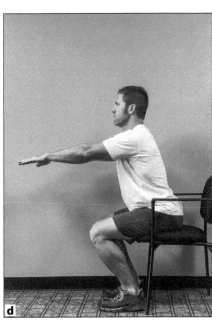
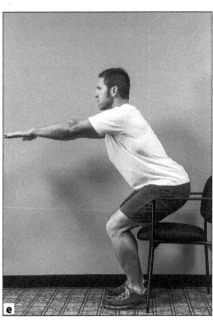
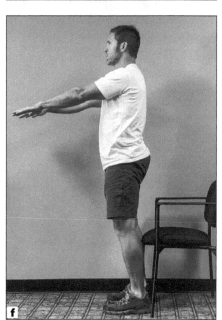

Sit to stand. Option 1: *(a)* Sit toward front of chair with arms folded across chest. *(b)* Flex (lean) forward at hips. *(c)* Stand up while keeping knees behind toes. Focus on using legs, not momentum. Slowly return to seated position. Option 2: *(d-f)* Perform same exercise with arms reaching forward. Choose which option works best for each patient. Consideration: For taller individuals, those with knee pain, or significant muscle weakness, use higher chair surface. Purpose of exercise: leg strengthening.

Photos courtesy of Kim Eppen.

This can be achieved by increasing the intensity (weight or resistance), total repetitions per set, repetition speed or rhythm, number of sets of each exercise, and/or decreasing the rest period between sets or exercises (16, 108, 109). Reassessment is required before any advancement of intensity or time and only one feature of intensity should be increased at a time.

# OTHER TESTS OF MUSCULAR FITNESS

The pulmonary rehabilitation practitioner may choose from any number of validated physical function tests to assess muscular strength and endurance prior to pulmonary rehabilitation

## ACSM FITT Resistive Exercise Recommendations for Patients with COPD or Asthma

The ACSM FITT (Frequency, Intensity, Time, and Type) principles are evidence-based resistive exercise recommendations for patients with COPD and asthma (table 3.7) (16). These guidelines may apply only to patients with either COPD or asthma, as further research needs to be performed on patients with other types of chronic lung disease before evidence-based guidelines may be presented for these populations. Some of the recommendations presented may not be applicable to specific patients depending upon their individual characteristics, comorbidities, and frailty. Certain patients may not be able to effectively perform sustained aerobic exercise during pulmonary rehabilitation sessions. Thus, low-level resistance exercise may be a good alternative for these patients. While the ACSM recommends two to four sets of exercises to improve muscular strength, other investigators have found that one set of resistive exercises provides comparable strength and physical function improvements in COPD patients compared to multiple-set protocols (7). Nevertheless, these recommendations may help to provide a framework for the pulmonary rehabilitation practitioner in the development of individualized resistive exercise prescriptions for patients with either COPD or asthma.

The ACSM FITT recommendations are also supported, in part, by the American Thoracic Society and the European Respiratory Society (1). The ATS/ERS guidelines recommend that resistance exercise guidelines should follow the same ACSM FITT principle for apparently healthy and older adults (1, 106). The AACVPR currently does not state a specific FITT recommendation for resistive exercise in pulmonary patients (29).

**Table 3.7    ACSM FITT Resistive Exercise Recommendations for COPD and Asthma**

| FITT | Resistance Exercise |
| --- | --- |
| Frequency | 2–3 days/week |
| Intensity | *Strength:* 60%-70% of 1-RM for beginners; ≥80% 1-RM for experienced weight trainers<br>*Endurance:* < 50% of 1-RM<br>Assessment of dyspnea or RPE using a validated scale may be considered. |
| Time | *Strength:* 2–4 sets, 8–12 repetitions<br>*Endurance:* ≤2 sets for 15–20 repetitions |
| Type | Weight machines, free weight, or body weight exercises |

Key: RM = repetition maximum, RPE = rating of perceived exertion

Adapted by permission from American College of Sports Medicine, *ACSM's Guidelines for Exercise Testing and Prescription*, 10th ed. (Philadelphia, PA: Lippincott Williams & Wilkins, 2018), 254.

participation. The patient can then be tested periodically at regular intervals throughout program participation for outcomes documentation and assessment of improvement or decline. Moreover, upper- and lower-body muscular power (e.g., watts) may be assessed from some of these tests. These tests include, but are not limited to, the following:

- Timed up and go (TUG) test (110–112)
- 30-second chair stand test (113)
- 6-minute pegboard and ring test (6PBRT) (114)
- Five-times-sit-to-stand test (115)

- 30-second arm curl test (111, 116)
- Handgrip dynamometer test (117–121)
- Seated medicine ball throw test (122)
- Gallon jug shelf transfer test (123)

While normative data currently does not exist for many of these tests for pulmonary populations, these normative values may provide a reasonable reference point for the pulmonary rehabilitation participant to determine their rate of decline or improvement over time, although consideration must be given to severity and type of lung disease, comorbidities, musculoskeletal abnormalities, and hypoxemia with regular subjective and objective assessment. This data also shows the patient how they compare to individuals in their age category.

The ACSM (16), ATS/ERS (1) and AACVPR (29) have presented varying but similar recommendations (106) on ways to incorporate resistive exercise progression within the formal pulmonary rehabilitation exercise prescription. The ACSM focuses on a gradual progression, increasing resistance, repetitions, or frequency per session over time (16). The ATS/ERS recommends increasing the weight, number of repetitions per set, and number of sets per session over time, or to reduce rest intervals when the patient can perform one or two repetitions over the desired number during two consecutive sessions (1). The AACVPR has stated that the pulmonary rehabilitation clinician should monitor the patient's RPE as well as muscle/joint fatigue, soreness, and pain over time to incorporate overload and progression. For those with osteoporosis, caution should be exercised with spine flexion or rotation and heavy weight training. For those with pulmonary hypertension, low-level resistance training with paced breathing is acceptable (29). Overall, each of these agencies offers prudent resistive exercise progression and overload guidelines and the pulmonary rehabilitation clinician may use a combination of the above approaches.

# INSPIRATORY MUSCLE TRAINING

With any continuous exercise over a period of several minutes, respiratory muscles, with normal mechanical dynamics, can increase minute ventilation (tidal volume × respiratory rate). Consequently, repeating this pattern over a period of weeks at regular intervals, a training effect occurs with improved strength and endurance of the respiratory muscles. This improvement does not occur among those with mechanical disadvantages of the respiratory muscles due to disease, such as a flattened diaphragm muscle because of COPD (1). Whether more specific inspiratory muscle training, using resistive breathing devices, enhances outcome is controversial (1, 17). Some studies have demonstrated that resistance breathing leads to an increase in respiratory muscle strength and endurance, a reduction in dyspnea, walking distance, and health-related quality of life. The British Thoracic Society's guidelines on pulmonary rehabilitation in adults evidence-based clinical practice guidelines do not support the routine

use of inspiratory muscle training as an adjunct to pulmonary rehabilitation (17). This therapy may be considered for respiratory patients with documented respiratory muscle weakness (e.g., due to cachexia or corticosteroid use) or persons who use an interval training technique to improve $P_I$max (maximal inspiratory pressure measured at the mouth).

Types of respiratory muscle training include flow resistive training (breathing through a progressively smaller orifice), threshold loading training (a preset inspiratory pressure, usually at some fraction of the maximal inspiratory pressure, is required), and isocapneic hyperventilation. Suggested guidelines for employing resistive inspiratory muscle training include a frequency of 4 or 5 days a week; intensities of 30% of $P_I$max and a duration of one 30-minute session per day or two 15-minute sessions over at least 2 months (29).

# FLEXIBILITY TRAINING

The majority of evidence of exercise effectiveness is based on aerobic and resistance training, yet flexibility training is commonly included as part of pulmonary rehabilitation programs (1) (table 3.8). Maintaining flexibility and good posture are very important components of a pulmonary rehabilitation program. Exercises such as yoga (124) and Tai Chi can help patients maintain needed flexibility and good posture. Range of motion improvement exercises should be incorporated into each warm-up and cool-down session to help overcome the effects of postural impairments that limit thoracic mobility and therefore lung function (1, 16). Flexibility exercises may also help to improve range of motion, prevent patient falls, and improve overall QOL, although more research is needed in this area before any steadfast conclusions may be formulated.

# PATIENT SAFETY

Safety, clinical stability, and prevention of muscle tears are of crucial importance, especially for persons on chronic steroid therapy who may be at risk of muscle or tendon rupture when exposed to high-intensity loads. Furthermore, strength training precautions are warranted for postsurgical pulmonary patients, those with osteoporosis, and patients diagnosed with pulmonary arterial hypertension (PAH) and moderate to severe pulmonary

## Table 3.8  ACSM Evidence-Based FITT Recommendations for Flexibility Training in Patients with COPD or Asthma

| FITT | Flexibility |
|------|-------------|
| Frequency | > 2–3 days/week, with daily being most effective |
| Intensity | Stretch to the point of feeling tightness or slight discomfort |
| Time | 10–30 seconds for static stretching; 2–4 repetitions of each exercise |
| Type | Static, dynamic, or proprioceptive neuromuscular facilitation (PNF) stretching |

Adapted by permission from American College of Sports Medicine, *ACSM's Guidelines for Exercise Testing and Prescription*, 10th ed. (Philadelphia, PA: Lippincott Williams & Wilkins, 2018), 257.

hypertension (PH). Light resistance exercise training using dumbbells has been shown to be safe (i.e., no severe adverse effects) in patients with PH (125). However, it is very important to instruct the patient to avoid lifting heavy weights and any breath holding or Valsalva to avoid abnormal increases in intrathoracic pressure and blood pressure during any type of resistive exercise. Until resistance guidelines are established for patients with PH, the pulmonary rehabilitation practitioner should take a prudent approach to incorporating resistance training in this population. Light hand weights, dumbbells, ankle weights, and elastic bands or tubes may be beneficial for upper- and lower-body strength development in this selected patient population.

The need for cardiovascular monitoring may be less of a priority for the pulmonary rehabilitation participant who performs resistance exercise compared to traditional aerobic exercise. While patients with COPD have been shown to work closer to their peak $\dot{V}O_2$ during upper- and lower-body resistance exercise training than age-matched healthy adults (126), resistance exercise training generally elicits a *lower* cardiorespiratory demand than that of aerobic exercise (127). This form of exercise demands a lower level of $\dot{V}O_2$ and minute ventilation and therefore evokes less dyspnea (123).

The pulmonary rehabilitation practitioner should monitor patients who are prone to hypertensive/hypotensive responses with periodic blood pressure checks, even during the resistance movement itself. If an exercise blood pressure can be taken, the rate-pressure product (double-product) can be determined with a measurement of HR for optimal patient safety and refinement of the resistance exercise prescription. If the pulmonary

rehabilitation participant is being monitored with continuous ECG telemetry, the practitioner should continue to monitor for arrhythmias and adverse ECG changes during periods of resistance exercise training.

Certain patients will require one-on-one guidance and supervision during resistive testing and training, depending upon their risk level and frailty. Each patient should be given proper training instructions, followed by the pulmonary rehabilitation practitioner demonstrating the exercise. Mild muscle soreness and fatigue are common 12 to 24 hours after testing and training. If the patient complains of persistent or significant soreness or joint pain (>1 week), the referring pulmonologist or physician should be notified. Holding off resistance and aerobic training of the affected area is warranted until discomfort has subsided. Patients with major orthopedic limitations, kyphoscoliosis, acute episodes of joint inflammation, uncontrolled metabolic disease, a resting $SpO_2 < 90\%$, acute systemic illness (e.g., influenza), recent significant increase in dyspnea, fatigue, or who report of experiencing a "bad breathing day" may be contraindicated from resistive testing and training and require further screening.

# PRECAUTIONS IN PULMONARY HYPERTENSION

The cardiovascular and ventilatory response to exercise is limited in pulmonary hypertension (PH) due to restriction in maximum cardiac output associated with increased right ventricle afterload (128–131). Persons with PH experience multiple physiologic abnormalities during exercise, including reduced peak $\dot{V}O_2$, oxygen pulse, and low anaerobic threshold (130, 131). Evaluation and management by skilled specialists, along with the advent and use of disease-targeted agents in appropriate patients, have been associated with improved symptoms, exercise capacity, and health-related quality of life in persons with PH. Exercise training is now a class IA recommendation for PH patients (131–134).

Well-designed trials have demonstrated improvement in exercise, functional capacity, and quality of life in people with PH participating in exercise training programs compared to untrained control groups, with exercise-based rehabilitation resulting in clinically relevant improvements in exercise capacity (135, 136). Evidence-based guidelines recommend accurate diagnosis, evaluation, and management by a PH specialist, supportive measures including oxygen, supervised exercise training, and avoidance of strenuous physical activity. Prior to exercise, patients should be referred for expert evaluation and treatment recommendations (132).

Optimal exercise training and prescription in PH have not been established, although gradual exercise protocols at low intensity and short duration are often used initially. Interval training should generally be avoided due to the associated rapid changes in pulmonary hemodynamics and risk of syncope. Based upon pulmonary and cardiovascular symptoms, HR, BP, and SpO2 response, the intensity and duration of exercise may be gradually advanced as tolerated with exercise training intensity and duration generally kept at submaximal levels (133). Moderate intensity resistance exercise is generally introduced only when the patient effectively uses appropriate controlled breathing techniques and avoids breath holding or the Valsalva maneuver. There is no evidence for restricting arm lifting above the head (with or without weights) as long as the patient consistently uses controlled breathing and the clinical response is within defined acceptable limits for dyspnea, $SpO_2$, HR, and blood pressure with absence of syncope or presyncope (137). Reducing or stopping exercise is recommended in the presence of chest pain, lightheadedness, palpitations, hypotension, severe dyspnea, presyncope, or syncope. Extreme caution must be used to avoid interruption of intravenous vasodilator therapy and to prevent falls for individuals taking anticoagulants.

# EXERCISE-INDUCED HYPOXEMIA

Hypoxemia during exercise is a common and clinically important finding in the pulmonary rehabilitation setting (138). The incidence of hypoxemia is unknown with very limited guidance or standards available to direct evaluation and management of hypoxemia during exercise. A subset of hypoxemic patients develop severe exercise-induced hypoxemia (SEIH) (139). SEIH is defined as the need for >6 L/min oxygen to yield an $SpO_2 \geq 88\%$ (139). Negative consequences of sustained hypoxemia include pulmonary hypertension, cor pulmonale, cardiac dysfunction, arrhythmias, erythrocytosis, cognitive abnormalities, decline in self-care, and increased mortality (139). Hypoxemia may be managed with supplemental oxygen therapy to improve oxygenation. A potential concern in persons with COPD is suppression of hypoxic ventilatory drive, resulting in hypoventilation and $CO_2$ retention. Most cases of $CO_2$ retention result from ventilation/perfusion mismatch rather than respiratory drive suppression (140–142). Clinically stable COPD patients are generally at low risk for significant or unstable hypercapnia, particularly when using low-flow oxygen, although some may experience clinically important respiratory drive suppression when using high-flow oxygen (142).

In cases of SEIH, evaluation and management should be based upon a systematic approach to determining the underlying cause(s) of SEIH, and development and use of appropriate management strategies. If the patient is clinically stable based on HR, symptoms, and BP, gradually progressive, incremental, supervised exercise in a pulmonary rehabilitation setting is reasonable as long as hypoxemia is controlled and the patient demonstrates both objective and subjective clinical stability and exercise tolerance.

Underlying cause(s) of hypoxemia during exercise may be multifactorial and may include ventilation/perfusion mismatch, diffusion defect, right-to-left shunt, or alveolar hypoventilation. Hypoxemia in persons with COPD is usually due to ventilation/perfusion (V/Q) mismatch (143). A diffusion defect is a potential contributing factor, especially at higher exercise intensities (144). Hypoxemia from diffusion defect is generally well controlled versus that due to a right-to-left shunt which may be associated with a more limited response to supplemental oxygen. As the shunt fraction increases, some patients may be refractory to up to 100% oxygen due to shunted blood bypassing alveoli required to transfer oxygen into the bloodstream (145–147). Hypoxemia due to depressed ventilatory drive resulting from oversedation is rare in the pulmonary rehabilitation setting and is typically accompanied by hypercapnia and low pH. Chronic respiratory failure is associated with hypercapnia, near normal pH, and elevated bicarbonate. Hypoxemia is often aggravated with exposure to high altitude or during disease exacerbation.

Evaluation of hypoxemia at a minimum begins with history and physical exam, pulse oximetry at rest and exercise, and evaluation of symptoms and vital signs. Evaluation for severe hypoxemia should include arterial blood gas determination and pulmonology evaluation, if not already in place.

## Hypoxemia during Exercise

In chronic lung disease, the ability of the lungs to maintain normal arterial oxygen is often impaired, with compromise of oxygen delivery particularly during exercise. Muscular demand for oxygen increases during exercise in proportion to the amount of work performed (138). Higher cardiopulmonary demand results in complex physiologic adjustments as well as significant potential for dysfunction or failure during activity (147).

## Managing Hypoxemia during Exercise

Supplemental oxygen is used to increase arterial oxygen levels, decrease carotid body stimulation (reducing pulmonary ventilation, respiratory muscle work, and dyspnea) and relieve pulmonary vasoconstriction (improving cardiac output restriction). Oxygen improves the effectiveness of short- and long-term exercise training in pulmonary rehabilitation by reducing dyspnea, hypoxic ventilatory drive, and hyperinflation, as well as delaying acidosis. Ambulatory oxygen has the potential to increase mobility, compliance, exercise tolerance, and autonomy in hypoxemic patients. The pulmonary rehabilitation clinician should address appropriate equipment selection, use, and flow rate; communicate these recommendations to the clinical team, including the referring clinician; and assess the patient during rest, activity, and exercise using the patient's portable system. Patients who

are unable to obtain appropriate oxygen for rest and ambulation due to lack of access or lack of provision from their medical equipment company should address these concerns with their prescribing clinician and insurance.

## Developing an Oxygen Prescription for Exercise-Induced Hypoxemia

A comprehensive assessment requires evaluation of desaturation and oxygen requirements during exercise testing. While a 6MWT or other exercise test may reveal significant hypoxemia associated with exercise, a separate assessment and titration should be conducted to determine severity of desaturation and oxygen needs during usual self-walking pace as well as "purposeful exercise" or other activities of daily life. Assessment must also occur using the patient's ambulatory oxygen source. Nighttime $O_2$ needs require a separate assessment based on the clinical judgment of the referring clinician. All testing revealing hypoxemia and oxygen titration should be promptly communicated to the referring clinician. Most guidelines recommend oxygen titration to an $SpO_2$ level of ≥88–93%. Community practice of management of SEIH describes oxygen flow rates of 7–15 L/min by several types of nasal cannula and/or delivering up to 100% oxygen by mask interfaces in one small study (139). Multiple interfaces are used in the pulmonary rehabilitation setting, including nasal cannula, Oxymizer cannula and pendant, non-rebreathing (NRB) mask, Oxymask, Venturi mask, transtracheal oxygen, and other interfaces in an attempt to meet the oxygen needs of this population during exercise.

Inpatient practitioners have extensive experience with various high-flow oxygen systems, including NRB masks and heated, humidified, high-flow oxygen. These modalities have historically had limited use or availability in the outpatient setting due to comfort concerns and lack of portability during exercise. Use, safety, and effectiveness of these systems during exercise are poorly understood.

## Oxygen Monitoring, Titration and Exercise Training

In hypoxemic COPD patients, long-term oxygen therapy has been found to improve survival, exercise, sleep, and cognitive performance with a therapeutic goal of $SpO_2$ level of ≥88–90% during rest, sleep, and exertion (1, 2, 16). Patients with ongoing desaturation despite use of high-flow oxygen require medical evaluation and management prior to resuming exercise. Optimal strategies for exercise training for SEIH patients have not been established (139). Progressive exercise routines should be based upon physiologic findings, such as an adequate $SpO_2$ determined from a pulse oximeter, symptom level including dyspnea and fatigue, stable heart rate and blood pressure, and the results of a 6MWT or CPET. If available, pulmonary rehabilitation programs should consider telemetry monitoring during the patient's first exercise session and ongoing telemetry monitoring in those with significant pulmonary hypertension or cardiac abnormalities. Patients with significant arrhythmias require medical evaluation and treatment before exercise is performed. Interval training should be avoided in persons with significant PH due to rapid changes in pulmonary hemodynamics and risk of syncope. Exercise should be stopped if the patient develops desaturation refractory to supplemental oxygen, significant tachycardia, arrhythmias, severe dyspnea, hypotension, severe hypertension, dizziness, or chest pain. Patients should have ongoing evaluation and management of their chronic lung disease and comorbidities by a pulmonologist, primary care provider, and other appropriate consultants.

Low-intensity exercise is recommended in the initial stages of exercise based upon evaluation of dyspnea, $SpO_2$, HR, blood pressure, and subjective symptoms. Guidelines support safe incremental increase in exercise intensity based on clinical stability. Exercise prescription and a home exercise program should be established and communicated to the patient as well as indications for stopping exercise and symptoms to report to their physician. Interval training exercise routines require further investigation in SEIH to determine safety and effectiveness.

# HOME EXERCISE CONSIDERATIONS

Patients participating in a formal pulmonary rehabilitation program should be provided with a home exercise prescription to support ongoing exercise. All patient recommendations should be tailored to the individual based upon their performance and achievements during the pulmonary rehabilita-

tion program. Aerobic exercise, muscular strength conditioning, range of motion exercises, and, in select patients, inspiratory muscle training should be included in the home exercise program. It is essential to consider the patient's future exercise setting when prescribing independent exercise to promote adherence to the program. For example, if the patient does not have access to weight-training machines, specific strength training exercises that the patient can perform with inexpensive modalities such as elastic resistance bands, light dumbbells, and hand or cuff weights should be recommended. The home exercise prescription should reflect activities performed during the rehabilitation program to allow the patient to proceed with confidence in their personalized independent program.

Participation in a pulmonary maintenance exercise program in a supervised setting promotes short- and long-term exercise adherence, patient and group support, clinical monitoring of cardiopulmonary signs and symptoms, and the opportunity for ongoing training and reinforcement of self-management strategies.

# Home-Based Pulmonary Rehabilitation

Although pulmonary rehabilitation is typically provided in supervised outpatient or inpatient settings, growing evidence suggests that home-based exercise training can be effective (148–150). Home exercise programs should encourage exercise as well as lifestyle modifications to promote improved health and functional status. While home-based pulmonary rehabilitation offers the potential for convenience, cost savings, and increased access, several potential barriers exist. Potential concerns and limitations of home-based pulmonary rehabilitation include safety, liability, supervision responsibilities, outcome measurement, grossly inadequate or absent coverage by insurance, limited group support, and lack of well-developed, evidence-based guidelines that are widely applicable for the home setting and an equally strong evidence base of effectiveness. Ongoing, direct clinical supervision, monitoring, and management of clinical abnormalities in the home is unlikely. Technology systems supporting home pulmonary rehabilitation are in their infancy and have not been extensively tested in this setting. Older patients, particularly those who are less affluent and more disabled, may be disconnected from e-health both physically and psychologically (151).

# Technology-Supported Home-Based Pulmonary Rehabilitation

Key principles to ensure that technology-supported home-based pulmonary rehabilitation is effective include evaluation for clinical efficacy as well as safety. Goals of care should include enhancement of function, patient independence, symptom control, and improvement in quality of life. Optimized exercise safety is a key requirement for unsupervised exercise. Whether technology-supported home-based pulmonary rehabilitation has the potential to reduce health care utilization and mortality in pulmonary populations requires further research (152–154). Key areas include mechanisms for:

- Evaluation of desaturation at rest and with exercise, and oxygen titration prior to home pulmonary rehabilitation
- Patient training and return demonstration of proper use of inhaled medications and, when appropriate, secretion clearance devices
- Insurance coverage or patient payment for home pulmonary rehabilitation
- Patient support to reinforce new behaviors

As with traditional pulmonary rehabilitation programs, a patient must undergo a complete history and physical examination, symptom assessment, and discussion of optimal control and management of chronic lung disease and comorbidities prior to initiating a home exercise program. The preevaluation includes evaluation of functional capacity typically using a 6MWT, shuttle walk test (endurance or incremental), or CPET (1, 16, 29, 35). Those patients unable to walk 50 feet either unassisted or with their usual walking aid should be referred to either physical therapy for improvement in functional capacity or to a supervised inpatient or outpatient pulmonary rehabilitation. Patients should have had an ECG within the past year. Those with an abnormal ECG, cardiovascular symptoms, or poorly controlled cardiovascular disease should be referred to a cardiologist for further testing, management, and clearance before beginning a home exercise program. Patients with significant ECG or echocardiogram abnormalities or New York Heart Association

class III-IV congestive heart failure require close supervision and monitoring not available in the home setting.

# Home Exercise Prescription

Guidelines are lacking for home exercise. The following sections provide a general framework for home exercise in stable patients with mild to moderate chronic lung disease.

## Dyspnea Control and Symptom Management

Patients should be trained in strategies for dyspnea control, including pursed-lip breathing, three-point posture, intermittent rest periods, use of electric or battery-operated fan, open window, and walking in a mall or large store while leaning on a shopping cart or using a rollator or rolling walker (avoiding peak crowds). Considerations for distraction from dyspnea include use of music, TV, scenic locations, and exercising with friends or family.

Moderate breathlessness and fatigue are common symptoms with exercise, particularly during the initial weeks of training. If symptoms increase to beyond 6–10 using a valid 10-point dyspnea or fatigue scale, the patient is advised to slow down or rest until at baseline, then resume walking or activity at a slower speed. If dyspnea does not improve or worsens despite dyspnea controls, the patient is instructed to promptly contact their clinician or seek emergency care.

## Adjuncts for Exercise

Tools that may support exercise include walking aids such as rollators that may improve balance, distance, dyspnea, and fatigue (155) and Nordic walking or trekking (156). Alternatively, the patient may use a usual walking aid if preferred.

Patients should be assessed for resting and exercise hypoxemia prior to home exercise along with development of an oxygen prescription and training on oxygen use and safety. Once home oxygen and prescription have been prescribed, the clinician should determine if the patient's portable ambulatory oxygen will adequately oxygenate the patient during activity by monitoring SpO2, heart rate, and dyspnea while performing 3 to 6 minutes of walking at the patient's usual pace. The patient should own an accurate oximeter and be trained in its use and goals for oxygen saturation during rest and exercise (157). If high-flow oxygen is required, consider evaluating use of a reservoir cannula or pendant to reduce continuous flow requirements. These devices require continuous flow oxygen for effective use. Patients with severe exercise-induced hypoxemia should be referred to outpatient or inpatient pulmonary rehabilitation.

Short- and long-acting bronchodilators play a key role in improving dyspnea and hyperinflation in obstructive lung disease (158). The clinician should determine if use of a short-acting bronchodilator such as albuterol alone or combined with ipratropium metered dose inhaler or nebulizer before exercise is warranted. Patients should be trained in and demonstrate proper inhaler use with regular follow-up evaluation.

The patient should be trained in self-monitoring of abnormal symptoms and appropriate management and reporting of abnormalities. The patient should have a mechanism to call for help, either with a family member or friend present, or use of a cellular phone. A summary of when to stop exercise is found in figure 3.13.

## Self-Management

Self-management training is a key element of pulmonary rehabilitation and therefore must be addressed as part of home pulmonary rehabilitation. The emphasis of self-management has moved from a formal, didactic approach to a focus on collaborative self-management, behavior change, and adaptation (159). Self-management includes goal setting, problem solving, decision making, and taking action based on a predefined action plan (160, 161). Specific models for providing home self-management training are few and have not been well evaluated. Figure 3.14 identifies topics for self-management training as part of pulmonary rehabilitation. Factors influencing activation of self-management may include anxiety, illness perception, body mass index, age, Global Initiative for Chronic Obstructive Lung Disease (GOLD) COPD stage, and comorbidities (161–165).

---

### Figure 3.13   When to not exercise and get help

- Breathlessness, fatigue, or weakness beyond normal levels that does not improve with rest or usual management (e.g., oxygen, rescue inhaler or nebulizer, tripod position, etc.)
- Chest pain or tightness
- Heart palpations, including very slow or fast heart rates
- Muscle pain that does not improve
- Feeling dizzy or faint
- Leg pain, weakness, or cramping
- Sweating more than usual with exercise

Reprinted by permission from C. Garvey et al., "Moving Pulmonary Rehabilitation Into the Home," *Journal of Cardiopulmonary Rehabilitation Prevention* 38, no. 1 (2018): 1.

---

### Figure 3.14   Educational topics concerning self-management

- Normal pulmonary anatomy and physiology
- Pathophysiology of chronic respiratory disease
- Communicating with the health care provider
- Interpretation of medical testing
- Breathing strategies
- Secretion clearance techniques
- Role and rationale for medications, including oxygen therapy
- Effective use of respiratory devices
- Benefits of exercise and physical activities
- Energy conservation during activities of daily living
- Healthy food intake
- Irritant avoidance
- Early recognition and treatment of exacerbations
- Leisure activities
- Coping with chronic lung disease

Reprinted with permission of the American Thoracic Society. Copyright © 2018 American Thoracic Society. M.A. Spruit et al., 2013, "An Official American Thoracic Society/European Respiratory Statement: Key Concepts and Advances in Pulmonary Rehabilitation," *American Journal of Respiratory Critical Care Medicine* 188:13–64. The *American Journal of Respiratory and Critical Care Medicine* is an official journal of the American Thoracic Society.

## Outcome Measures

At a minimum, home exercise programs should include measurement of dyspnea and physical activity. A tracking and reporting system should include the patient's resting and exercise heart rate, oxygen saturation, activity tracking using an accurate activity monitor, and oxygen flow rates if oxygen is used. For very slow walking patients, recording walking time or distance is acceptable. Pretesting and posttesting should include measurement of functional capacity such as 6-minute walk testing or shuttle walk testing, health-related quality of life, and mood (e.g., depression and possibly anxiety symptoms). A clinician should be identified to be responsible for tracking outcomes and addressing abnormal findings in home exercise (159).

# EMERGENCY PROCEDURES

Appropriate emergency procedures and supplies must be immediately accessible and used appropriately in the pulmonary rehabilitation exercise and patient training areas (1, 16). All staff should regularly demonstrate competency with these emergency procedures. Minimum emergency equipment should include an oxygen source adequate for use during patient resuscitation and delivery apparatus, resuscitation mask, first-aid supplies, bronchodilator medications, and defibrillator (either clinical defibrillator or automated external defibrillator) (figure 3.15). In addition, all staff should have at a minimum current certification in basic life support for health care providers. Personnel who work with pulmonary patients should be familiar with panic and dyspnea control techniques.

In the patient with acute dyspnea, the following interventions are recommended:

- Monitor $SpO_2$.
- Assess cardiovascular status with HR, blood pressure, and, when available, ECG rhythm strip.
- Have the patient stop the activity and assume a comfortable breathing position.
- Encourage the patient to use pursed-lip breathing and relaxation techniques.
- Administer supplemental oxygen, if indicated.
- Use a rapid-onset bronchodilator medication, if indicated.

### Figure 3.15 Emergency equipment for pulmonary rehabilitation

- Telephone in the room
- Sphygmomanometer
- Stethoscope
- Pulse oximeter
- Clinical defibrillator or automated external defibrillator (AED)
- Oxygen with delivery apparatus
- Resuscitation mask (Ambu bag)
- First-aid supplies

**If available:**

- Fully equipped crash cart with emergency drugs, including bronchodilator medications*
- IV pole for fluid administration*

*A ongoing system is required for proper training and use of equipment, medications, and supplies.

Immediately summon the supervising physician, rapid response team, or code blue team if the patient continues to deteriorate despite the above emergency measures or when indicated.

# DOCUMENTATION OF THE EVALUATION AND TREATMENT SESSION

As part of initial and ongoing patient pulmonary rehabilitation evaluation and reevaluation, every skilled clinician treating patients in pulmonary rehabilitation should perform an independent evaluation of each patient specific to the clinician's particular scope of practice. For example, the respiratory therapist would evaluate a patient's use of MDIs and (when appropriate) secretion clearance devices, whereas a physical therapist or clinical exercise physiologist should evaluate a patient's functional mobility. Cross-training of clinicians is appropriate and reasonable to further strengthen the competency of the clinical team and patient rehabilitation interventions. Within this evaluation, the clinician should identify the patient's problems, set goals to address these problems, and create a plan of care directed toward the defined goals. Overall, the patient initial assessment and evaluation should include the following: history of pulmonary and nonpulmonary disease; comorbidities and clinical manifestations; physician's review of pulmonary function tests, arterial blood gases (if available), and other relevant diagnostic tests; past medical history; current medications and oxygen liter flow (if used); baseline functional level; psychosocial status; ADL and mobility functional deficits; and an assessment of the patient's rehabilitation potential.

Documentation from treatment sessions should include the time and date; frequency, intensity, time, and type of exercise; education provided to the patient; patient's response to treatment; patient progress; and, importantly, rationale for continuing skilled intervention. Documentation of patient problems or deficits and the above information is summarized on the individualized treatment plan (ITP) in collaboration with the supervising physician at start of care, every 30 days, and at discharge.

# SUMMARY

The importance of an exercise training program cannot be overemphasized. However, before a safe exercise program can be provided, a thorough patient assessment is required to evaluate exercise tolerance, formulate an appropriate exercise training prescription, detect exercise-induced hypoxemia or bronchospasm, and detect occult cardiac or other pulmonary and nonpulmonary limitations to exercise. The benefits of exercise training are well documented and include improved aerobic capacity, decreased dyspnea, increased physical capability, increased muscular strength and endurance, and improved quality of life. Areas requiring further research regarding effectiveness and use in the pulmonary rehabilitation setting include add-on or adjuncts to exercise (166), home- or community-based pulmonary rehabilitation (159), and use of high-flow oxygen systems (139).

**VISIT THE WEB RESOURCE** ————————————————————————
for links to additional resources and various tools, checklists, and forms.

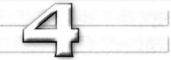

# Collaborative Self-Management and Patient Education

**Gerene Bauldoff, PhD, RN, MAACVPR**
The Ohio State University College of Nursing

**Jane Knipper, RN, MA, AE-C, MAACVPR**
University of Iowa Hospital and Clinics

**Debbie Koehl, MS, RRT-NPS, AE-C, FAARC**
Indiana University Health Methodist Hospital

Expert opinion and systematic reviews support the inclusion of education as an essential component of a comprehensive pulmonary rehabilitation program (1–7). As discussed in chapter 2, evaluation of the education needs of the patient and family or caregiver is the base on which an individualized education program is designed. Traditionally, education in pulmonary rehabilitation has been presented by a health care provider, one on one or in a group lecture setting, with the content being a disease-specific but not necessarily patient-specific focus. This approach has been shown to have low overall effectiveness (2). Rather than present information in the traditional didactic format, the education process that is currently recommended is to utilize the model of collaborative self-management training. This promotes learning by doing, which increases knowledge, enhances skills mastery, and increases self-efficacy (2). Traditional didactic education is insufficient to promote health behavior change

and optimize disease control. Self-management training changes a patient's behavior by teaching individualized problem-solving skills that improve self-efficacy, which is defined as the patient's confidence to perform a behavior required to reach a specific goal. Continued development of innovative self-management programs is ongoing (2–5). Collaborative self-management training benefits both the patients and the caregivers. The patients become active partners in the management of their chronic lung disease. Patients gain the ability to assess their progress and problems, set goals, and problem solve (4, 5). Strategies that integrate self-management training and enhance communication between the patients and their health care providers have been shown to improve adherence to their treatment plans (7–9), reduce health care utilization, and reduce the probability of hospitalizations and readmissions (7). An important benefit of self-management strategies is reduction in non-adherence (2).

# DEVELOPING AN INDIVIDUALIZED SELF-MANAGEMENT PROGRAM

Self-management interventions must be individualized to each patient's needs and concerns, diagnosis, disease severity, and comorbidities. Self-management training may be presented one on one or in a group setting, but the content must be sufficient to meet the specific needs of each patient. In addition, the interventions must focus on the patient's motivation to change (2).

Important characteristics to include in self-management training are as follows:

- Encourage active rather than passive learner participation (e.g., include group discussions instead of all classes in lecture format).
- Utilize a variety of presentation styles: visual, auditory, models and demonstrations, and active participation with return demonstrations (see, hear, do).
- Evaluate patient and family comprehension and skill mastery (e.g., use of teach-back, direct questioning, and observation).
- Provide repetition and reinforcement.
- Supply written material for reinforcement and for sharing with the family and caregiver.
- Encourage interaction between participants (fellow classmates and pulmonary rehabilitation professionals).
- Take advantage of teachable moments (e.g., discuss prevention of exacerbations and when to call the doctor when a patient returns after a hospitalization for an exacerbation).

# IMPLEMENTING SELF-MANAGEMENT TRAINING

The most effective form and content of self-management intervention has not been standardized and is an ongoing challenge. However, the goal is clear, to target behavior change by assisting the patient in achieving the knowledge, self-confidence, and skills to effectively self-manage their disease. The training should enhance the patient's ability to

- engage in activities that promote health and prevent adverse sequelae,
- effectively interact with health care providers,
- adhere to treatment protocols, and
- self-monitor physical and mental status to inform appropriate management decisions.

Interdisciplinary team members with special training or expertise in a particular content area should present the relevant information at training sessions. Many excellent resources are available for content development. The COPD Foundation serves as the repository for the U.S. copyrighted COPD Assessment Test (see chapter 7). To access the COPD Assessment Test, register for a free account at www.copdfoundation.org.

Depending on the patient's individual needs, any or all of the topics listed in figure 4.1 may be appropriate for inclusion in a self-management training program. Education content should also be included in the Individual Treatment Plan (ITP) (see chapter 10). The content is not listed by order of importance but rather in a sequence that builds on previous information presented.

## Normal Pulmonary Anatomy and Physiology

A basic understanding of the normal anatomy and physiology of the respiratory system is the foundation on which an understanding of respiratory illness can be built. It is particularly useful to use demonstration models and other teaching aids when discussing this material because laypersons frequently have difficulty envisioning the pulmonary anatomy.

## Pathophysiology of Chronic Lung Disease

Content discussed regarding the pathophysiology of the patient's disease should be tailored to mirror the diagnosis that the patient has received from the health care provider. With a basic understanding of their specific respiratory disease, patients may be more willing to adhere to their prescribed therapeutic interventions.

For example:

- Link medication actions to lung physiology and symptoms, bronchodilation, airway swelling.
- Show oxygen transport through the lungs and how it varies with the different disease states and its effect on the heart.

**Figure 4.1   Educational topics (as indicated for the individual patient)**

1. Normal pulmonary anatomy and physiology
2. Pathophysiology of chronic lung disease
   a. COPD
      i. Chronic bronchitis
      ii. Emphysema
   b. Asthma
   c. Bronchiectasis
   d. Restrictive lung disease
   e. Pulmonary fibrosis
   f. Pulmonary hypertension
   g. Cystic fibrosis
   h. Other
3. Description and interpretation of medical tests
   a. Spirometry
   b. Lung volumes
   c. Sleep study
   d. Pulse oximetry
      i. Rest
      ii. Exercise
      iii. Nocturnal
   e. Arterial blood gas
   f. Other
4. Breathing strategies
   a. Pursed-lip breathing
   b. Active expiration
5. Secretion clearance
   a. Coughing techniques, cough assist
   b. Postural drainage, percussion, vibration
      i. Traditional
      ii. Vest
   c. Positive expiratory pressure
      i. With vibration
      ii. Without vibration
   d. Autogenic drainage
6. Medications
   a. Oxygen
      i. Indications
      ii. Delivery systems
   b. Bronchodilators
      i. Inhaled
      ii. Oral

c. Steroids
   i. Inhaled
   ii. Oral
d. Proper inhaled medication technique
   i. Metered-dose inhaler
   ii. Dry powder inhaler
   iii. Use of spacer chamber
   iv. Nebulizers
e. Antibiotics
   i. Prophylactic macrolide
   ii. Prescribed for treatment of infection
f. Mucolytics
g. Antitussives
h. Other
7. Respiratory devices
   a. Metered-dose and dry powder inhalers
   b. Nebulizers, compressors
   c. Peak flow meters
   d. Oxygen delivery systems (concentrators, liquid, compressed gas, pulse)
   e. Oxygen-conserving devices
   f. Transtracheal oxygen
   g. Inspiratory muscle trainer
   h. Positive expiratory pressure (PEP)
   i. Sleep assessment equipment (oximetry, apnea monitors)
   j. Continuous positive airway pressure (CPAP), bi-level airway pressure (BiPAP) and non-invasive ventilation (NIV)
   k. Suctioning in the home
   l. Tracheostomy care
   m. Ventilator management in the home
8. Benefits of exercise and maintaining physical activities
   a. General principles
      i. Aerobic
      ii. Strength
   b. Home exercise program/maintenance exercise program
9. Activities of daily living (ADLs)
   a. Breathing strategies during ADLs
   b. Energy conservation
   c. Work simplification

*(continued)*

**Figure 4.1**    *(continued)*

10. Eating right
    a. General nutrition guidelines
    b. Strategies for weight loss
    c. Strategies for weight gain
    d. Type II diabetes
11. Irritant avoidance
    a. Smoking cessation
        i. Importance and benefits
        ii. Techniques
        iii. Resources
    b. Hazards of secondhand smoke
    c. Environmental and occupational irritant avoidance
12. Early recognition and treatment of exacerbations
    a. Signs and symptoms of a respiratory infection
    b. When to call your health care provider
    c. Self-management strategies for increased symptoms
        i. Action plan
    d. Vaccination

13. Leisure activities
    a. Travel
        i. Availability of supplemental oxygen
        ii. Planning for travel
    b. Sexuality
14. Coping with chronic lung disease
    a. Depression and anxiety
    b. Application of breathing strategies to panic control
    c. Relaxation techniques
    d. Stress management
    e. Care for the caregiver (as indicated)
15. Advance directive planning
    a. Importance of patient–physician–family discussion
    b. Durable power of attorney for health care
    c. Living will
    d. Prehospital medical care directive
16. Palliative care
    a. Patient–caregiver relationship
    b. Role and timing of hospice

## Description and Interpretation of Medical Tests

The description and interpretation of medical tests can be very confusing to the patient, so explanations should be kept simple. Many times patients have never seen their test results, nor have they understood how their results compare to the normal range. The patient's ability to understand the medical tests and their results can facilitate adherence with treatment plans.

### Here are some examples:

- Increased adherence to the use of inhaled bronchodilators after being shown spirometry that demonstrates a significant degree of postbronchodilator reversibility
- Increased adherence to the use of nocturnal oxygen or CPAP after review of pulse oximetry results during a sleep study or nocturnal oxygen study

## Breathing Strategies

Every patient in pulmonary rehabilitation should be instructed in breathing strategies. If the strategies are found to reduce symptoms, the patient will adopt the strategy. Pursed-lip breathing and active expiration (contraction of abdominal muscles during exhalation) may help patients control and relieve breathlessness as well as reduce panic by improving their ventilatory dynamics and pattern. These breathing strategies may prevent dynamic airway compression and (in COPD) improve gas exchange by decreasing dynamic hyperinflation through slowing the respiratory rate. It is important to recognize that not all patients respond positively to pursed-lip breathing, and the non-responders may develop asynchronous breathing with use of the technique (10). Patient response to use of pursed-lip breathing should be observed closely. Instruction in abdominal breathing has fallen out of favor because of the lack of evidence to support its use. One effective teaching technique to demonstrate the effectiveness of pursed-lip breathing in increasing oxygen saturation is to have your patient monitor oxygen saturation while walking and performing pursed-lip breathing. Breathing strategies should not be presented as "exercises" but rather as techniques that utilize the lungs more efficiently. The strategies are effective not only for decreasing dyspnea when in a panic situation but also as a preventative measure to reduce dyspnea and forestall panic. The sense of being in control of breathing when utilizing pursed-lip and active expiration increases the patient's self-efficacy.

Figure 4.2 provides an example of program documentation for educational interventions and outcomes.

## Secretion Clearance

Instruction in secretion clearance techniques is important in patients who have difficulty raising sputum. Instruction should begin with controlled coughing, the least complicated technique, and progress to more complex techniques if clinically indicated. Recommendations for patients who produce excessive amounts of sputum (e.g., bronchiectasis, cystic fibrosis) are to instruct in the technique that the patient is most apt to use, since no one technique has been found to be more beneficial than any other. Emphasis should be placed on the use of inhaled bronchodilators before secretion clearance, followed with inhaled steroids and inhaled antibiotics, if prescribed. Instruction in secretion clearance techniques should utilize return demonstrations. If supplemental oxygen is used with exercise, it should also be used during secretion clearance techniques. The goal to maintain secretion clearance, without the need for hospitalization, is important in self-management and enhancing self-efficacy. It is important that the pulmonary rehabilitation professional not only be able to teach cough techniques but also understand the many devices available for secretion clearance. Devices range from Positive Expiratory Pressure (PEP) therapy, vibratory devices, and high frequency chest wall oscillation devices (the "vest"). Patients should additionally be instructed on the importance of hydration and (if needed) expectorant use.

## Medications

Pulmonary rehabilitation is an excellent venue to assess a patient's oxygen needs at rest and with activity and to determine the delivery system that best meets their needs. Although the primary care or referring physician is responsible for prescribing medications, it is the role of the pulmonary rehabilitation staff to train patients in the proper use of their respiratory medications, including oxygen. Patients should be aware of what their medicines are supposed to do and what they are not supposed to do. For example, the simple explanation that oxygen is being prescribed to treat a low blood oxygen level, and that oxygen alone may not prevent shortness of breath, can improve adherence to supplemental oxygen therapy.

Individualized medication education should include the usual prescribed dosage, frequency, side effects, indications, contraindications, and potential interactions. Although the primary emphasis in pulmonary rehabilitation is on respiratory medications, a review of all medications may be clinically beneficial and improve adherence. Patients should understand the importance of maintaining a list of all medications, including complementary, alternative, and over the counter, and of telling all their health care providers what medications they are taking. This can reduce the possibility of harmful drug interactions and duplication. Medication instruction should include return demonstrations of proper inhaler technique and cleaning of the inhalation device. The use of a spacer chamber with a metered-dose inhaler is recommended if coordination of actuation and inhalation is impaired. By having a solid understanding of the proper use of their medications, the patient's self-management is enhanced.

With so many different inhaled devices on the market, nebulizers, MDI, DPIs, MDIs with built-in spacers, it is vitally important that pulmonary rehabilitation professionals ensure that patients use these devices correctly and in the proper order of administration. Many patients do not understand that an inhaler is not just an inhaler. Knowing a SABA from a LABA and a rescue medication from a controller medication is equally as important. It is the responsibility of the pulmonary rehabilitation professional to keep up to date on current medication delivery systems.

## Respiratory Devices

Patients with chronic respiratory disease frequently use various types of respiratory therapy devices. Specific treatments are based on the patient's disease and individual needs. Reinforcement and additional education and training may

**Figure 4.2   Sample documentation for self-management education**

Patient name: _____

**Pursed-Lip Breathing and Active Expiration (PLB/AE)**

| | Intervention | Goal | Assessment | Outcome |
|---|---|---|---|---|
| Session 1 | Review anatomy and physiology of a normal lung. Discuss consequences of airway collapse and dynamic hyperinflation. Distribute written information for reinforcement. | Awareness of effects of airway collapse | Verbalization | Met _____<br>Not met _____<br>Date _____<br>Comments:<br>_____<br>_____<br>Signature:<br>_____ |
| Session 2 | Verbally instruct and demonstrate pursed-lip breathing and active expiration. Provide written instructions for reinforcement. | Ability to properly perform pursed-lip breathing and active expiration | Return demonstration of pursed-lip breathing and active expiration | Met _____<br>Not met _____<br>Date _____<br>Comments:<br>_____<br>_____<br>Signature:<br>_____ |
| Session 3 | Verbally instruct and demonstrate the application of pursed-lip breathing and active expiration to activities of daily living (ADLs). Provide written instructions for reinforcement. | Ability to properly perform pursed-lip breathing and active expiration during ADLs | Return demonstration of pursed-lip breathing and active expiration during ADLs | Met _____<br>Not met _____<br>Date _____<br>Comments:<br>_____<br>_____<br>Signature:<br>_____ |
| Session 4 | Verbally instruct and demonstrate the application of pursed-lip breathing and active expiration to control panic. Provide written instructions for reinforcement. | Ability to properly perform pursed-lip breathing and active expiration for panic control | Return demonstration of pursed-lip breathing and active expiration to control panic | Met _____<br>Not met _____<br>Date _____<br>Comments:<br>_____<br>_____<br>Signature:<br>_____ |

be necessary to ensure that patients are correctly using their equipment and are adherent to their physician's instructions. The discussion of proper use of devices should begin by asking the patient to bring in *all* the "gizmos and gadgets" they have received from various health care interactions. Instruction should include appropriateness of use, indications, contraindications, and proper cleaning of each device.

## Benefits of Exercise and Maintaining Physical Activities

The benefits of exercise and increased physical activity for patients with chronic pulmonary disease are well established (see chapter 3). Teaching this information underscores the importance of adherence to individualized exercise programs and participation in activities of daily living. To facilitate continued adherence and promote physical activity, each patient should receive an individualized home exercise program before the completion of pulmonary rehabilitation. An exercise log or diary may be useful for patients to self-record their home exercise and physical activity. The benefits of lifelong exercise should be stressed, and patients should be encouraged to continue in a maintenance exercise program in addition to remaining physically active.

## Activities of Daily Living (ADLs)

Independence in activities of daily living is a primary goal for patients with chronic respiratory disease. By applying breathing strategies to ADLs and using energy conservation and work simplification techniques, patients find they have the self-confidence and breathing capacity to participate in many activities. Return demonstrations while performing ADLs are imperative. Patients who have the confidence to perform an activity in the rehabilitation setting are more apt to attempt the activity elsewhere. This confidence is an example of increased self-efficacy and improved self-management skills.

## Eating Right

General nutrition principles apply to all patients who have chronic respiratory disease (see chapter 2). The pulmonary patient can fall anywhere along the weight spectrum, from severe nutrition depletion to morbid obesity. Patients should be educated on the reasons for their nutrition abnormalities, such as the increased metabolic cost of breathing resulting in weight loss, a sedentary lifestyle or oral corticosteroids resulting in weight gain, risk for the development of Type 2 diabetes and osteoporosis. Instruction should be geared to the individual needs of the patient, as determined on initial and follow-up assessments. In some instances, it may be beneficial to refer the patient for intensive nutrition counseling.

## Irritant Avoidance

The major intervention in reducing the progression of respiratory disease is avoidance of inhaled irritants. Patients must learn to avoid all environmental and occupational irritants, especially firsthand and secondhand cigarette smoke. Current smokers and ex-smokers benefit from receiving information on becoming and remaining nonsmokers. Many excellent resources for smoking cessation programs are available online.

## Early Recognition and Treatment of Exacerbations

The importance of teaching early recognition and treatment of exacerbations in pulmonary rehabilitation cannot be overstated. Open communication and collaboration between patients and their health care providers is essential in the early treatment of exacerbations. Strategies that teach patients to recognize an impending exacerbation and promptly initiate treatment may reduce severity and complications as well as decrease hospitalizations. The use of an action plan (figure 4.3) is a promising strategy to improve collaborative self-management. Action plans can simply instruct the patient to contact his health care provider when symptoms increase, as in figure 4.3, or if the patient has mastered a higher level of self-management, action plans can be personalized with specific medication and dosage recommendations. The appropriateness of receiving influenza and pneumonia immunizations, along with the importance of frequent hand washing and covering the mouth when coughing, should also be covered when discussing exacerbations.

## Leisure Activities

The ability to participate in leisure activities is a goal of many patients attending pulmonary

## Figure 4.3   COPD action plan

Name: _____    Date: _____

Health care provider: _____    Phone: _____

Pharmacy: _____    Phone: _____

**Green Zone**

My sputum is clear/white/usual color and easily cleared.

My breathing is no harder than usual.

I can do my usual activities, including exercise.

I am able to think clearly.

I am eating well.

I am sleeping well.

Take your usual medicines, including oxygen, as you are told to do by your health care provider. Avoid cigarette smoke, second-hand smoke, and other inhaled irritants.

**Yellow Zone**

My sputum has changed (color, thickness, amount).

I am more short of breath than usual.

I cough or wheeze more.

I weigh more and my legs/feet swell.

I have less energy and cannot do my usual activities or exercise without resting.

My sleeping is bad, and my symptoms wake me up

I am not eating well, I have lost my appetite.

I am using my rescue inhaler or nebulizer more often.

Continue your daily medications. Call your health care provider. You may be told to begin taking an antibiotic and prednisone. Have your pharmacy phone number available.

**Red Zone**

I cannot cough out my sputum, it is thicker, the color has changed, or there is blood in it.

I am really short of breath, even when I rest.

I need to sit up to breathe.

I cannot sleep.

I cannot do my usual activities or exercise.

I am unable to speak more than one or two words at a time.

I cannot think clearly, and I feel sleepy.

I have chest pains.

Call your health care provider as you need medical care right away. You may be asked to come in to be seen, be told to go to the emergency room, or be told to call 9-1-1.

rehabilitation. Forfeiting the ability to travel is a loss that is difficult for many patients to accept. Information on the availability and use of supplemental oxygen when traveling is readily available on the Internet. Traveling with lung disease is not easy; patients need to understand how to plan for that travel. The COPD Foundation has many great resources to assist the patient with travel preparations. The inclusion of a discussion on sexuality can be intimidating for some rehabilitation staff, but with preparation, the topic can be thoughtfully presented and well accepted. There are resources available via the COPD Foundation's website to assist health care providers and patients. Registration is free on the foundation website (www.copdfoundation.org). Once registered, information such as the Slim Skinny Reference Guide (SSRG) provides detailed information for the health care provider.

## Coping with Chronic Lung Disease

Chronic lung disease is often accompanied by comorbidities. Psychosocial comorbidities are common and are detailed in chapter 5. Pulmonary rehabilitation is an excellent setting for group discussions on panic control, where patients can appreciate that they are not alone in their fears. Shortness of breath during exercise sessions provides the opportunity to demonstrate to patients the effectiveness of breathing strategies to slow their respiratory rate and help them remain in control of their breathing. Relaxation techniques and stress management strategies should also be offered to assist the patient in preventing panic and in coping effectively with their chronic lung disease. As with breathing strategies, if the patients find relaxation techniques or stress management effective, they will adopt their use. It is also important that pulmonary rehabilitation staff recognize the burden placed on caregivers. Family and social roles often change when someone has a chronic illness. Pulmonary rehabilitation professionals should recognize when caregivers feel overwhelmed, stressed, and helpless. Referring the caregiver for support and informing them of resources is important as well. This can include friends, counselors, family physician, or even clergy.

## Care Transitions: Hospital to Home

The pulmonary rehabilitation staff are important members of the care transition team. There is increasing evidence of the benefits of pulmonary rehabilitation in the acute setting, either during or shortly after hospitalization for acute exacerbation of COPD (11). The immediate posthospitalization period is a high-risk time for a new exacerbation to occur. Persistent inactivity following a hospitalization has been shown to increase the likelihood of readmission with a subsequent exacerbation. In addition, self-reported daily physical activity in patients with severe COPD has been shown to be independently associated with hospitalizations for acute exacerbation (12). Pulmonary rehabilitation staff have a responsibility to design programs to allow enrollment in pulmonary rehabilitation as soon as possible following a hospitalization. This can assist the patient in improving their functional activity tolerance and disease self-management skills, which may then prevent readmission.

## End-of-Life Planning

Palliative care is an example of collaborative self-management, in which the goal is to relieve suffering and improve quality of life. Pulmonary rehabilitation can provide a forum to institute palliative care for patients with chronic pulmonary diseases. For example, end-of-life discussions and decision making require communication among the patient, family, and caregivers that can be facilitated in the pulmonary rehabilitation setting.

Palliative care may transition into hospice care. Most patients believe when the term *palliative care* is used that the end of life is looming, and the mention of *hospice* means death is imminent. Dispelling these notions by initiating discussions on these topics in pulmonary rehabilitation is appropriate and encouraged (13). Providing the opportunity to discuss options for end-of-life care leads to an increase in adoption of advance directives (durable power of attorney for health care, living will, and prehospital medical directive), and patients will become more comfortable initiating discussions with their families and physicians regarding their care.

## SUMMARY

Collaborative self-management training is an essential component of comprehensive pulmonary rehabilitation. Self-management training promotes learning by doing and taking advantage of teachable moments. The recommended content should be patient-specific, yet it is imperative to include for all patients training in early recognition and treatment of exacerbations, including the use of an action plan, proper medication use with emphasis on adherence and technique for inhaled medications, and the importance of daily exercise. Educational sessions are an opportunity to facilitate the discussion of end-of-life decision making.

**VISIT THE WEB RESOURCE**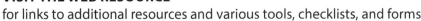
for links to additional resources and various tools, checklists, and forms.

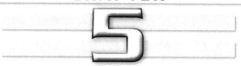

# Psychosocial Assessment and Intervention

*Psychosocial Assessment and Intervention*

**Maria Buckley, PhD, FAACVPR**

The Miriam Hospital/Brown Medical School, Providence, RI

**Kent Eichenauer, PsyD, FAACVPR**

Cardiopulmonary Rehabilitation Consultant, Urbana, OH

Pulmonary patients often present with multiple psychosocial issues while in the midst of managing chronic lung disease. Psychological distress, treatment nonadherence, unhealthy lifestyle habits, and cognitive dysfunction often co-occur and interact in individuals living with pulmonary disease. These issues may adversely affect quality of life and pulmonary rehabilitation outcomes. Pulmonary rehabilitation is an ideal setting in which to design and implement individualized treatment plans that incorporate psychosocial status in order to reduce patient distress and to improve outcomes. The multidisciplinary pulmonary rehabilitation team can play a pivotal role in significantly improving patient confidence and motivation to work toward important and meaningful patient goals. This chapter begins with a discussion of the relevance and requirements around psychosocial assessment in pulmonary rehabilitation. The prevalence and impact of psychosocial symptoms on function, adherence, and outcomes are described. Screeners for evaluation of psychological symptoms, social support, and cognitive dysfunction as well as lifestyle habits

are provided. Evidence-supported interventions are offered to guide appropriate treatment planning. In conclusion, strategies for partnering with psychosocial providers are suggested.

## ASSESSMENT OF PSYCHOSOCIAL FUNCTIONING

Psychosocial morbidity is common in patients with chronic respiratory disease. A psychosocial assessment is an integral component of the overall patient evaluation. The psychosocial assessment provides an individualized evaluation of each patient's psychosocial functioning as well as the cognitive and social factors that may impact adherence to pulmonary rehabilitation and treatment outcomes. The psychosocial findings are incorporated into the patient's individualized treatment plan. Additional information regarding specific pulmonary rehabilitation staff competencies can be found in the Clinical Competency

Guidelines article published by Collins and colleagues (1). Also, listed here are the specific Medicare requirements for a psychosocial assessment for patients enrolled in a pulmonary rehabilitation program.

### Medicare Requirements:

42 CFR §410.47 Pulmonary rehabilitation program: conditions for coverage (2)

*Psychosocial assessment* means a written evaluation of an individual's mental and emotional functioning as it relates to the individual's rehabilitation or respiratory condition (3). *Psychosocial assessment.* The psychosocial assessment must meet the criteria as defined in paragraph (a) of this section and includes:

(i) An assessment of those aspects of an individual's family and home situation that affects [sic] the individual's rehabilitation treatment.

(ii) A psychosocial evaluation of the individual's response to and rate of progress under the treatment plan.

## Depression

Approximately 40% of COPD patients present with depressive symptoms (3). Higher rates have been reported in those patients with advanced disease and with supplemental oxygen use (4). Depression is underrecognized and undertreated in COPD (5, 6). Pulmonary rehabilitation treats patients presenting with a variety of lung diseases in addition to COPD. Table 5.1 provides prevalence rates for depressive symptoms in patients presenting with other respiratory illnesses. It is suggested that clinicians caring for COPD patients be aware of the impact of psychosocial conditions on the treatment of COPD patients and its outcomes (7).

## Symptoms

Common symptoms of depression include persistent depressed mood, anhedonia (lack of pleasure), feelings of worthlessness, difficulty with concentration, as well as sleep or appetite disturbance. Patients may present with multiple symptoms which may or may not meet criteria for a psychiatric diagnosis. For more information regarding diagnostic criteria and related issues, the reader may refer to the *Diagnostic and Statistical Manual of Mental Health Disorders, Fifth Edition* (DSM-5) (11). Although it is useful to be aware of these criteria, a psychiatric diagnosis must be made by a qualified licensed professional. The critical role of the pulmonary rehabilitation program is to adequately screen for depression, identify those in need, and refer, when necessary, for professional assessment and treatment. Additionally, given that depressive symptoms may be owing to a medical condition, it is paramount that a medical condition is ruled out to ensure appropriate diagnosis and treatment.

## Impact on Function, Adherence, and Outcomes

Depressive symptoms independently predicted worse 6-minute walk distance (6MWD) performance in the ECLIPSE study, which included 1,795 COPD patients (12). In the general population, depressed individuals are three times less likely to adhere to their medication regimen (13). Depression impedes progress in pulmonary rehabilitation and results in worse outcomes, over and above medical burden and disease severity (14). Keating and colleagues found that depression was associated with dropout (15). In a more recent study, depression predicted dropout in women but not men (16). Depression is also associated with extended hospital stay, mortality, and persistent smoking (17). Fan and colleagues found that depression was

### Table 5.1　Prevalence of Depressive Symptoms in Interstitial Lung Disease, Pulmonary Hypertension, and Bronchiectasis

| Pulmonary Disease | Depression Prevalence Rate |
|---|---|
| Interstitial lung disease | 23% (8) |
| Pulmonary hypertension | 55% (9) |
| Bronchiectasis | 20% (10) |

associated with risk of 3-year mortality in patients diagnosed with severe COPD (18).

## Screening Tools

Depression screening tools that may be administered at baseline, during, and following pulmonary rehabilitation include:

- Single factor screeners
  - Beck Depression Inventory—II (BDI–II) (19)
  - Physician Health Questionnaire (PHQ-9)* (20)
- Multiple factor screeners
  - Hospital Anxiety and Depression Scale (HADS)* (21)
  - Psychosocial Risk Factor Survey (PRFS) (22)

The Beck Depression Inventory is endorsed by National Institutes for Health and Clinical Excellence to evaluate depression and responsiveness to treatment in primary care (23).

More detail around these scales can be found on the AACVPR Pulmonary Outcomes Resource Guide (24) (formerly referred to as the Pulmonary Outcomes Toolkit). These tools can be used as outcomes measures to evaluate the effects of pulmonary rehabilitation programs. These tests may include an item pertaining to suicidal ideation. A word of caution regarding management of patients presenting with suicidal ideation: Patients endorsing suicidal ideation should be considered as having an emergent need for further assessment. Immediate follow-up by a qualified professional is necessary to ensure patient safety. It is imperative for pulmonary rehabilitation program staff to know and follow approved program policies around management of suicidal ideation. Additional resources such as the Columbia Suicide Severity Rating Scale (25), the VA Suicide Risk Assessment Guide (26), and the Joint Commission Sentinel Event Alert, Issue 56 (27) are available for review and consideration.

## Anxiety

Anxiety is common in patients with respiratory disease. COPD patients have a 36% prevalence rate, and 32% of pulmonary rehabilitation patients present with significant anxiety symptoms (28). Panic disorder rates are approximately 10 times higher in the COPD population than the general population (1.5% to 3%) (29). The extant literature provides anxiety prevalence rates in patients with other respiratory disorders as presented in table 5.2.

### Symptoms

Several anxiety disorders are included in the DSM-5 (11). For example, generalized anxiety disorder is manifested by significant worry across multiple domains. Specific phobia is a fear of a particular experience that is often avoided. For example, patients may avoid exercise due to fear of dyspnea. Panic disorder involves recurrent panic attacks, which are intense episodes of anxiety. Posttraumatic disorder is an anxiety disorder experienced following a traumatic event with significant fear related to that event. Individuals with social phobia are fearful of being judged by others, which may be of concern for patients with supportive oxygen needs. For more detailed review of the diagnostic criteria for these disorders, the reader is referred to the DSM-V.

As with depression, it is important to be aware of the criteria for anxiety disorders, without diagnosing the disorder. Screening is necessary, and monitoring patients' symptoms and receiving collateral reports from family members as appropriate may provide important clinical data as well. Since respiratory patients commonly experience symptoms such as fatigue and dyspnea, their interpretation in the context of anxiety assessment can be difficult. Given the potential overlap between

| Table 5.2  Prevalence of Anxiety Symptoms in Interstitial Lung Disease, Pulmonary Hypertension, and Bronchiectasis ||
| --- | --- |
| **Pulmonary Disease** | **Anxiety Prevalence Rate** |
| Interstitial lung disease | 31% (8) |
| Pulmonary hypertension | 46% (9) |

anxiety and various medical conditions, a medical condition must be ruled out to ensure appropriate assessment and intervention around the patient's signs and symptoms.

### Impact on Function, Adherence, and Outcomes

The National Emphysema Treatment Trial (30) reported worse 6MWT results in patients with elevated anxiety scores after controlling for age, gender, $FEV_1$, DLCO, and Beck Depression Inventory scores. Additionally, anxiety is a risk factor for rehospitalization in patients of low health status (31). Consistent with depression, anxiety impedes progress and results in poor outcomes on key indicators beyond the impact of medical burden and disease severity (14).

Figure 5.1 illustrates adaptation of the fear-dyspnea cycle first offered by Ries (32). This figure illustrates the role of fear and anxiety in dyspnea and further deconditioning. Essentially, as a patient with dyspnea performs an exertional activity, the resultant natural increase in dyspnea generates increased anxiety and fear about further exertion. As such, the patient is more likely to avoid exercise and therefore become further deconditioned. As such, instances of further exertion fuel even more dyspnea, reinforcing the anxiety, fear, and avoidance in a vicious cycle. It is therefore understandable why some pulmonary patients are reluctant to join pulmonary rehabilitation programs or are reticent about physical exertion within the program.

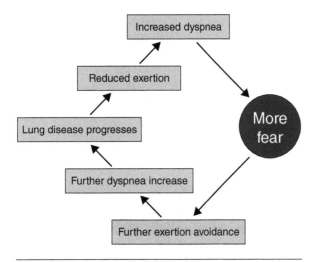

**Figure 5.1**  Model of development of avoidance in COPD.
Based on Ries (1990).

### Screening Tools

Anxiety screening tools that may be administered at baseline, during, and following pulmonary rehabilitation include:

- Single factor screeners
  - Beck Anxiety Inventory (BAI) (33)
  - Generalized Anxiety Disorder 7-Item (GAD-7) (34)
- Multiple factor screeners
  - Hospital Anxiety and Depression Scale (HADS) (21)
  - Psychosocial Risk Factor Survey (PRFS) (22)

Scoring and interpretation around these scales can be found on the AACVPR Pulmonary Outcomes Resource Guide (24) (formerly referred to as the Pulmonary Outcomes Toolkit). These questionnaires can be used as outcomes measures to evaluate the effects of pulmonary rehabilitation program on anxiety symptoms.

## Hostility

The term *hostility* is frequently used as an umbrella for anger (the affective or emotional component), aggression (the behavioral or acting out component), and hostility (the attitudinal or cognitive component). Hostility can exist without anger or aggression and consists of a negative attitude toward others, including cynicism, mistrust, and a tendency to view others' actions as having a negative intent. Unfortunately, this is an area where there is often minimal insight and therefore is often less detectable when relying on self-report or superficial observation.

### Impact on Function, Adherence, and Outcomes

While the evidence base of the relationship of hostility and pulmonary functioning is limited, there is indication in the literature that younger persons with higher levels of hostility obtain poorer results on pulmonary $FEV_1$ and FVC (35). Furthermore, while a separate study of older men discovered similar baseline results in $FEV_1$ and FVC, the investigators followed up and found an additional decline in the pulmonary functioning of subjects with higher hostility scores (36).

### Screening Tools

Hostility screening tools that may be administered at baseline, during, and following pulmonary rehabilitation include:

- Single factor screener
  - State Trait Anger Expression Inventory-2 (STAXI-2) (37)
- Multiple factor screener
  - Psychosocial Risk Factor Survey (PRFS) (22)

These questionnaires can be used as outcomes measures to evaluate the effects of pulmonary rehabilitation program on anxiety symptoms.

## Social Support

The pulmonary patient's subjective sense of social support appears to impact the patient's overall functioning. There is evidence that interventions targeted at enhancing social support may improve and maintain the overall functioning of these patients (38, 39). With proper attention to this fundamental aspect of care of the pulmonary patient, pulmonary programs are well positioned to offer some enhancement to the patient's social support during the patient's attendance in the program.

### Building Support Systems

Staff support, consisting of caring professionals displaying counseling skills, is key to successful programs. Such services often entail active listening and crisis management skills as well as patient advocacy and facilitation of resource acquisition. Additional support may be derived from family members, friends, and other program participants.

Social support within the pulmonary rehabilitation program can be enhanced through educational presentations and patient involvement in support groups that encourage the sharing of personal experiences. The group environment is conducive to participant sharing of disease-related information and successful coping skills. It also provides an outlet for emotional release and elicitation of emotional support. Further opportunities for patient interaction can be developed in waiting areas and during social events. To enhance their sense of self-worth, some patients may also choose to serve as volunteers for the rehabilitation program or other community activities. It is important to note that some patients do not do well in a group

setting; the pulmonary rehabilitation staff must respect each patient's sense of privacy.

Social support can also be fostered through the involvement of the patient's spouse or support person. Significant others should be encouraged to participate in support groups in which family dynamics and interpersonal skills can be observed, information can be shared, misperceptions can be clarified, and fears and concerns can be addressed. Rehabilitation staff should be sensitive to caregivers and spouses because they are often receiving little support themselves. Particularly important are discussions and skill development activities focusing on how family members can provide support to the patient without promoting dependency. Collaboration between the patient and support person is fostered when both parties can come to terms with the illness; commit to working together to manage the illness; be sensitive to cues signaling the needs, desires, and feelings of the other; compromise; and seek out choices and resources for managing their lives. In order to assist patients in the observation of spousal dynamics and skills development, it is strongly recommended that a psychosocial provider is directly involved with this aspect of patient care. This may involve directly providing the patient service or careful coordination of this service with rehabilitation staff. Furthermore, for the patient having significant interpersonal or family conflict, referral to a clinical social worker, psychologist, or other counselor for family or relationship counseling is recommended.

### Screening Tools

Social support screening tools that may be administered at baseline, during, and following pulmonary rehabilitation include:

- Single factor screeners
  - MOS-Social Support Survey (MOS-SSS) (40)
  - ENRICHD Social Support Instrument (ESSI) (41)
- Multiple factor screeners
  - Psychosocial Risk Factor Survey (PRFS) (22)

Scoring of these questionnaires can be used as outcomes measures to evaluate the effects of pulmonary rehabilitation program on social support.

# Intimacy

Limited research exists in the area of sexuality in patients with chronic respiratory disease. In one study of 53 COPD outpatients, 76% reported erectile dysfunction; the severity of dysfunction was determined by pulmonary function (42). A recent study from Portugal (43) revealed a higher rate (87%) of erectile dysfunction in COPD patients.

Female patients have reported reduced frequency of sexual intimacy compared to age- and gender-matched control subjects. Males experience worse sexual quality of life compared to the healthy comparison group. Self-esteem interferes with sexual experience for men. Despite the impact of reduced sexual functioning on their lives, patients do not discuss sexual health issues with their physicians (44). Health care providers may contribute to the lack of communication due to embarrassment around discussing sexual health issues with their patients. Pulmonary rehabilitation staff have the opportunity to improve patient quality of life by discussing strategies such as timing, sexual positions, energy conservation, and environmental factors with patients who are willing to discuss this area of their life (45). The ATS/ERS Pulmonary Rehabilitation Statement provides the practitioner with practical strategies to approach this discussion (46).

Intimacy screening tools that may be administered at baseline, during, and following pulmonary rehabilitation include:

- The Respiratory Experiences with Sexuality Profile (RESP) (47)
- Intimate Physical Contact Scales (48)

# Substance Abuse

Substance abuse can impact the pulmonary patient in several ways. Alcohol increases exacerbations and mortality in lung diseases (49). Alcohol and drug abuse are independently associated with higher all-cause 30-day readmission rates for persons with COPD (50, 51) with indications that these readmission rates are substantially higher for smokers of illicit drugs than smokers of tobacco (52). Suicidal ideation and attempts are higher in substance-abusing COPD patients (53). Alcohol abuse is significantly associated with COPD (54) and COPD patients with a history of alcohol abuse are less likely to adhere to pharmaceutical treatments (55).

Substance abuse screening tools that may be administered at baseline, during, and following pulmonary rehabilitation include:

- The CAGE Questionnaire (56)
- The CAGE-AID (57)
- Alcohol Use Disorders Identification Test (AUDIT) (58)

# Cognitive Impairment

Cognitive impairment is prevalent in COPD and can be complicated by chronic hypoxemia (59, 60). Furthermore, the degree of hypoxemia influences the level of cognitive impairment (61). Cognitive impairment increases as COPD progresses. Additionally, cognitive functioning declines more rapidly in COPD patients than non-COPD patients (62). Some have suggested that cognitive impairment should be considered a primary component of hypoxemic COPD and not a mere comorbidity of this disease (63).

Cognitive impairment is common in patients with respiratory disorders. The literature suggests a prevalence rate of 16% to 20% (64). However, the NOTT trial found 42% of COPD patients suffered moderate to severe cognitive dysfunction compared to 14% of controls (65).

Depression and anxiety, which are frequently comorbid with pulmonary disease, also appear to be associated with diminished cognitive functioning. Verbal memory impairment is associated with comorbid anxiety and depression (66), and depression is related to decreased hippocampal volume, which can be associated with memory difficulties (67).

## Impact on Function, Adherence, and Outcomes

The outcomes data regarding the impact of pulmonary rehabilitation on cognitive functioning is mixed. It has been suggested that even a short course of pulmonary rehabilitation can demonstrate improvements in depression, verbal memory, and visuospatial functioning (68). As well, exercise has improved executive function, such as purposive behavior, self-control, and ability to shift attention (69, 70). It has also been suggested that exercise training has little or no benefit in cognitive function in hypoxic COPD (63), and it may be necessary to adapt and tailor the program to maximize the patient's acquisition and carry-over of pulmonary rehabilitation instructions. If cognitive impairments are such that judgment and retention of information are compromised, then a significant other or caregiver needs to be an integral partner in the rehabilitative process.

In a systematic review by Schou et al. (71), cognitive impairment was present in patients with severe COPD. The review included 15 studies with inconsistent neuropsychologcial tests which limited the conclusion drawn from the findings. The authors also assert that the clinical implications of this dysfunction have not been determined. The reviewers discuss the need to further study this issue to ascertain a clearer understanding of the impact of cognitive impairment in patients with COPD and the implications for intervention. In 2014, Cleutjens' group published a review paper (72) that noted an association between cognitive impairment and daily functioning. Thus, they recommend a cognitive assessment of COPD patients in order to provide interventions tailored to suit the patient's needs.

### Screening Tools

The Montreal Cognitive Assessment (MOCA) (73) and the Mini-Mental Status Exam (MMSE) (74) are two widely used cognitive screening tools. Both tests require training by a qualified professional. If a cognitive deficit is suspected, the patient should be referred for this specialized screening. Patients who screen positive on cognitive screeners should also be monitored around task performance at pulmonary rehabilitation and in the home environment by reliable support persons. Follow-up neuropsychological testing should be considered. While this referral process might be seen as complex or burdensome, the ultimate success for the patient in the pulmonary rehabilitation program is likely to be enhanced with recommendations to compensate for cognitive deficits.

It is important to be aware of how to respond to the results of psychosocial screeners. As mentioned earlier, a depression screener should first be checked for the patient's response to a question about suicidal ideation and address this as appropriate.

When sharing the screening results, it is advantageous to engage the patient and reduce potential defensiveness. One example of an introduction is, "Your responses to the items on the psychosocial screening tool suggest you are feeling . . ." Upon sharing the result and defining the psychosocial area that is screened, the patient can be asked, "How close, or not, does this score seem to fit for

you?" It can also be helpful to review specific items the patient endorsed that contributed to the elevated score. This can offer a springboard to share more of his or her psychosocial circumstances.

Most screeners offer levels of severity (mild, moderate, severe) of the construct being screened. When a patient obtains a positive score in the mild range or above, the pulmonary rehabilitation professional should be prepared to respond in several ways.

- The clinician needs to be able to offer knowledgeable verbal feedback regarding the characteristics of the psychosocial factor and its potential impact on the patient's treatment.
- The professional needs to be able to offer printed material that reinforces this information to enhance the patient's acquisition of the information.
- The pulmonary rehabilitation program needs to have a relationship with a psychosocial provider and be prepared to offer a referral to address the concerns.
- The patient's primary care physician needs to be notified of a positive result.

## Patient Nonadherence

Nonadherence to medication and lifestyle modification is common in COPD patients. Lack of adherence to medication regimen, regular physical activity, or exercise prescription, continued smoking, low enrollment and increased dropout in pulmonary rehabilitation, and reduced self-management can lead to more rapid worsening lung function, increased health care utilization, and mortality (75).

George and colleagues (76) found that the following conditions were independent predictors of nonadherence: "I vary my recommended management based on how I am feeling" and "I get confused about my medications." Pulmonary rehabilitation programs are well poised to provide education specific to the barriers to patients and their support persons as needed. Another study found that nonadherent patients who either refused or prematurely terminated their pulmonary rehabilitation program were dissatisfied with their level of disease-specific social support. In this investigation, the nonadherent group was not more likely to be depressed or anxious, to hyperventilate, or to have had a history of psychotherapy (77). This study may suggest the need to further explore the contract of social support with patients and to address and intervene to the extent that is feasible in the pulmonary rehabilitation setting. A recent study by Oates and colleagues (78) indicated that lower socioeconomic status, smoking, and worse performance on the 6MWT were associated with worse adherence to pulmonary rehabilitation.

Clearly, pulmonary rehabilitation can intervene using behavior changes around smoking cessation and exercise capacity. The staff may also be able to provide resources for patients with limited resources.

# INTERVENTIONS TO IMPROVE PSYCHOSOCIAL FUNCTIONING

Psychosocial interventions in pulmonary rehabilitation fall into several categories, including exercise, mind/body interventions, cognitive, behavioral therapy, pharmaceutical therapy, motivational interviewing techniques, and smoking cessation. In addition to managing psychosocial concerns, psychosocial interventions can also improve physical outcomes such as lung function, dyspnea, exercise capacity, and fatigue in COPD patients with psychological concerns (79).

## Exercise

The 2017 GOLD writing group recognizes the benefits of exercise in improving depression in the general population (79). Likewise, recent meta-analysis findings support the antidepressant effects of regular exercise (80). Emery posits that exercise may reduce proinflammatory cytokines as a mechanism of improvement (81). Furthermore, even a short course of pulmonary rehabilitation has demonstrated improvements in depression, verbal memory, and visuospatial functioning (68). Exercise improves executive function, such as purposive behavior, self-control, and ability to shift attention (69, 70).

## Mind/Body Interventions

Mind/body interventions such as mindfulness-based therapy, yoga, and relaxation have been demonstrated to reduce anxiety and depression and to improve physical outcomes such as lung function, dyspnea, exercise capacity, and fatigue in individuals with COPD and psychological distress (79).

- Progressive muscle relaxation is a structured relaxation exercise that involves alternating between tensing and relaxing specific muscle groups one at a time (82).
- Diaphragmatic breathing involves consciously ensuring diaphragm use to breathe deeply. Ideally, patients can be instructed while lying down to place one hand on the chest and one hand on the abdomen. The patient is instructed to breathe in through the nose such that the abdomen rises while the chest does not. The abdominal muscles contract, forcing the exhaled air through pursed lips.
- Yoga is a system of physical positioning that can employ breathing techniques and meditation derived from Eastern philosophy but often practiced separately from these roots to enhance physical and emotional health.

## Cognitive Behavioral Therapy

Cognitive behavioral therapy (CBT) has proven efficacy for reducing anxiety and depression (79). There is emerging evidence supporting the benefits of this approach in improving psychological symptoms in patients with COPD (83, 84). CBT is a method of therapy that focuses on developing an awareness of our cognitive distortions, including unrealistic perspectives or expectations of ourselves or others, and then developing and practicing tools to correct these distortions (85). This model of therapy also prescribes behavioral activities to reduce depression, such as scheduling pleasurable events and completing tasks that aim to produce a sense of mastery. To reduce anxiety, exposure to an avoided activity (such as exercise due to fear of dyspnea) may be employed with medically appropriate supervised exposure to the feared situation, such as walking on a treadmill (86). The practice of CBT requires extensive training and is outside the scope of practice for most pulmonary rehabilitation professionals.

## Pharmacotherapy

These guidelines provide general information around pharmacotherapy and are not intended to be construed as medical advice around a specific medication regimen for any patient. Pharmacotherapy should be prescribed by the patient's personal physician in conjunction with the patient. Various psychopharmacological medications are prescribed to treat psychological symptoms such as anxiety and depression. To date, the effects of antidepressants specifically on COPD patients have been inconclusive, which may be owing to methodological issues (79).

Benzodiazepines comprise one class of psychotropic medications frequently prescribed for pulmonary patients for conditions including insomnia, depression, anxiety, and refractory dyspnea (87). Common examples include lorazepam (Ativan), alprazolam (Xanax), diazepam (Valium), and clonazepam (Klonopin) (88). Pulmonary rehabilitation staff needs to be aware of potential side effects, including increased adverse pulmonary events and fall risk (87, 89). Of note, an increased fall risk was associated with CNS-active medications, including antidepressants, benzodiazepines, and anticonvulsants in a large sample of community dwelling elderly women (90).

As discussed earlier, in addition to referral to a psychosocial provider, the patient's primary care physician should be notified of elevated scores in psychosocial screening. The patient can discuss the appropriateness of medication with his or her physician. The combination of psychotherapy and psychotropic medication may be prescribed for certain patients.

## Motivational Interviewing

When patients enter pulmonary rehabilitation, they are offered an opportunity to make multiple behavior changes to improve their functioning, such as exercise, pacing, energy conservation, smoking cessation, and adherence to supplemental oxygen and other medications to improve overall functioning. While these changes are beneficial, they can be overwhelming for patients to change habits that they have been practicing for years and sometimes decades. Patients are usually aware that they could benefit from behavior change such as smoking cessation and weight management, yet find it very difficult to commit to changing their pattern of behavior. Sometimes individuals are engaging in the only habit that brings relief from stress even though they are aware of the long-term risks. Patients may sometimes feel angry and disappointed in themselves and remain stuck in the cycle of unhealthy habits.

Fortunately, an effective method is available for health care providers to assist patients with resolving their ambivalence and committing to making behavior changes. Specifically, motivational interviewing effectively improves adherence

around multiple behaviors, such as alcohol use, weight management, blood pressure (91, 92), and physical activity (93). The impact of motivational interviewing in COPD patients has recently been explored (94). According to Miller and Rollnick, motivation exists within the individual as well as within the context of the relationship between the patient and the health care provider. Having respect for the patient and his or her own values is a key component of motivational interviewing. Advice giving and ordering are appropriate in the acute care environment but not with respect to longer-term behavior change issues. Communication styles such as warning, criticizing, and persuading are incongruous with the spirit of motivational interviewing.

One of the basic motivational interviewing tools is OARS (open-ended questions, affirming, reflecting, and summarizing) (91). Some examples of OARS statements include:

- Open-ended questions:
  - "What would you like to set as a goal for pulmonary rehabilitation?"
  - "How is your breathing when you don't use your inhaler?"
  - "What is it about pacing that is difficult for you?"
- Affirmations
  - "You are doing great with pacing your activity."
  - "It is really impressive that you are willing to come to rehab to help you get stronger."
  - "Your efforts are paying off as you are doing more since you started rehab."
- Reflections
  - "So it sounds like you want to breathe better and you are willing to try to pace your activity even though it's hard."
- Summarizing
  - "You are saying that you want to keep moving to get out on your own, take care of your house, and be able to play golf."
  - "So you are having difficulty breathing and feel uncomfortable wearing the oxygen when out in public. At the same time, you want to be able to do as much as you can without putting stress on your body. You've made a decision to

use your oxygen because you value your health and you want to be here for your family."

Training in motivational interviewing requires considerable time to obtain sufficient conceptual knowledge and practical skills taught by a qualified trainer. Like any skill, such as learning a new language, it takes time and practice. Due to confusion regarding the tenets of their approach, Miller and Rollnick published a paper titled, "The 10 Things that Motivational Interviewing Is Not" (95) in order to clarify their method, promote treatment fidelity, and distinguish their approach from other paradigms.

# Tobacco Dependence

Tobacco use is the leading preventable cause of death and disease in the United States. Smoking results in more than 480,000 deaths annually (96, 97) and is the major risk factor for COPD (94).

Electronic cigarettes, also known as e-cigarettes or electronic nicotine delivery systems, were introduced to the U.S. market in 2004 and have skyrocketed in awareness, use, and controversy over the past decade. E-cigarettes mimic traditional cigarettes in design and are battery powered to heat liquid nicotine and other chemicals and produce a vapor that is inhaled. They are often assumed to be "safer" than traditional cigarettes or to help smokers quit. The U.S. Surgeon General has concluded that e-cigarettes can expose users to several potentially harmful chemicals, including nicotine, carbonyl compounds, and volatile organic compounds (98). The health effects are unknown, and much research is underway to determine the health impacts and to help inform regulations. In addition to tobacco, e-cigarette use is common in current (58.8%), former (29.8%), and never (11.4%) smokers (99). E-cigarettes are not currently FDA approved as a smoking cessation aid (100).

## *Impact on Function, Adherence, and Outcome*

Nicotine dependence interventions can rapidly reduce the risk of smoking-related diseases and their consequences (101). Tobacco use and dependence are chronic disorders in which repeated cessation attempts and sporadic relapses are common. Successful long-term cessation without assistance is unlikely but improves with optimal clinical support. A chronic disease model empha-

sizes the importance of continued patient education, counseling, and advice over time, particularly given that half of the individuals who quit smoking will relapse in the first year (102). Clinicians in the pulmonary rehabilitation setting play a key role in motivating patients to quit and assisting them with proven methods to facilitate long-term successful cessation.

Smoking stimulates neurochemical pathways associated with cognitive stimulation, memory, pleasure, mood control, anxiety reduction, relaxation, and appetite suppression. Smoking's pleasurable effects are reinforced by the conditioned response associated with environmental triggers, including alcohol use. Conversely, nicotine withdrawal is associated with anxiety, restlessness, irritability, impaired concentration, depressed mood, insomnia, headache, increased appetite, and weight gain.

## *Screening Tools*

The Fagerstrom Test for Nicotine Dependence (103) incorporates the patient's desire to quit, the number of cigarettes smoked daily, whether the patient smokes within 30 minutes of awakening, as well as previous quit attempts, including methods, effectiveness, and relapse triggers.

## *Pharmacotherapy and Behavioral Interventions*

The focus of pharmacological and behavioral management of nicotine dependence is to reduce withdrawal symptoms and promote behaviors linked with successful long-term cessation. Use of combined pharmacological and behavioral interventions improves the chances of successful long-term cessation. Persons who are pregnant should be encouraged to quit without medication. Specific treatment planning around pharmacotherapy needs to be provided by the patient's personal physician to review the risks and benefits of medications in order to determine the appropriate treatment plan for the individual patient.

**Pharmacological Strategies** Approved first-line pharmacological management for nicotine dependence includes nicotine replacement, bupropion (Zyban, Wellbutrin), and varenicline (Chantix). Nicotine replacement therapy (NRT) is available in patch, lozenge, and gum form without a prescription and as a nasal spray and oral inhaler with a prescription. NRT normally begins on the identified quit date and usually continues for 2 to

3 months. Acidic beverages such as coffee, juices, and soft drinks reduce oral nicotine absorption and should be avoided for 15 minutes before and during use of nicotine gum, lozenges, and inhalers. Patient preference, affordability, and medical considerations should dictate pharmacological therapy.

- Transdermal patches provide extended release of nicotine over 24 hours. Patches are applied daily to nonhairy skin, and the sites are rotated regularly to avoid irritation. Symptoms of insomnia and vivid dreams may be controlled by removal of the patch at bedtime.
- Nicotine gum provides rapid relief from craving, with peak serum nicotine levels achieved in 20 minutes. The gum is chewed until flavor is tasted and then is parked between the cheek and gums.
- Nicotine lozenges offer an alternative to gum for those with dentures or poor dentition. The lozenge is dissolved in the mouth over 30 minutes by wetting and parking it between the cheek and gums.
- Nicotine inhalers offer the advantage of addressing both physical and emotional nicotine dependence.
- Nicotine nasal spray provides a rapid rise in nicotine concentration, with a peak concentration 10 minutes after use.
- Bupropion is thought to reduce craving by enhancing CNS noradrenergic and dopaminergic release. Bupropion generally begins 1 week before the quit date.
- Varenicline is a partial nicotine receptor agonist that binds to and partially stimulates nicotine receptors. It acts to reduce both nicotine withdrawal symptoms and the rewarding sensations of cigarette smoking. Varenicline is typically started 1 week prior to the quit date.

**Patient Counseling**   Nonpharmacological approaches include individual and group counseling as well as self-help materials. Effective counseling includes cognitive behavioral strategies such as problem solving and increasing social support (104). Additional strategies such as self-monitoring, gradual reduction in smoking in anticipation of an established quit date, and relapse prevention strategies may also be utilized. Counseling helps patients problem solve barriers to quitting and use

## Special Considerations for Pharmacological Therapy

With any medication, the risks and benefits must be weighed carefully between physician and patient in determining the appropriate treatment plan. Of note, with Chantix and Zyban, patients should stop taking these medications and contact their health care provider immediately if they experience agitation, hostility, depressed mood, or atypical changes in thinking or behavior. If they are experiencing suicidal thoughts or suicidal behavior, patients must seek immediate emergency treatment by calling 9-1-1 or going to a local emergency room.

social support for successful cessation. There is a dose-response relationship between the amount of counseling time or number of counseling sessions and the success rate of smoking cessation. In fact, counseling up to 300 minutes or 8 sessions increases the likelihood that a smoker will become and stay smoke-free (105). Motivational interviewing may help patients to resolve their ambivalence around quitting. Patients need to be offered alternatives and options for managing cravings such as distraction, deep breathing, postponing smoking and rethinking the need to smoke, and calling a supportive person. Toll-free numbers are available for counseling, including 1-800-QUIT-NOW in the United States. Encourage persons concerned about increased hunger to use oral substitutes for cigarettes such as gum, cinnamon sticks, sugar-free hard candy, toothpicks, water, and low-calorie drinks. Symptoms of irritability may improve with a walk, a bath, or a pleasurable activity. Patients should be encouraged to reinforce their successes with short-term and longer-term rewards.

Critical factors for smoking cessation include a patient's desire to quit as well as skills and assistance to quit. AHCPR guidelines (105) provide a framework for health care providers to help patients stop smoking vis-à-vis the five As:

**1. Ask**—Identify all tobacco users at every visit.

**2. Advise**—Deliver a clear, strong, and personalized message: "As your [respiratory therapist, nurse, physical therapist], I need you to know that quitting smoking is the most important thing you can do to protect your health now and in the future. Smoking will make your lung disease worse. I will help you with quitting. It is important that you quit smoking now. Occasional or light smoking is still dangerous."

**3. Assess**—Determine the patient's willingness to quit. "Are you willing to try to quit?"

**4. Assist**—Provide counseling and medication. Help the patient develop a quit plan and set a quit date, ideally within 2 weeks. The patient should discuss his plan with family and friends and ask for understanding and support. Challenges should be anticipated, particularly during the first 2 weeks of withdrawal symptoms. Instruct the patient to remove tobacco products from his environment. Recommend approved medication, except when contraindicated or when there is insufficient evidence of effectiveness, such as for pregnant women, smokeless tobacco users, light smokers, and adolescents. Evaluate what has helped and hindered past attempts at quitting, and build on past successes. Discuss challenges and triggers and how to successfully overcome them. Alcohol is associated with relapse, and the patient should consider not drinking or limiting alcohol while quitting. Quitting is more difficult when there is another smoker in the household. Other smokers at home should be encouraged to quit or advised to not smoke around the patient. Provide the patient with ongoing support, including written information from the national quitline network in the United States (1-800-QUIT-NOW) and other organizations. Materials should be appropriate for the patient's culture, race, education, and age. Provide practical counseling including problem solving and skills training. Strive for total abstinence.

**5. Arrange**—Ensure follow-up contact. Follow-up contact should begin soon after the quit date, preferably during the first week. A second follow-up contact is recommended within the first month. Identify concerns encountered, and anticipate future challenges. Assess medication use and problems. Congratulate nonsmokers on their success. If the patient is smoking, review the circumstances of relapse and work with the patient on complete cessation. Consider use of more intensive treatment.

If a patient has little or no interest in quitting, asking what the person likes and dislikes about smoking may help the clinician to understand the patient's perspective and the patient to consider possible negative aspects of smoking.

Intensive behavioral interventions are the most effective. Adjunct strategies include recommending exercise, proper nutrition, and spiritual support for those who express interest. Those who struggle with persistent smoking despite use of guidelines strategies may benefit from referral to a nicotine dependence specialist.

# PARTNERING WITH A PSYCHOSOCIAL PROVIDER

Pulmonary rehabilitation programs should have a partnered relationship with a psychosocial provider. Ideally, this provider would be able to provide at least some limited services within the program. Generally, these providers will fall into the following disciplines: psychologist, social worker, counselor, or addictions counselor, all of whom possess a master's degree or above.

If the pulmonary rehabilitation program is located in a hospital or university setting, the most convenient avenue is to contact the institution's department of psychology or psychiatry to seek assistance from staff within this department. Another option is to seek referrals of private practitioners in the local community. One might consider methods to be selective in determining whom to contact. In order to be selective in finding the best fit of a psychosocial provider for a pulmonary rehabilitation program, primary care physicians can be utilized to determine a pool of potential referral resources.

These providers can be contacted to determine their receptiveness to referrals from the pulmonary rehabilitation program. Additionally, it would be advantageous to personally meet with the provider to offer information about psychosocial concerns that may be more common for patients with pulmonary disease. While the ability to make direct referrals is a benefit to the pulmonary patient, in some cases, it may be possible to make arrangements for the provider to offer services directly in the pulmonary rehabilitation program.

# SUMMARY

A strong, trusting bond is important to establish early in pulmonary rehabilitation to promote patient engagement, improvement, and successful outcomes. Assessment of psychosocial issues should be routinely performed at the outset of pulmonary rehabilitation and at regular intervals during the pulmonary rehabilitation program. Brief screening tools can be used to assess anxiety, depression, anger, hostility, social support, and emotional guardedness. For patients who may have cognitive impairment, the MOCA or Mini-Mental State Examination performed by a trained professional is an appropriate screening evaluation. Patients experiencing substantial impairments in psychosocial and cognitive functioning should be referred to a mental health provider for further evaluation and treatment. Intervention for psychosocial problems of lesser degrees can be integrated into the comprehensive pulmonary rehabilitation treatment plan with appropriately trained staff. Psychosocial interventions, offered in either individual or group formats, can be effective in reducing distress and facilitating adaptive coping. Breathing retraining, relaxation training, and stress management training can also be beneficial in reducing anxiety and the dyspnea cycle and should be an integral part of the overall treatment plan.

A combination of behavioral and pharmacological approaches is recommended to maximize success with long-term smoking cessation. Reassessment of psychological status and refinement of interventions are helpful in formulating a postrehabilitation plan. Fostering those activities that promote and reinforce the strategies learned will be useful in the long-term maintenance of physiological and psychosocial gains.

**VISIT THE WEB RESOURCE** ————————————————
for links to additional resources and various tools, checklists, and forms.

# Nutritional Assessment and Intervention

## Ellen Aberegg, LD, MA, RDN, FAACVPR
Private Consultant, Columbus, OH

Awareness of the impact that dietary habits, nutritional status, and nutritional interventions have upon COPD incidence, progression, and outcome is an important component of multifactorial health care in pulmonary rehabilitation. The complexity of nutritional needs can be driven by pulmonary events but also by systemic consequences (e.g., cachexia and muscle weakness) and comorbidity (e.g., osteoporosis, diabetes, and cardiovascular disease) (1). The heterogeneity of pulmonary disease requires a multidimensional approach to identifying compromised nutritional status, poor diet habits, and the impact of diet upon clinical outcomes in pulmonary patients (1). Schols et al. have suggested that there are different phenotypes of pulmonary patients, independent of lung function. Once these phenotypes of patients are identified by anthropometric and clinical measures, increased risk can be predicted and nutrition guidance implemented (1).

## COMPROMISED NUTRITIONAL STATUS IN PULMONARY DISEASE

Nutritional status reflects the balance between nutrient supply (via diet or endogenous sources) and nutrient demand. Negative consequences result if supply is diminished by decreased food intake or if demand increases. In pulmonary disease, food intake may be limited by breathing status and changes in appetite. Nutrient demand may increase by changes in metabolism, energy expenditure, and pulmonary disease process. Macronutrients, which provide energy as well as building blocks of protein, affect body composition status. Requirements for micronutrients such as vitamins, minerals, and other phytochemicals may be heightened by the pulmonary disease process, and whereas patients may not express clear deficiencies, evidence suggests diets high in vitamin D, vitamin C, fruits, vegetables, and fiber may reduce risk.

## Body Composition and Macronutrient Status

Body composition, the proportions of fat mass (FM) and fat-free mass (FFM), is a reflection of macronutrient status. In order to develop targeted nutritional interventions to address specific metabolic phenotypes, an understanding of the pathophysiology and interrelatedness of muscle loss and adiposity in COPD is essential. Thus, included in this chapter is a brief summary relevant to alterations in nutritional status and nutritional intervention. For a more detailed overview of pathophysiology of skeletal muscle wasting in COPD, the reader is directed to the American Thoracic Society/ERS statement on lower-limb muscle dysfunction in COPD (2).

## Low Body Weight

It is well understood that body weight loss (loss of fat-free mass or loss of fat mass) results when energy expenditure exceeds energy intake. The normal adaptive response to an energy deficit is preferential loss of FM to "spare" loss of the metabolically and functionally active FFM. But in COPD patients, weight loss is accompanied by significant loss of fat-free mass, out of proportion to the loss of fat mass (1). Catastrophic weight loss was once considered a consequence of inevitable and terminal progression of the pulmonary disease process (3). Now convincing evidence demonstrates unintended weight loss is not an adaptive mechanism to decreased metabolic rate in advanced COPD (4), but is an independent determinant of survival. Thus, the priority of weight maintenance should be made throughout the care process. Anorexia and subsequent lower caloric intake is not the cause of unbalanced energy metabolism in COPD. In fact, adequate or excessive caloric intake has been observed in underweight pulmonary patients (5). In COPD patients, the resting metabolic rate (RMR) and whole-body protein turnover is increased (6–8), as compared to a reduction in RMR observed in normal individuals. The daily energy requirements in COPD patients increase because of altered inefficient breathing mechanics, higher ATP cost of muscular contraction, and the decreased mechanical efficiency of lower-limb exercise (9–10). Evidence to support the understanding of this relationship is observed when COPD patients can and do gain weight after improved breathing mechanics following lung reduction surgery (11). A decrease in the proportion of slow-twitch type 1 fibers and a relative increase in fast-twitch type 2 fibers are reported in the peripheral skeletal muscle of patients with stable severe COPD, indicating a relative shift from oxidative to glycolytic capacity. Glycolytic metabolism is less energy efficient because it produces less ATP per mole of glucose than oxidative metabolism. The functional consequences of these changes are reflected in significant changes in skeletal muscle energy metabolism of patients with COPD (12).

Unintentional weight loss of >5% over 6 months places the COPD patient at increased clinical risk (13, 14). In COPD patients, low body weight is related to the severity of disease (15). BMI <25 kg/m$^2$ is consistently associated with increased mortality (13, 14). COPD patients who are underweight (or low FFM) are more likely to experience bone mineral loss than overweight patients (15).

## Diminished Fat-Free (Lean Body) Mass

Loss of FFM is an independent predictor of mortality irrespective of fat mass (16). Muscle loss and decreased muscle oxidative metabolism have a critical role in impaired physical performance. The response to semi-starvation is an increase whole-body protein turnover (6) as it is increased in RMR (17, 18). Muscle loss occurs when catabolism exceeds anabolism. FFM mass is not "spared," and the decrease is likely due to the increased muscle protein degradation (19) while muscle-building pathways are stable or even increased (20). These lower plasma levels of branched chain amino acids (AA) are observed in COPD patients (21) and may be a result of low dietary intake or diminished absorption in the small intestine (22). Regulatory pathways of protein breakdown are the subject of future research, but metabolic efficiency of feeding does not appear to be impaired, thus adequate provision of protein and AA is a therapeutic goal (23).

## Excess Body Weight

The prevalence of obesity in COPD populations is variable and ranges from 18%-54% (24). Obese (>30 kg/m$^2$) individuals experience more dyspnea and exercise intolerance than the nonobese regardless of airflow limitations (25). The number of inhaled medications and fatigue is greater in obese COPD patients compared to normal weight individuals (26, 27). Obesity in COPD patients negatively affects performance of weight-bearing exercise. Obese COPD patients experience greater morbidity and mortality from CV disease. Leone found in a large population-based study that abdominal obesity was the strongest predictor of lung function impairment and that the risk of metabolic syndrome was 40% greater in these patients (28). But in the ANTADIR study and others, obese COPD patients had higher survival rates and lower hospitalization rates (29). This observation ("the obesity paradox") may be due to the relative reduction in static lung volumes in obese COPD patients or to concomitant increases in lean body mass associated with larger girth (30, 31) It is thought that obesity influences each COPD patient based upon patient characteristics and disease severity. It may protect against mortality in patients with advanced COPD whereas in earlier stages of COPD the negative impact of obesity (via low-grade inflammation and metabolic syndrome) accentuates CV risk and increases CV and all-cause mortality (24).

## Micronutrient Status

Micronutrients are nutrients that do not contribute to energy balance but are required for health. They sustain metabolism and maintain tissue function. Vitamins are organic compounds that fulfill many roles in the body such as co-enzymes, antioxidants, and hormone-like regulators. Nutritive minerals are needed in small or trace quantities to fulfill structural and functional roles, as well as electrolytes. The body does not synthesize essential vitamins and minerals and thus regular exogenous sources are required in the diet. Nonessential vitamins and minerals are needed for health but can be synthesized from endogenous sources from within the body during times of health. Phytochemicals are organic compounds that include carotenoids (some of which are plant precursors of vitamins A and E) and polyphenols (including phenolic acids, flavonoids, and stilbenes/ligans). Among their many functions, some of which are still being discovered, is the antioxidant activity important in the homeostatic response to inflammation.

Serum levels of micronutrients generally reflect diet intake but are confounded by age, gender, smoking, alcohol intake, and race as well as by heightened local demand (32). Most studies demonstrate the direct positive relationships between $FEV_1$ and specific diet components such as calcium, vitamin C, vitamin A, and vitamin E. Higher serum values of vitamins A, C, and E, calcium, and iron were associated with higher $FEV_1$ values (33) and conversely lowest serum values of vitamins C, E, and B-carotene had the lowest $FEV_1$ and FVC (34). Table 6.1 summarizes the roles certain nutrients play in lung health.

Vitamin D acts either directly upon muscle fiber contractility or by vitamin D receptors (via calcium) (36). Vitamin D deficiency impairs calcium uptake, down regulates protein synthesis, and increases cell death (37). Prevalence increases with disease severity (38). Vitamin D deficiency is associated with muscle weakness, increased risk for falls, decreased physical performance, impaired functional capacity, and reduced training benefits (39) in the elderly and in COPD patients. The Normative Aging Study showed more rapid rates of decline in $FEV_1$ per pack year of smoking in vitamin D deficient individuals compared to those who were not deficient (40).

Calcium imbalance is a frequent risk in pulmonary patients because of increased osteoporotic risk with steroid therapy, poor diet intake, and decreases in FFM. Poor bone density is often a concomitant finding in cachexic pulmonary patients and those with poor vitamin D status. Steroid therapy also increases risk of weight gain, increased triglycerides, increased HDL, and increased serum glucose.

Iron deficiency often occurs in COPD, which may be caused by several factors including systemic inflammation, malabsorption of iron from the gut, renal failure (as a consequence of concomitant chronic kidney disease or diabetes mellitus), and medications such as angiotensin-converting enzyme inhibitors and corticosteroids (42).

# DIET INTAKE AND COPD

Seventy-five percent of entry pulmonary rehabilitation patients have reported diets low in vitamin D and calcium, and more than one-third have low intake of protein and vitamins A, E, and C. Patients with a low fat-free mass index (FFMI) (see table 6.1) more often have low intake of protein, while abdominally obese patients more often have low intakes of protein and most micronutrients (P<0.05). Patients with both low FFMI and abdominal obesity appeared most often to be consuming a poor-quality diet (43).

## Diet Patterns and COPD

Dietary intake may be described as absolute quantities of macro- and micronutrients. Nutrient need is confounded by the intake of other nutrients or availability, thus intake is better described and prescribed by use of food patterns or food groups. Epidemiological evidence of long-term increase in fruit and vegetable intake is related to smaller declines in lung function in COPD patients (44). Diet patterns that do not include fruit, vegetables, oily fish, and whole grains are associated with lower $FEV_1$ in English men. Those who were in the lowest quintile for diet quality were 54% more likely to have COPD than the top quintile (45).

In women and men, a diet rich in fruits, vegetables, and fish may reduce the risk of COPD, whereas a diet rich in refined grains, cured and red meats, desserts, and french fries may increase the risk of COPD (46, 47). A recent large longitudinal study in Sweden showed that high consumption of fruits and vegetables is associated with reduced COPD incidence in both current and ex-smokers but not in never-smokers. Individuals eating five daily servings of fruits and vegetables had a 35%

## Table 6.1 Selection of Nutrients of Relevance in Lung Health

| Nutrient | Role in Lung Health | Status |
|---|---|---|
| Protein/Amino Acids | COPD disease process favors increased whole-body protein turnover, plus catabolic triggers negatively affect muscle remodeling. | |
| Carbohydrate | Changes in proportion of Type 1 muscle fiber and mitochondria result in decreased fat oxidative capacity and preference for carbohydrates. Rapid source of energy without satiety. | |
| Polyunsaturated fatty acids (PUFA) | Calorie dense micronutrient. N-3 PUFA associated with anti-inflammatory process. Both N-3 and N-6 PUFA helpful in reducing CVD risk. Promotes quick satiety. | |
| Vitamin A | Plays a role in the differentiation of epithelial cells. | Serum concentrations of retinol do not appear to be related to observed levels of usual intake; hepatic vitamin A stores may be more reflective of nutrient adequacy. |
| Carotenes | Vitamin A precursors. The antioxidant activity of carotenes may be more important than vitamin A and is used as a biologic marker of intake of fruits and vegetables. | Correlation between intake and serum concentrations has been shown to range from 0.21 to 0.52 (P 0.05). |
| Vitamin C | Appears to be the most abundant antioxidant substance in extracellular lung fluid; scavenges superoxide radicals; contributes to the regeneration of membrane-bound oxidized vitamin E. | Body tissue sites are maintained at higher concentrations than serum concentrations; correlation between intake and serum concentrations has been shown ($r = 0.28 - 0.56$ $P<0.05$). |
| Vitamin E | Breaks the lipid peroxidation chain reaction, representing the primary defense of cellular membranes against oxidative damage. | Intake of vitamin E correlates with serum vitamin D ($r = 0.07$, $P < 0.001$) dietary vitamin E correlated with serum vitamin E to cholesterol ratio after adjustment for age, sex, BMI, alcohol, and gamma-tocopherols correlated with serum levels of tocopherols ($r = 0.03 - 0.55$ $P < 0.05$). |
| Vitamin D | May regulate the expression of genes in bronchial smooth muscle cells; deficiency may increase levels of matrix metalloproteinases, which aggravate inflammatory injury and contribute to changes in lung structure. | Serum levels of 25(OH)D have been established as the marker of vitamin D intake in the form of diet or sun exposure. |
| Calcium | Risk of osteoporosis increases with corticosteroid use, inflammatory process, and poor diet. Adequate intake of calcium and vitamin D essential for bone health. | DEXA bone density studies reflect long-term adequacy. Few biochemical markers reflect calcium status accurately. |

| Nutrient | Role in Lung Health | Status |
|----------|---------------------|--------|
| Iron | Iron status impacts production of red blood cells and respiratory enzymes. Prevalence of anemia reported to be between 4.9%-38%. Nonanemic iron deficiency is common in COPD and appears to be driven by inflammation (41). | Soluble transferrin receptor >28.1 nmol/L; (2) transferrin saturation <16% and (3) ferritin <12 µg/L (41). |
| Sodium | Hypertension frequent comorbidity. Snack or convenience foods are high in sodium yet may be the primary foodstuffs. | Blood pressure better indicator than serum sodium. |

Adapted from Hanson et al. (2013).

reduced risk of developing COPD compared with those eating two or fewer portions. Each extra serving of fruits and vegetables was associated with a 4% lower risk of COPD in former smokers and an 8% lower risk in current smokers (48).

## Impediments to Healthy Eating Behavior

Physical limitations of pulmonary disease negatively affect eating behavior. Breathlessness and fatigue reduce appetite and meal duration. Postprandial shortness of breath functionally limits the volume of food consumed. Swallowing problems limit food choices to soft, tender, homogenous, or liquid foods. Limited social and financial supports constrain selection of well-tolerated nutrient-dense foods. Further, limited knowledge and reduced motivation in the face of other consequences of the disease process hamper making a higher quality diet a priority (49). Fatigue limits the desire to prepare meals or shop for food, and convenience foods high in sodium and saturated fat and low in nutrients may be preferred. Changes in taste acuity due to medications or illness discourage pulmonary patients from selecting formerly preferred foods.

Smoking is a strong confounder when examining the positive relationship between diet and lung function. The increased general oxidant burden and inflammation associated with smoking increases the need for antioxidants. In the B-carotene Cancer Study, high baseline intakes and high serum levels of vitamin E in male smokers were associated with a low incidence of bronchitis and dyspnea (35).

# ASSESSMENT OF NUTRITIONAL STATUS

Nutritional status is an important determinant of COPD outcome (1). Evaluation of nutritional status includes analysis of body composition and diet intake. Nutrient status deemed at risk from these two assessments may require further detailed serum analysis. Schols and others have identified different metabolic phenotypes of COPD that are useful in patient counseling as well as in future clinical trial design. Refer to table 6.2 for an overview of the described phenotypes and health risks.

## Body Composition Assessment

Incorporation of body composition analysis into nutritional assessment has been a major step forward in understanding systemic COPD pathophysiology and nutritional potential (1). Identification of patients at risk of diminished fat-free mass increases the potential for improvement in clinical outcomes by subsequent appropriate supplementation. Measurements of height and weight, weight history, and specific anthropometric measurements are assessable in most pulmonary rehabilitation settings. The most accurate methods are not suitable for common daily use in pulmonary rehabilitation due to their high cost and time burden. Skinfolds may overestimate FFM, although many studies found no significant difference by method (50). Clinical indications of each individual will determine the necessity of more

## Table 6.2 Metabolic Phenotypes and Clinical Risk

| Metabolic Phenotype | Definition | Clinical Risk |
|---|---|---|
| Obesity | BMI >30 kg/m² | ↑ CV Risk |
| Morbid obesity | BMI >35 kg/m² | ↑ CV Risk<br>Physical performance impairment |
| Sarcopenic obesity | BMI >30 to 35 kg/m²<br>and MAMC <15; SMI <2 | ↑ CV Risk<br>Physical performance impairment |
| Sarcopenia | MAMC <15; SMI <2 | ↑ Mortality Risk<br>Physical performance impairment |
| Pre-cachexia | BMI within normal limits<br>Unintended weight loss >5% over 6 months | ↑ Mortality Risk |
| Cachexia | Unintended weight loss >5% over 6 months<br>and FFMI <18 kg/m² (males)<br>FFMI <15 kg/m² (females) | ↑ Mortality Risk<br>Physical performance impairment |

Reprinted by permission from A.M. Schols et al. "Nutritional Assessment and Therapy in COPD: A European Respiratory Society Statement," *European Respiratory Journal* 44 (2014): 1504-1520.

expensive or precise serial methods of assessment, particularly in osteoporotic, pre-cachexic, and cachexic patients. See table 6.3 for assessment information.

Training and competency are essential for pulmonary rehabilitation professionals to ensure accuracy and validity of measures. For specific instructions on methods of measurements, see *Fitness Professionals Handbook*, 2016 (51). Specific anthropometric measures are listed in table 6.3. Calculations of BMI, FFM, FM, FFMI, and FMI are made using standard reference equations. The major shortcoming of the BMI is that the actual composition of body weight is not taken into account: excess body weight may be made up of adipose tissue or muscle hypertrophy, both of which will be judged as "excess mass." On the other hand, a deficit of BMI may be due to an FFM deficit (sarcopenia) or a mobilization of adipose tissue or both combined (52). In a study of European Caucasian males and females aged 18 to 98 years, using the 25th and 75th percentiles as cutoffs, Shutz proposed the following FFMI and FMI ranges as normal. The 25th and 75th percentiles correspond well to the cutoff of BMIs of 20 and 25 kg/m² respectively (53). Thus, skinfold measures have been demonstrated as an accessible tool for determination of FFM and FM utilizing the Durnin Womersley equation (54), the Siri

equation (55), or the Jackson-Pollock equations for men (55) and women (56). Revised equations for obese individuals have been proposed (57).

Risk increases as FFM decreases, FM increases, involuntary weight loss occurs, or BMI varies high and low from the norm. As these parameters vary along a continuum, four clusters of risk become apparent. Schols (1) identifies these clusters as metabolic phenotypes: obesity and morbidly obesity, sarcopenia and sarcopenic obesity, normal WNL, plus cachexic and pre-cachexic.

## Cachexia and Pre-Cachexia

Cachexia is a complex syndrome frequently present in patients with chronic severe illnesses, including COPD, cancer, and congestive heart failure. Cachexia is associated with increased mortality (16), impairments in health-related quality of life, and muscle weakness (62). The clinical phenotype of cachexia ranges from minimal or no weight loss with signs of muscle wasting to severe weight loss with signs of muscle depletion, fatigue, and reduced mobility (62). The anthropometric measure of FFMI is an indication of risk. An FFMI <10th percentile (<17 kg/m² for men and <15 kg/m² for women) is a strong predictor of mortality (16), thus an urgent flag for nutrition intervention. Weight stabilization and gains in FFM will be clear indicators of improvement attainable

## Table 6.3 Measures of Body Composition Available in Clinical Practice (adapted from 58–61)

| Variable | Clinical Measurements | Complications | Normal |
|---|---|---|---|
| Height, weight, BMI* | Height and weight* | Weight (kg)/height (m²) | 20 < BMI <25 |
| Fat-free mass/fat mass* | Sum of four skinfolds: Triceps, biceps, subscapular, suprailiac* DEXA | Sum of skinfolds, then reference table FM = % fat × weight (kg) FFM = weight − FM | Body fat Men 12%-19% Women 16%-25% |
| Fat-free mass index (FFMI) Fat mass index (FMI) | | FFMI = FFM × BMI FMI = FM × BMI | FFMI Men 18.2–20 kg/m² Women 15–16.6 kg/m² FMI Men 3.5–5.9 kg/m² Women 4.9–7.8 kg/m² |
| Muscle mass (MM)* | Mid-arm circumference (MAC) in cm* Trifold skinfold (mm)* | Muscle circumference (MAMC) calculation MAC − (3.1415 × TSF/10) | |
| | Biomarkers Creatine height markers (CHI) DEXA appendicular lean mass (ALM) | CHI = (Patient creatine × 100/ideal creatine for height) | |
| Visceral mass* | Waist-hip ratio (WHR)* DEXA Ultrasonography sagittal diameter | Waist (cm)/Hip (cm) | Men < 0.90 Women < 0.85 |
| Bone density/mass | DEXA HRCT | | |
| Muscle strength Related physical performance* | 6-minute walk (gait speed)* 1 repetition max* Handgrip strength* Get up and go test* Stair climb power test* | | |

*Indicates tests commonly performed in pulmonary rehabilitation.

Reprinted by permission from A.M. Schols et al. "Nutritional Assessment and Therapy in COPD: A European Respiratory Society Statement," *European Respiratory Journal* 44 (2014): 1504-1520.

while the patient is in the pulmonary rehabilitation program. The pre-cachexic patient is in a state of >5% unexplained BW loss over 6 months without measurable deficits in FFM. Nutrition intervention is warranted due to increased risk and weight stabilization and improvement in diet quality will be the indicator of improvement.

## Sarcopenia and Sarcopenic Obesity

Sarcopenia is a deficit in skeletal muscle, and thus FFM, resulting in weakness. While the clinical relevance of sarcopenia is widely recognized, there is currently no universally accepted definition of the disorder. Sarcopenia may be optimally defined (for the purposes of clinical trial inclusion criteria, as well as epidemiological studies) using a combination of measures of muscle mass and physical performance.

Sarcopenia is prevalent in patients eligible for pulmonary rehabilitation throughout all ranges of BMI. A deficit of FFM may occur regardless of FM status. Schols (6) recommends using appendicular skeletal muscle index (SMI) (appendicular lean mass as measured by DEXA)/height2) <2. DEXA measurements may be most precise, but mid-arm muscle circumference (MAMC) and waist circumference (WC) have been used in large sarcopenia mortality studies successfully. Figure 6.1 utilizes both anthropometric and strength measures as suggested by Cruz-Jentoft (58) in order to identify normal patients at risk for sarcopenia and then alert physicians to the potential for more precise studies.

Sarcopenic obese men had the highest risk of all-cause mortality but not CVD mortality. Efforts to promote healthy aging should focus on preventing obesity and maintaining muscle mass (63, 64). Abdominal obesity seems to have protective effects on physical functioning. Sarcopenia and central adiposity were associated with greater cardiovascular mortality and all-cause mortality. Atkins found that composite anthropometric measure of MAMC and WC is more effective in predicting all-cause mortality than measures of FFMI and FMI. Traditionally, the nutritional interest in COPD, cystic fibrosis (CF), and lung cancer has been on management of weight loss and muscle wasting (cachexia) in advanced disease stages, while obesity was predominantly investigated in relation to onset and progression of asthma and obstructive sleep apnea syndrome. Obesity has now been identified as a risk factor across all respiratory diseases. Furthermore, combined with aging-induced changes in muscle mass (sarcopenia), the clinical significance of sarcopenic obesity has been highlighted in COPD (54) and lung cancer (64).

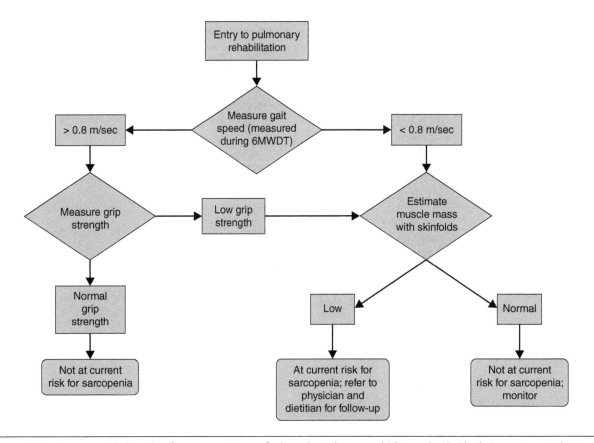

**Figure 6.1** A suggested algorithm for sarcopenia case finding. Consider comorbidity and individual circumstances that may influence each finding.

In a large longitudinal study, the Cardiovascular Health Study (54) found that sarcopenic obesity that was characterized using muscle strength was modestly associated with CVD risk. In men with decreased endurance, WC and low muscle mass, as measured using MAMC, were associated with all-cause mortality. Sarcopenia (MAMC ≤25.9 cm) and obesity (WC >102 cm) were associated with CVD mortality and all-cause mortality risk, but did not have an excess risk of CVD mortality beyond that associated with sarcopenia or obesity alone. Sarcopenic obesity was more strongly related to non-CVD mortality, independent of inflammation, than CVD mortality. Despite the sarcopenic obese group having the highest risk of mortality, there was no evidence of interaction between sarcopenia and obesity, suggesting that the presence of obesity does not modify the effect of sarcopenia.

## Normal BMI and FFM

Refer to reference ranges for normal BMI, FFM, FM, FFMI, and FMI in table 6.2. Inquiries regarding weight history, including recent changes that were unintended or not desired, should be made in addition to body composition to ensure any "normal" values were not achieved at the expense of FFM loss. Serial measures taken early in the course of pulmonary disease or, at least at the beginning of pulmonary rehabilitation, are helpful in accessing body composition changes over time and as the disease progresses.

## Obesity and Morbid Obesity

Obesity, defined as a BMI >25 kg/m$^2$, and morbid obesity, >30 kg/m$^2$, are associated with higher mortality and morbidity due to increase in CVD risk. In nonpulmonary, nonsmoking individuals, a BMI between 20–25 kg/m$^2$ had the lowest all-cause mortality risk. But in COPD patients with moderate to severe obstruction, a BMI <25 kg/m$^2$ was associated with higher risk than those whose BMI >25 or even >30 kg/m$^2$ (1). Although weight loss is routinely recommended for all obese individuals, caution should be exercised in recommending weight loss in COPD patients with moderate to severe obstruction. No studies have systematically investigated the effects of weight loss interventions on adiposity, functionality, and systemic inflammatory profile in patients with COPD (1). Modest reductions in weight can reduce the cardiovascular disease risk through improvements in body fat distribution. A combination of moderate hypocaloric, moderate to high protein diet and aerobic exercise may achieve this goal best because aerobic exercise training improves insulin sensitivity, induces mitochondrial biogenesis in skeletal muscle, and induces loss of visceral fat mass. Rapid weight loss is frequently associated with loss of FFM and thus is not recommended in pulmonary individuals.

See table 6.4 for metabolic phenotypes and the related nutritional instructions and considerations during pulmonary rehabilitation.

# Diet Intake Assessment

The effectiveness of various dietary assessment tools depends on which diet component is being measured, the ability of the assessor to interpret findings, and patient factors, such as literacy, stage of illness, and readiness to change. Different dietary instruments all have unique strengths and weaknesses. Diet histories, diet records, and 24-hour recalls, if administered by trained personnel, will yield an accurate analysis of nutrient content that can guide counseling or referral to a registered dietitian. However, producing meaningful pre- and post-diet assessment data depends on well-standardized tools. Diet histories are obtained by interviews with trained personnel and can reflect a patient's "usual" food intake, including characteristics, frequency, and amount of the foods consumed. The patient keeps diet records over three to four days (accuracy decreases with longer duration). The accuracy of the data collected is dependent upon patient motivation, training in food volume assessment, and ease of use (i.e., free written, forms, or electronic means). Twenty-four-hour recall can be an interview-driven or self-administered tool. Food intake over a 24-hour period is quantified but may not be truly reflective of foods consumed (65). These tools are helpful for clinical assessment and counseling guidance but are not useable as pulmonary rehabilitation outcomes or group comparisons as pre/post measures because of their nonstandardized methodologies.

Food frequency questionnaires (FFQ) are standardized checklists of foods and beverages with a frequency response section for patients to report how often each item was consumed over a specified period of time (65). Brief FFQs may have only 12 to 22 targeted questions and take far less time, yet yield only information regarding high, medium, or low ranges of food groupings. Screening tools are brief FFQs that assess consumption of singular

## Table 6.4    Metabolic Phenotypes and Implications in Nutrition and Lifestyle

| Metabolic Phenotype | Nutritional Recommendations | Pulmonary Rehabilitation Implications |
|---|---|---|
| Obesity | Gradual weight loss with high-quality, adequate protein and modest calorie reduction. Emphasize increased fruits, vegetables, and high fiber intake. | Increase calorie deficit with exercise |
| Morbid obesity | Gradual weight loss with high-quality, adequate protein and modest calorie reduction. Emphasize increased fruits, vegetables, and high fiber intake. | Consider intermittent exercise High-intensity, non–weight bearing exercise |
| Sarcopenic obesity | Inquire about recent weight loss. Ensure diet higher in protein. Postpone calorie reduction recommendations until FFM restored. Refer to dietician for malnutrition. | Increase calorie deficit with exercise |
| Sarcopenia | Increase caloric and high-quality protein intake with diet or whole food "supplementation." Refer to dietician for malnutrition. | Load-bearing exercise |
| Pre-cachexia | Moderate increase in caloric and high-quality protein intake with diet or whole food "supplementation." Modify food format as necessary. If weight loss doesn't cease, refer to physician and dietician. | Load-bearing exercise |
| Cachexia | Increase caloric and high-quality protein intake with diet or whole food "supplementation." Utilize smaller, frequent feedings as tolerated. Multivitamin supplementation. Refer to dietician for malnutrition. | Consider intermittent exercise High-intensity non–weight bearing exercise |

nutrients or patterns. These tools can measure just fruit and vegetable intake or focus, for example, on just fat intake. Brief FFQs need validation in a variety of populations and literacy levels and are helpful as a means to evaluate need for further diet counseling or for referral to a dietitian. Brief FFQs are not appropriate for pre- and post-change measurements. An extended FFQ can be 50 to 150 questions and able to collect data on both macro- and micronutrients. Published results for reliability and validity must be evaluated and validity comparisons made to the patient population. Computerized versions of FFQs may improve reliability and accuracy of the measure.

Diet indices are the means to evaluate the results from FFQ, diet histories, and 24-hour recalls and to systematically score the diet according to defined parameters. The Healthy Eating Index (HEI) was developed to measure how well diets conform to federal dietary guidelines (USDG) regarding food groups and patterns. The total HEI scores were positively associated with $FEV_1/FVC$, whereas associations with component scores were inconsistent (66). The alternative HEI (aHEI) rates the diet based on absolute intake quantity in contrast to a nutrient density basis of the HEI (per 1,000 kcal). A higher AHEI-2010 diet score (reflecting high intakes of whole grains, polyunsaturated fatty acids, nuts, and long-chain omega-3 fats, and low intakes of red or processed meats, refined grains, and sugar-sweetened drinks) was associated with a lower risk of COPD in both women and men. These findings support the importance of a healthy diet in multi-interventional programs to prevent COPD (74). The Dietary Approaches to Stop Hypertension (DASH) score is used frequently in studies in CVD. Clinical trials have demonstrated that the DASH dietary pattern was associated with substantially lower blood pressure, one of the leading risk factors for CVD (67). An overall healthy diet, regardless of index used, is associated with higher lung function and reduction in all-cause morbidity and mortality (67).

# NUTRITION SUPPORT

Given the emergent pivotal role of sarcopenia, osteoporosis, visceral adiposity, and poor dietary quality in COPD risk and progression, dietary awareness and intervention become integral parts of disease management (1). In 2003, a Cochrane report could not demonstrate a relationship between nutrition support and improvement in anthropometric measures or functional exercise capacity due to lack of homogeneity in study populations. Confusion in the literature regarding the benefit of nutritional support resulted from lack of a clear definition of nutritional support (alimentation, nutraceuticals, or food) as well as previous lack of RCT data demonstrating benefit. In 2012, the report was updated and concluded moderate-quality evidence that nutritional supplementation promotes significant weight gain among patients with COPD, especially if malnourished. Nourished patients may not respond to the same degree to supplemental feeding. Recent studies have found a significant change from baseline in fat-free mass index/fat-free mass, fat mass/fat mass index, MAMC (as a measure of lean body mass), 6-minute walk test, and a significant improvement in skinfold thickness (as a measure of fat mass) for all patients receiving nutrition supplementation. In addition, there were significant improvements in respiratory muscle strength (maximum inspiratory pressure and maximum expiratory pressure) (68).

Overall, the evidence indicates that a well-balanced diet is beneficial to all COPD patients, not only for its potential pulmonary benefits, but also for its proven benefits in metabolic and cardiovascular risk (1). Nutrition therapy for COPD

has transitioned from a focus on supposed adverse effects of carbohydrate overload on the ventilatory system to beneficial effects of nutritional intervention on body composition and physical functioning as an integral part of disease management (69). Past concerns regarding high CHO intake and increased $CO_2$ production have not been substantiated or duplicated using normal foods (70–72). There is a strong rationale for prioritizing carbohydrate oxidation during exercise training in COPD. Structural and metabolic abnormalities in the skeletal muscles of patients with COPD include reductions in the proportion of type 1 fibers and mitochondrial density, resulting in decreased fat oxidative capacity and increased glucose production. Early muscle fatigue is associated with early lactic acid rise and adenine nucleotide loss, even at the low absolute exercise intensities that COPD patients can achieve. Provision of higher-carbohydrate, lower-fat foods and beverages may be beneficial as a rapid energy source for the muscle without leading to satiety precluding normal food intake. Carbohydrate-rich supplements induce less postprandial shortness of breath than do fat-rich supplements in RCTs (73). Thus, the additional calories that might be needed by underweight COPD patients can come from high-quality carbohydrate sources as well as from PUFA.

Protein intake generally is recommended to be 0.8gm/kg BW. Individuals who have reduced FFM should increase their protein intake in order to provide adequate AA building blocks for muscle anabolism. Essential amino acids stimulate anabolism and combat catabolism (suspected) secondary to COPD disease process effect upon whole-body protein turnover. The protein synthesis depends upon amino acid availability in the blood stream. Greater quantities of amino acids may need to be provided because of impaired branch chain amino acid extraction in some COPD patients. The goal of nutrition intervention is to provide enough protein and amino acids but also adequate calories in order to ensure those amino acids are used to promote muscle synthesis and not as an energy source to maintain homeostasis.

The balance between potentially toxic substances and the protective actions of antioxidant defenses, including those derived from diet, may play a role in the loss of lung function over time and the eventual development of COPD. These prospective findings support the importance of a healthy diet in multi-interventional programs to prevent COPD. The results encourage clinicians to consider the potential role of the combined effect of foods in a healthy diet in promoting lung health (74).

Yet there have been studies that have demonstrated reduced COPD risk with individual food components. Dietary fiber is independently associated with better lung function and reduced prevalence of COPD (75). A diet high in fiber, and possibly specifically cereal fiber, may reduce risk of developing COPD (76). Six hundred IU of vitamin E led to a 10% reduction in the risk of chronic lung disease in women (77). Vitamin D deficient COPD patients supplemented long term with vitamin D have improved muscle strength, skeletal muscle mitochondrial oxidative phosphorylation, $FEV_1$ volumes, and decreased number of falls (78, 79). This benefit was not observed in short-term supplementation (80, 81) or in COPD patients who were not vitamin D deficient. Use of steroids in the treatment of lung disease raises the risk of development of osteoporosis. The risk is compounded by malnutrition, sedentary lifestyle, smoking, and systemic inflammation common in COPD patients. Intakes of calcium and vitamin D higher than normal should be recommended for individuals who take corticosteroids, but preference should be given to food options rather than supplementation.

# SUMMARY

Opportunities for dietary and nutrition interventions in COPD management should be explored, aiming at early detection, prevention, and early treatment of involuntary weight loss. This means expanding the target group to include COPD outpatients and primary care patients before they become underweight, and putting more emphasis on dietary change than on medically prescribed supplementation. Successful intervention assumes (voluntary) adjustment of dietary behavior, and health professionals play an essential role in encouraging patients to make and maintain these changes. Achieving dietary change among COPD patients may require a combination of diet counseling and self-management (82).

Medical nutrition therapy is recommended for any patient who is deemed malnourished. Referral to a dietitian is a required standard of care. The dietitian can tailor protein recommendations appropriately as well as give specific guidance regarding supplementation versus real food preparation. Recommendation of small, frequent (every 2–3 hours) feedings of highly nutritious foods for any patient who suffers from poor appetite or inability to consume adequate calories is usually well tolerated and appreciated. Liquid versions of meals or blenderized smoothies minimize distention and discomfort.

Education classes have traditionally focused upon didactic information that is too generalized and often is not remembered. Practical information and hands-on experiences aid retention and enhance interest. Sharing the documented effects of fruits, vegetables, and foods high in antioxidants upon $FEV_1$ may persuade patients to select more of these foods daily. Targeting class topics to patients who need to either gain weight or lose weight limits embarrassment and frustration.

**VISIT THE WEB RESOURCE** ————————————————————— 
for links to additional resources and various tools, checklists, and forms.

## 7

# Patient-Centered Evidence-Based Outcomes

**Gerene Bauldoff, PhD, RN, MAACVPR**
Ohio State University College of Nursing

**Eileen Collins, PhD, FAACVPR**
University of Illinois-Chicago College of Nursing

Outcome measures are tests to evaluate if a desired end is met. In pulmonary rehabilitation, there are two broad areas of outcome analysis: patient-centered clinical outcomes and program performance measures. The former evaluates how effective the intervention was in areas of importance to the respiratory patient. The latter evaluates how effective the program was in meeting its quality goals. Both are necessary for pulmonary rehabilitation and essential for certification from AACVPR.

As established by AACVPR, patient-centered outcomes address, at a minimum, three essential areas: functional status/exercise capacity, dyspnea, and health-related quality of life (health status). Other outcome assessments such as measures of other symptoms (fatigue), psychosocial screening, or exercise capacity may also be indicated, depending on the needs of the patient and the resources of the program. Psychosocial and nutritional outcome screening, assessment, and intervention are discussed in chapters 5 and 6. A list of required outcome areas and currently AACVPR-approved measurement tests/instruments are outlined in table 7.1.

Outcome measures are useful for a variety of reasons. They can be used to evaluate individual patient progress (patient-centered outcomes), to

determine overall effectiveness of the program (performance measures), for clinical research, for program certification, and for reimbursement.

Patients are unique and obtain varying degrees of benefits from a program. The evaluation of individual patient progress is a core component of pulmonary rehabilitation. However, many standardized outcome measures tell providers how groups of people performed, not how an individual patient performed. For this reason, statistical measures of outcomes such as minimal clinically important differences (MCID) are used as a broad guide for program achievement, not as a gold standard of the minimal level that *a particular patient* must achieve. However, MCID is an appropriate benchmark when establishing program performance. See chapter 9 for program performance discussion.

Assessment of individual patient progress ultimately depends on a one-on-one clinical assessment, aided by standardized tests. The overall effectiveness of the program is best assessed using outcome assessment tools. The certification process of AACVPR mandates that the program utilize outcome data to evaluate its effectiveness (see chapter 10 on certification).

This chapter discusses the timing of outcome assessment, followed by a discussion of AACVPR-required patient-centered outcomes

## Table 7.1    Required Outcome Areas for Pulmonary Rehabilitation

| Outcome | Evidence-Based Tests and Instruments (available in the public domain) |
| --- | --- |
| Functional status/exercise capacity | 6-minute walk test* |
| Dyspnea<br><br>Select one instrument; additional instrument use optional | Modified Medical Research Council Scale (mMRC)* |
| | University of California, San Diego Shortness of Breath Questionnaire (UCSD SOBQ) |
| | Baseline Dyspnea Index (BDI) |
| | Transitional Dyspnea Index (TDI) |
| Health-related quality of life (HRQL)<br><br>Select one instrument; additional instrument use optional | St. George's Respiratory Questionnaire (SGRQ) |
| | Chronic Respiratory Disease Questionnaire (CRQ) |
| | COPD Assessment Test (CAT)* |

*Indicates instrument available in the public domain

as well as other outcomes that may be of interest to programs. It should be noted that some patient-centered outcome measures may not be appropriate for all respiratory disorders. However, AACVPR-required patient-centered outcome measures have been reported as valid and reliable for patients with COPD and interstitial lung disease (ILD). For instance, some health-related quality of life questionnaires have been validated only for COPD and ILD, and their use in other diseases has not yet been described in the literature. Therefore, patients with conditions other than COPD or ILD may need different outcome assessments. Some of these outcome assessments are discussed in further detail in chapter 8.

# TIMING AND ANALYZING OUTCOMES

Outcome assessment requires a minimum of two time points: one before pulmonary rehabilitation (baseline) and one immediately after completing rehabilitation. Optional postrehabilitation outcome measurements can also be taken at further intervals such as 3, 6, or 12 months; however, these frequencies are not always practical since some patients are lost to follow-up or may be unwilling to return for testing.

AACVPR program certification requires only a pre- and postrehabilitation measure of outcomes. The pulmonary rehabilitation program must include at least 10 pulmonary rehabilitation sessions within a 3-month period. However, the pulmonary rehabilitation program can run longer than 3 months. Change in performance is generally evaluated by comparing the post–pulmonary rehabilitation program measure with the corresponding baseline measure. Some measures, such as the 6-minute walk test distance, are best expressed by documenting the absolute value (e.g., in feet or meters). For comparison of pre- and postaggregate outcome data, paired t-tests or nonparametric tests can be used for statistical analysis (1).

The immediate post–pulmonary rehabilitation time, although very practical, may or may not be the best time to evaluate postrehabilitation changes. While improvement may continue well after the program has been completed (2–3), possibly because patients may take weeks to months to incorporate health behavior changes learned in pulmonary rehabilitation into their everyday lives, a defined time period or number of sessions is recognized for measurement to allow consistent evaluation.

# PATIENT-CENTERED OUTCOME MEASURES

Patient-centered outcome measures in pulmonary rehabilitation consist of evaluating an individual's ability to exercise, symptoms, and health-related quality of life. This section describes the standard outcome measures used in the clinical setting to evaluate pulmonary rehabilitation. Based on published evidence, AACVPR identified a limited set of valid and reliable instruments for each patient-centered outcome, including at least one instrument found in the public domain. Other outcome measures can also be used but are often more practical in a research setting. Detailed information on all patient-centered outcome measures and valid and reliable instrument descriptions are available to members of AACVPR at the www.AACVPR.org website by searching for "Pulmonary Rehabilitation Outcome Resource Guide." This guide is updated regularly by pulmonary rehabilitation experts.

## Functional Status and Exercise Capacity

Measures of functional status and exercise capacity range from simple field tests to cardiopulmonary exercise stress tests. The most commonly used field tests of exercise capacity are the 6-minute walk test (4–5) and the incremental (6) or endurance (7) shuttle walk test (SWT) (8). Tests used for exercise assessment are discussed further in chapter 3.

## Symptoms

The most common symptoms experienced by patients with respiratory diseases are dyspnea and fatigue. These can be measured with dyspnea- and fatigue-specific instruments or as domains of other questionnaires. The quality of either sensation can be measured as *frequency* of occurrence, its *intensity*, degree of *distress* it creates, or its *impact* on activities. For example, the frequency of dyspnea (how many times a day, how many days a week) can be measured by asking the patient to report a frequency score. Intensity of dyspnea is an important outcome during exercise or field testing, using a numerical scale (0 to 10 or 100). While dyspnea intensity is an important tool, this dimension does not reflect the global impact of dyspnea. The distress of dyspnea can be described as fear of being active or fear of breathing's worsening, while the impact of dyspnea can be described as limitation in a particular activity or activities. Dyspnea should be monitored during exercise and its values reported before and after (such as during a walk test) as well as measured before and after rehabilitation (e.g., baseline level of dyspnea

before enrolling in rehabilitation and baseline level of dyspnea after completing rehabilitation).

The simplest and most common ways to rate dyspnea intensity during exercise are the Borg CR10 Scale or a numerical rating scale. The Borg CR10 rating scale (9) is a category-ratio scale. Users should be aware that the Borg CR10 Scale requires permission from the author for use. Equally important is that users understand and accurately follow Dr. Borg's instructions for correct use of the scale.

A numerical rating scale—the example here is the visual analog scale (VAS) (10, 11)—asks the patient to rate her degree of dyspnea on a 100mm scale (line). Descriptive anchors are included on either end of the scale, with 0 representing no breathlessness and 100 representing greatest breathlessness (refer to figure 3.12). Variations of the scale differ in measured length and use numerical descriptors.

Table 7.2 lists dyspnea outcome measures that can be used to assess changes in this symptom. Based on the strength of evidence of these instruments and their usefulness in the clinical setting, AACVPR requires one of the following three instruments be used in programs seeking certification: the modified Medical Research Council scale, the University of California, San Diego Shortness of Breath Questionnaire, and the Baseline Dyspnea Index (BDI) and Transition Dyspnea Index (TDI). All these measures evaluate the *impact* of dyspnea on the performance of activities, while the UCSD scale also measures the *distress* of dyspnea. Additional/optional questionnaires are listed in table 7.2 and in the AACVPR Pulmonary Rehabilitation Outcome Resource Guide (available at www.aacvpr.org for members). These instruments measure both dyspnea and functional status and include the Pulmonary Functional Status and Dyspnea Questionnaire (PFSDQ) (16), Pulmonary Functional Status and Dyspnea Questionnaire-Modified (PFSDQ-M) (17), and Pulmonary Functional Status Scale (PFSS) (18).

Dyspnea is also measured in respiratory-specific HRQL questionnaires. The symptom domain of the St. George's Respiratory Questionnaire (SGRQ) (19) evaluates dyspnea in combination with other symptoms such as cough, sputum, and wheeze. This domain of the SGRQ is therefore not specific to dyspnea. The SGRQ's activity domain also reflects activity limitation resulting from dyspnea. The dyspnea domain of the Chronic Respiratory Disease Questionnaire (20) evaluates the intensity of dyspnea with five activities the patient identifies as important. The Seattle Obstructive Lung

## Table 7.2 Dyspnea Measures (AACVPR-required in italics)

| Name of measure | Number of items | Time to complete (min) | Dimension of dyspnea measured | Domains evaluated | Comments |
|---|---|---|---|---|---|
| **Programs *must* use *one* of the following three dyspnea impact measures.** | | | | | |
| *Modified Medical Research Council (mMRC)* (12) | *5* | *<1* | *Impact* | *1 score* | *Public domain* |
| *University of California, San Diego Shortness of Breath Questionnaire (UCSD SOBQ)* (13, 14) | *24* | *5* | *Impact, distress* | *A total score* | *Requires licensing* |
| *Baseline Dyspnea Index (BDI), Transitional Dyspnea Index (TDI)* (15) | *3* | *3* | *Impact* | Functional impairment, magnitude of task, magnitude of effort, and a *total score* | • *Requires licensing*<br>• *TDI ratings change from BDI* |
| **Intensity measures (used during exercise to evaluate time point symptom)** | | | | | |
| Borg CR10 Scale (9) | 1 | <1 | Intensity | 1 score of categorical-ratio rating of dyspnea or other symptom | • Requires licensing<br>• Evaluates symptoms |
| Visual Analog Scale (VAS) (10, 11) | 1 | <1 | Intensity, distress, impact | 1 score rating dyspnea or fatigue (by substituting the term *breathlessness* with *tiredness*). Depending upon the phrasing, the VAS may evaluate 3 dimensions. For example, one scale can evaluate the intensity of dyspnea (on a 0 to 10 scale), another evaluate the distress the person experiences with dyspnea, etc. | • Public domain<br>• Evaluates dyspnea and fatigue |
| **Optional questionnaires** | | | | | |
| Chronic Respiratory Disease Questionnaire (CRQ) (16) | 20 | 15–25 | Intensity, impact | Dyspnea, fatigue, emotional function, mastery | • Requires licensing<br>• Has a fatigue scale |
| Dyspnea-12 (17) | 12 | 10 | Intensity, impact | Dyspnea only | No MCID reported |
| Dyspnea Management Questionnaire-Computer Adaptive Test (DMQ-CAT) (18) | 71 | 25 | Intensity, symptom anxiety, self-efficacy | | No MCID reported |

| Name of measure | Number of items | Time to complete (min) | Dimension of dyspnea measured | Domains evaluated | Comments |
|---|---|---|---|---|---|
| The Functional Assessment of Chronic Illness Therapy—Dyspnea (FACIT—Dyspnea) (19) | 33 or 10 short form | 15 or 5–10 | Intensity, impact | | MCID 5 points reported in heart failure; no MCID for COPD |
| Global Chest Symptoms Questionnaire (GCSQ) (20) | 19 | 10 | Daily intensity | | |
| Multidimensional Dyspnea Profile (MDP) (21) | 11 | 5–10 | Impact | Sensory and affective dimensions of dyspnea | Copyrighted by authors, free with permission |
| Pulmonary Functional Status and Dyspnea Questionnaire (PFSDQ) (22) | 164 | 15 | Frequency, intensity, impact | Functional status, dyspnea | Contact author (Suzanne Lareau) |
| Pulmonary Functional Status and Dyspnea Questionnaire-Modified (PFSDQ-M) (23) | 40 | 7 | Frequency, intensity, impact | Functional status, dyspnea, fatigue | • Contact author (Suzanne Lareau)<br>• Has a fatigue scale |

Disease Questionnaire (SOLQ) (21) evaluates several dimensions of dyspnea; however, there is no specific score that captures dyspnea.

All the features of dyspnea (frequency, intensity, impact, and distress) also apply to the symptom of fatigue. Fatigue can therefore be measured with a brief evaluation such as a VAS, substituting the word *dyspnea* with a comparable word for fatigue (e.g., tiredness, exhaustion). The Borg scale can also be used in this regard with word substitution. Fatigue-specific questionnaires have also been developed to more extensively evaluate fatigue. These questionnaires include the Multidimensional Fatigue Inventory (MFI) (22) and the Multidimensional Assessment of Fatigue (MAF) (23–24). Fatigue can also be a dimension of other questionnaires, such as the vitality dimension of the SF-36, the fatigue dimension of the CRQ, the fatigue dimension of the PFSDQ-M, and the fatigue/inertia and vigor/activity subscales of the Profile of Mood States (POMS) (25).

## Health-Related Quality of Life (HRQL)

Health-related quality of life scores (also referred to as health status) reflect domains of importance to a patient's quality of life in the context of a health issue. HRQL measures can be generic or disease- or condition-specific questionnaires (table 7.3). Scores can be expressed as a total score (i.e., a composite score of several domains) or as individual domain scores. The total score reflects overall quality of life. Most, but not all, HRQL questionnaires include measures of physical function, symptoms (although not always dyspnea), and emotional function. Reporting of individual component scores is also useful and complementary. For instance, the dyspnea domain of the CRQ can fulfill the requirement for dyspnea assessment, while the total score of this instrument can fulfill the requirement for HRQL assessment.

## Table 7.3 Disease-Specific HRQL Measures (AACVPR-required in italics)

| Name of measure | Type of measure | Number of items | Time to complete (min) | Dimensions | Comments |
|---|---|---|---|---|---|
| **Programs _must_ use _one_ of the following three dyspnea impact measures** | | | | | |
| _Chronic Respiratory Disease Questionnaire (CRQ) (16)_ | _Disease specific_ | _20_ | _15–20_ | _Dyspnea, fatigue, emotional function, mastery_ | • _Requires licensing_<br>• _Dyspnea score cannot be compared to other patient scores_ |
| _COPD Assessment Test (CAT) (24)_ | _Disease specific_ | _8_ | _5_ | _Cough, mucus congestion, chest tightness, exertional dyspnea, ADL limitations, independence, sleep quality, energy_ | _Public domain_ |
| _St. George's Respiratory Questionnaire (SGRQ) (25)_ | _Disease specific_ | _76_ | _10_ | _Symptoms, activities, impact, and a total score_ | • _Requires licensing_<br>• _Measures three domains: symptoms, function, impact_ |
| **Optional questionnaires** | | | | | |
| Medical Outcomes Survey Short-Form (SF-36) (26) | Generic | 36 | 5 | Physical functioning; role limitations due to physical health problems; bodily pain; social functioning; general mental health; role limitations due to emotional problems; vitality (energy or fatigue); general health perceptions | • Requires licensing<br>• Does not have dyspnea measure<br>• Measures fatigue in vitality domain |
| Ferrans and Powers Quality of Life Index—Pulmonary Version III (QLI) (27) | Disease specific | 36 | 10 | Total quality of life score; subscales include: health and functioning; social and economic; psychological/spiritual; family | Public domain |
| Dartmouth Primary Care Cooperative (COOP) (28) | Disease specific | 6–9 single-item charts | 10 | Physical function, emotional function, daily activities, social activities, social support, change in health, overall health, pain, quality of life | Requires licensing |
| Pulmonary Functional Status Scale (PFSS) (29) | 53 | 15–20 | Impact | Daily activities, social function, psychological function, sexual function, and a total score | • Contact author (Terry Weaver, PhD, RN)<br>• Has a dyspnea subscale |
| Seattle Obstructive Lung Disease Questionnaire (SOLQ) (30) | Disease specific | 29 | 5–10 | Physical function, emotional function, coping skills, treatment satisfaction | Contact author (Shin-Ping Tu, MD) |

Among the disease-specific questionnaires frequently used to evaluate the HRQL of pulmonary patients are the St. George's Respiratory Questionnaire (SGRQ), the Chronic Respiratory Disease Questionnaire (CRQ), and the COPD Assessment Test (CAT).

The SGRQ evaluates activities, the impact of disease (social function and psychological disturbance), and symptoms (dyspnea, cough, sputum, and wheeze) (25). As mentioned previously, the symptom domain of the SGRQ is not specific to dyspnea. The SGRQ has been validated for several obstructive lung diseases. A new shorter version of the SGRQ, the SGRQ-C specific only to COPD, is now available but is not the recommended version per AACVPR as the tools are not equivalent according to the developers.

The CRQ includes the domains of dyspnea, fatigue, emotion, and mastery (16). The composite (total) score of these domains reflects health-related quality of life. To complete the CRQ dyspnea domain, the patient must identify five dyspnea-producing activities that are important and have caused dyspnea recently, then rate each on a 7-point scale. Although this patient-specific approach in the dyspnea domain increases the CRQ's ability to detect change after interventions such as pulmonary rehabilitation, it increases its complexity and requires interviewer administration. Subsequently, standardized versions of the CRQ are now available (31–33).

The CAT is an 8-item questionnaire that uses a 6-point Likert-type scale asking questions about cough, mucus congestion, chest tightness, exertional dyspnea, ADL limitation, confidence in leaving the home, sleep quality, and energy level (24). It is scored from 0 to 40, with higher scores indicating greater levels of limitation. The CAT has been initially validated in prospective studies conducted in the United States, Europe, and China but is globally applicable. The CAT U.S. version is available as an educational material download by registering for a free account with the COPD Foundation (www.copdfoundation.org). Outside the United States, the CAT is available online.

The most frequently used non–disease-specific HRQL measure is the Medical Outcomes Study (MOS) short form (called the SF-36 because it is made up of 36 questions). This self-administered questionnaire measures general domains of interest in people with health problems. The two major domains are physical and emotional function; several subcategories exist under these domains. These subcategories evaluate symptoms of fatigue as well as limitations in activities and psychological distress. Being a generic instrument, the SF-36 can be used to assess various respiratory diseases and comorbidities. However, it does not address dyspnea, which is a major area of importance to the pulmonary patient.

# Other Outcomes of Importance

Numerous other outcomes may be important to measure in pulmonary rehabilitation. Functional performance and home-based activity, psychological outcomes such as anxiety and depression, adherence (dropout or attendance rate), disease-specific knowledge and self-efficacy, smoking cessation, weight modification, health care utilization, mortality, and patient satisfaction are all of interest. Many programs elect to measure several of these outcomes as a means of evaluation.

## Functional Performance and Home-Based Activity

The primary purpose of improving a patient's strength and endurance with exercise training is to enable the patient to engage in daily activities. Although exercise is evaluated as an outcome (e.g., walk distance), the ultimate outcome is to have the patient be more active. The goal is that patients will resume activities they may have abandoned because of dyspnea and increase their level of participation in work, school, social, and recreational activities. Enabling a patient to resume activities after pulmonary rehabilitation is related not just to strength and endurance but also to increased confidence and self-efficacy.

Activity levels can be evaluated with monitoring devices or self-report measures. It is reasonable to use monitoring devices to assess activity before and after pulmonary rehabilitation as an outcome measure if not cost-prohibitive for the program. These devices focus mostly on walking activities and, to a lesser extent, upper-body activities. Functional status questionnaires, on the other hand, evaluate a wide range of activities that reflect changes after pulmonary rehabilitation. Common functional status measures are the PFSDQ, PFSDQ-M, and PFSS, described earlier.

## Psychosocial Outcomes

Anxiety and depression are common psychological symptoms in patients with chronic respiratory disease. Questionnaires used to screen for anxiety or depression can help identify patients who need referral for psychological evaluation. Instruments used for psychological screening and assessment are described in chapter 5.

## Patient Adherence

Patient adherence, assessed as an outcome, can be used to evaluate program attendance (exercise sessions, education sessions, or both) and dropout rate. Factors that affect adherence include program factors (cost, hours of operation), travel distance, transportation, climate and seasonal variations, and disease exacerbations.

Although it may be valuable to identify patients who may not adhere to pulmonary rehabilitation, there is no consistently identified variable that can determine the likelihood of adherence. Tracking dropouts may provide insight on adherence within individual programs. This can be accomplished by following up with patients about their reasons for withdrawal.

## Knowledge and Self-Efficacy

Self-management education during pulmonary rehabilitation improves disease stability and health care utilization (see chapter 4). To document the benefits of such education, patients must demonstrate a change in knowledge. This can be determined by return demonstration or knowledge tests. There are few well-tested measures of knowledge used in pulmonary rehabilitation. Few measures of self-efficacy are available for the patient with chronic respiratory disease. The measure most commonly used for the COPD patient is the COPD self-efficacy scale (34). The psychometric properties, however, are weak for all self-efficacy measures in COPD (35).

## Smoking Cessation

Although data is not available, smokers enrolled in pulmonary rehabilitation may reduce their tobacco use or stop smoking as a result of support from the program. Smoking cessation may be used as an outcome measure after pulmonary rehabilitation. Evaluation of smoking can occur by measuring quit rates or number of cigarettes smoked. Some programs are of the opinion that enrolling smokers may adversely affect former smokers. There is no data to support this contention. On the other hand, pulmonary rehabilitation is the ideal time for patients to stop smoking because of the education and support offered by the program.

## Weight Modification

Changes in weight or body composition can occur during pulmonary rehabilitation. For some, weight loss may be a desired goal, and for others, weight loss may be problematic. Weight loss may reflect a change in distribution of fat mass, or the loss may indicate increasing malnutrition and muscle loss. Weight gain can therefore be an intentional objective for some patients. Body weight, body mass index (BMI), or other measures of body composition can be used as outcome measures before and after the program.

## Health Care Utilization

Chronic respiratory diseases are often complicated by exacerbations associated with an increase in symptoms and a decline in functional status. Exacerbations often require escalation of medical care. Patients with frequent exacerbations are considered candidates for pulmonary rehabilitation referral. The self-management education and exercise in pulmonary rehabilitation can help stabilize the disease. Unplanned office or emergency room visits, hospitalizations, and duration of hospitalizations are all outcomes that can be studied to assess the impact of pulmonary rehabilitation on exacerbations.

## Mortality

Higher levels of dyspnea and greater impairments in exercise capacity, functional status, and quality of life have been shown to predict mortality in groups of patients with chronic obstructive pulmonary disease (36–41). Pulmonary rehabilitation has not been convincingly shown to affect survival as available studies are small and often underpowered to demonstrate a survival benefit (42, 43). Since pulmonary rehabilitation has proven of benefit in each of the outcome areas listed previously, it is reasonable to assume it may favorably affect survival in a reasonably powered clinical trial.

## Patient Satisfaction

Patient satisfaction surveys can clarify issues that potentially influence program success and patient adherence. These surveys can also help programs modify their content according to the needs of the participants. Brief postrehabilitation questions can target the areas of satisfaction by simply asking the following: Are you satisfied with the pulmonary rehabilitation program? Are you satisfied with the exercise program? Are you satisfied with the education component? Do you think you benefited from the program? Would you recommend the program to others? The answers will provide information about patient satisfaction.

# SUMMARY

Outcome assessment across several patient-centered areas, including functional status, exercise capacity, dyspnea, and health-related quality of life, is an important component of pulmonary rehabilitation. Psychological outcome assessment is also important given the prevalence and impact of psychosocial problems in patients with chronic pulmonary disease, as outlined in chapter 5. However, realistic time constraints may limit the zeal of the rehabilitation staff in capturing all outcomes. With these issues in mind, clinical programs should use the required patient-centered outcomes as a minimum data set, with data collection at baseline and at completion of the pulmonary rehabilitation program.

**VISIT THE WEB RESOURCE**
for links to additional resources and various tools, checklists, and forms.

CHAPTER

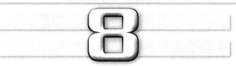

# Disease-Specific Approaches in Pulmonary Rehabilitation

**Charlotte C. Tenebeck, MD**
University of Vermont Medical Center

**Katherine Menson, DO**
University of Vermont Medical Center

**Jonathan Raskin, MD, FAACVPR**
Mount Sinai Hospital, New York, NY

**Brian Carlin, MD, MAACVPR**
Sleep Medicine and Lung Health Consultants, Pittsburgh, PA

Chronic obstructive pulmonary disease (COPD) remains the most common condition for which people are referred for pulmonary rehabilitation. However, the systemic manifestations of chronic respiratory disease and the resultant dyspnea, fatigue, exercise intolerance, anxiety, depression, and functional disability are by no means unique to this disease. Since the disablement processes are often similar, there is a strong scientific rationale for administering pulmonary rehabilitation for respiratory diseases other than COPD. A listing of some of these disease states and conditions is given in figure 8.1.

Although the outcomes of pulmonary rehabilitation for non-COPD diagnoses are less studied than those for COPD, the benefits of pulmonary rehabilitation for patients with disorders other than COPD have been acknowledged in the recent ACCP/AACVPR evidence-based guidelines (1) as well as the American Thoracic Society/European Respiratory Society statement on pulmonary rehabilitation (2). In recent years, studies of patients with a variety of disorders in pulmonary rehabilitation programs have shown that patients with non-COPD diagnoses can achieve benefits in exercise tolerance and quality of life comparable to those made by patients with COPD. These findings will be discussed in detail in the sections that follow. Based on existing data and ongoing research and the recognized benefits of pulmonary rehabilitation for patients with COPD, patients with a wide variety of respiratory disorders are increasingly being referred to pulmonary rehabilitation programs.

Despite the fact that patients with chronic respiratory diseases other than COPD stand to benefit from pulmonary rehabilitation, they also pose new challenges for the rehabilitation professional. Pulmonary rehabilitation care providers must be familiar with the physiology, clinical features, and

---

**Figure 8.1** Conditions other than COPD for which pulmonary rehabilitation may be helpful

**Obstructive lung diseases**

Asthma

Cystic fibrosis (CF)

Non-CF bronchiectasis

**Restrictive lung diseases**

Interstitial lung disease (including survivors of adult respiratory distress syndrome)

Restrictive chest wall disease

Neuromuscular disease

**Pulmonary vascular disease**

Pulmonary vascular disease and pulmonary hypertension

**Other pulmonary rehabilitation populations**

Before and after lung volume reduction surgery

Before and after lung transplantation

Lung cancer and thoracic or abdominal surgery

Coexisting respiratory and cardiac disease

---

unique aspects of treatment for these patients. Close partnering among pulmonary rehabilitation staff and referring health care providers remains crucial. It may be a challenge incorporating the non-COPD patient into pulmonary rehabilitation groups still largely made up of COPD patients, since disease-appropriate education and age- and disease-appropriate symptom and health-status assessment tools must be utilized. Although a substantial portion of the assessment, self-management education, exercise, psychosocial intervention, and outcome measurement are the same as for COPD, some modification will be necessary to ensure patient safety and meet individual needs. An individualized, disease-appropriate approach to pulmonary rehabilitation geared to achievement of realistic goals remains necessary for all patients. This section will review the approaches to pulmonary rehabilitation for patients with obstructive lung diseases other than COPD, restrictive lung diseases, pulmonary hypertension, and postoperative and lung cancer patients.

# OBSTRUCTIVE LUNG DISEASES

As discussed, there is a vast body of research supporting the use of pulmonary rehabilitation in patients with chronic obstructive lung disease. This data is the backbone of the recommendations throughout this book, except when otherwise noted, and thus will not be further elaborated on in this chapter. In this section, we'll cover research focused on asthma, cystic fibrosis, and non–cystic fibrosis bronchiectasis.

## Asthma

Asthma is a chronic inflammatory disorder of the airways characterized by episodic bronchoconstriction, airway hyperresponsiveness, and intermittent exacerbations of airflow obstruction. As in COPD, dynamic hyperinflation during exercise may occur in those with active airflow obstruction. The airway obstruction is more reversible than that of COPD, and patients generally have more variability in symptoms. While most asthma patients experience dyspnea, cough, and wheezing, there can be marked variation in measures of disease severity, including lung function and exacerbations, namely frequency and triggers. In general, patients with asthma tend to be less physically fit than those who are unaffected (3, 4), and obesity and depression have both been independently linked with poor asthma control (5). Some patients can progress to chronic airflow limitation that may become difficult to distinguish from COPD. Fear of exercise, deconditioning, and steroid-induced myopathy commonly contribute to exercise intolerance, and some patients can progress to chronic airflow limitation that may become difficult to distinguish from COPD.

General goals of asthma management include preserving normal lung function, minimizing symptoms and exacerbations, preserving physical fitness, and preventing mortality. These goals are realized through pharmacological management, education, and promotion of physical activity.

Although all asthma patients stand to benefit from education and promotion of a healthy lifestyle, those with well-controlled asthma and without significant functional impairment generally do not need referral to a pulmonary rehabilitation program. Pulmonary rehabilitation should be reserved for those who remain dyspneic despite maximal medical therapy or have individualized educational needs. A systematic review performed in 2014 showed that structured physical activity showed a statistically significant improvement in cardiopulmonary fitness by measure of maximum oxygen uptake (6). Additionally, recent studies have shown that exercise training can improve anxiety, depression, and quality of life in moderate to severe asthmatics (7). There has been no evidence that exercise improves spirometric measurements; however, this is most likely due to the dynamic and reversible nature of asthma.

Some program modifications that may be necessary for patients with asthma are listed in figure 8.2 (8).

Many asthmatics do not use their maintenance inhalers correctly or adherently, often due to lack of education and training. Improving adherence is associated with a reduction in symptoms and improved quality of life in patients with asthma; as such, the goal of pulmonary rehabilitation in this patient population should focus on these factors (9). Additionally, because recurrent corticosteroid use contributes to obesity and metabolic syndrome, nutrition counseling should be provided.

People with well-controlled asthma can have normal cardiopulmonary responses to exercise. Unlike other pulmonary disorders, resting lung function is a poor predictor of exercise ventilation, and therefore cardiopulmonary exercise testing is particularly helpful in determining the causes of exercise intolerance, ascertaining the risk of exercise-induced bronchospasm, and formulating the exercise prescription for individuals (10). Strategies to prevent or manage bronchospasm must be incorporated into the rehabilitation plan, such as administration of an inhaled beta-agonist, warm-up exercises, and breathing techniques (8, 11). A 2013 systematic review showed that a variety of structured exercise programs, both aerobic and weight-training, improved cardiopulmonary fitness and quality of life. In patients with well-controlled asthma, training intensity may be set near the anaerobic threshold or at a high percentage of the maximal heart rate or peak $VO_2$. Low-intensity exercise, isometric exercise, or both may be suitable for severely disabled people unable to exercise at higher intensity. Endurance training of the upper and lower extremities can

---

## Figure 8.2   Pulmonary rehabilitation program modifications for patients with asthma

**Exercise assessment**

- Cardiopulmonary exercise testing (CPET) when possible
- Evaluation for exercise-induced bronchoconstriction (EIB)

**Exercise training**

- Preexercise warm-up and postexercise cool-down
- Medication before exercise to prevent EIB
- Upper- and lower-extremity strength and endurance exercise

**Age-appropriate patient and family education topics**

- Recognition and avoidance of triggers
- Role of medical therapy

  - Disease-modifying versus symptom-controlling medications
  - Importance of medication compliance
- Peak expiratory flow monitoring
- Variable symptoms of an asthma exacerbation
- When to contact your care provider: developing an effective communicative relationship
- Self-management plan
  - Management of baseline symptoms
  - Management of exacerbations
  - Stress, anxiety, and coping techniques
  - Nutritional evaluation and counseling
- Dietary evaluation for patients requiring chronic systemic steroids

promote weight loss and possibly reverse some of the muscle weakness caused by chronic steroid use.

There are no formal recommendations for assessing outcomes in asthmatics, but studies have often measured 6-minute walk distance, spirometry, maximal oxygen uptake, and maximal heart rate (6). Symptoms can be assessed with the Juniper Asthma Quality of Life Questionnaire (12), Pediatric Asthma Quality of Life Questionnaire (13), and St. George's Respiratory Questionnaire (14). Psychosocial symptoms can be evaluated with the Beck Depression Inventory and the State-Trait Anxiety Inventory (7).

# Cystic Fibrosis

Cystic fibrosis (CF) is an autosomal recessive disorder in which abnormal epithelial ion transport leads to excessively thick, viscous mucus throughout the body. Respiratory consequences include diffuse bronchiectasis, progressive airflow obstruction, hyperinflation, and recurrent respiratory infections characterized by increased sputum production, bronchoconstriction, and worsening functional limitation. Nutritional failure often results due to the exocrine pancreatic insufficiency and resultant poor absorption of fat and fat-soluble vitamins. Other manifestations include chronic sinus disease, liver and biliary disease, osteoporosis, and CF-related diabetes. Although the course of CF is variable, manifestations typically begin in infancy or early childhood, and significant pulmonary function abnormalities may be present by adolescence. Advances in medical management of CF have led to improved survival such that many patients live into adulthood. In fact, patients born today are likely to have a life expectancy well into their 30s or older (15), even without taking into account recent disease-altering small molecule therapies. With these new therapies, life expectancy is likely to be more than 50 years. Nevertheless, CF leads to major morbidity, with symptoms of cough, sputum production, dyspnea, intermittent hemoptysis, exercise intolerance, functional impairment, and impaired quality of life. As the disease progresses, hospitalizations become more frequent. More than 85% of CF mortality relates to lung involvement, although double lung transplantation may be an option for some patients.

Exercise capacity tends to be maintained until patients have moderate-to-severe disease (16). Exercise tolerance is most limited during and after exacerbations. Airflow obstruction, hyperinflation,

increased ventilatory requirements resulting from dead space and gas exchange disturbances, cardiocirculatory disturbances (including pulmonary hypertension), nutrition depletion, and skeletal muscle dysfunction contribute to the exercise impairment of patients with CF (17–19). Patients with moderate-to-severe CF have ventilatory limitations to exercise. Resting or exertional hypoxemia or both are common in later stages of the disease, and some patients may be affected by exercise-induced bronchospasm. Many CF patients also have significant dynamic hyperinflation with exercise, even in mild to moderate disease. Dynamic hyperinflation is associated with increased dyspnea and with reduced lung function and exercise tolerance (20). Inspiratory muscle strength is decreased in some individuals with moderate-to-severe disease and is related to dyspnea (21). In asthma, as in COPD, leg fatigue or discomfort limit exercise for some patients (16). The cardiovascular response to exercise is normal in mild disease, but as the disease progresses and pulmonary hypertension develops, right ventricular stroke volume may be impaired (17). Higher levels of physical activity are associated with a slower decline in lung function (22), and physical fitness has been shown to be an independent predictor of survival (23).

Therapy for CF is individualized to the needs of the patient; interventions may include the following:

- Regular exercise and increased levels of physical activity
- Maintenance of adequate nutrition
- Pancreatic enzyme and vitamin supplementation
- Regular use of airway clearance techniques
- Inhaled DNase to decrease mucus viscosity
- Antibiotic therapy, inhaled, oral, or intravenous
- Bronchodilators
- CFTR modulator therapy
- Aggressive exacerbation management strategies

The need for pulmonary rehabilitation in CF increases as the disease progresses and symptoms and functional limitations become pervasive. Most patients with CF are followed in specialized centers, and thus close collaboration between the rehabilitation staff and the CF care team is essential.

Exercise training in a number of different settings has been shown to be highly beneficial and result in increased aerobic fitness and endurance, increased strength and muscle mass, decreased exertional breathlessness, and improved quality of life (16, 24–26). Some studies, especially those including exercise training over a longer period of time (1 to 3 years), have demonstrated that exercise training is associated with better maintenance of lung function over time (16, 24, 26), although the mechanisms for the noted improvement are not clear. Enhanced sputum expectoration related to physical training (in conjunction with chest physical therapy) may account for some of this improvement (27). Physical training alone should not, however, be considered a replacement for conventional airway clearance measures (28).

Maintenance of stable pulmonary function (i.e., prevention of decline) and exercise tolerance are crucial for patients with CF to prevent long-term worsening disability. The long-term effects of pulmonary rehabilitation on functional status, quality of life, frequency of exacerbations, hospitalizations, prognosis, outcomes of lung transplantation, and survival are not yet known in the CF population.

Close partnering with health care providers and maintenance of regular long-term exercise are important educational topics in CF. Additional areas of importance to the CF patient include the following:

- Pacing and energy conservation
- Pursed-lip breathing
- Strategies to remain active in work, school, social, recreational, and sport activities
- The role of antibiotics and other medications (such as steroids and bronchodilators) in managing infection and optimizing lung function

The rationale, importance, and techniques of airway clearance should be reinforced to CF patients. There are several options for airway clearance, and the technique(s) chosen should fit the patient's needs, lifestyle, and resources. Mechanical secretion clearance devices such as the vibration vest and positive pressure breathing devices can be used to augment manual chest physical therapy. Most adult patients will be well versed in this and have likely already developed a preference for their optimal airway clearance techniques. In spite of this, many will benefit from reinforcement of additional techniques such as huff-cough and active cycle breathing.

Exercise tolerance cannot be predicted from resting measures of pulmonary function in patients with CF (29); therefore, cardiopulmonary exercise testing may help in assessing exercise capacity. It may also help in determining the relative contributions of cardiovascular, ventilatory, and deconditioning limitations to maximal exercise and may detect exercise-induced bronchoconstriction or oxygen desaturation. This information can help in formulating a safe, effective aerobic training regimen for the patient with CF (24, 30).

The goals of exercise training in patients with CF are to maintain and optimize leg and arm function and minimize the decline in strength, endurance, or functional capacity. Additional demonstrated benefits include improved exercise tolerance, lung function, and quality of life (24–26, 30). Supervised exercise training should be undertaken for at least 20 minutes but ideally 30 to 60 minutes, 3 to 5 days per week, for 12 to 16 weeks (16, 24–26). The intensity of training must be tailored to disease severity and patient tolerance. For medically stable patients, moderate-intensity training (50% of maximal work rate, 65 to 85% of maximal heart rate, or a moderate perceived exertion level) is recommended. Those unable to exercise at this level may start at a lesser intensity or duration and increase exercise as tolerated.

The intensity of training will need to be adjusted after disease exacerbations. Symptom-limited exercise may be appropriate for patients with more severe disease. Warm-up and cool-down periods should be provided. When possible, the exercise program should be tailored to include activities that the patient enjoys because motivation is important in promoting adherence to exercise over the long term. Ventilatory muscle training may also be included (resistive or threshold, conducted 10 to 30 minutes per day for several weeks) can increase inspiratory muscle strength and endurance in patients with CF (31). The effect of ventilatory muscle training on overall endurance is inconsistent, but exercise capacity has been noted in some patients (31, 32).

Oxygen saturation should be monitored and supplemental oxygen titrated to keep the $SpO_2$ greater than or equal to 90%. CF patients with $FEV_1$ less than 50% or DLCO less than 65% predicted are most likely to desaturate with exercise (17). In addition to the safety issue, supplemental oxygen can also improve exercise capacity and decrease dyspnea for hypoxemic patients (19).

Patients and staff members must pay rigorous attention to hygiene techniques during rehabilitation to avoid cross-infection of patients with bacterial pathogens that may be antibiotic resistant. Cross-infection of antibiotic-resistant organisms as well as pathogenic organisms among patients with CF is an extremely serious consideration that may alter the course of disease (33). *Burkholderia cenocepacia* is of particular concern, as it is associated with acute, life-threatening illness and is also often considered a contraindication for transplantation (34). Options for patients with this organism may include attending the last exercise sessions of the day or exercising in a non-group setting. Close attention must be paid to hand washing, standard precautions, and hospital-based aseptic techniques. Regardless of which organisms they harbor, patients with CF should always be separated by at least 6 feet (2 meters) in a health care setting. In a non–health care or community setting, only one person with CF should attend an event at any given time (35). While not strictly a community setting, most centers have interpreted these guidelines to mean that only a single patient with CF should use an exercise facility at any one time. Consideration should also be given to isolating exercise equipment (such as dumbbells or elastic bands) of patients with resistant organisms.

Nutrition intervention is crucial to maintain growth and restore and maintain weight in patients in with CF (36). Caloric and protein intake must be adjusted to meet the increased demand posed by exercise training, so that weight loss is avoided. Importantly, patients with CF have excess salt and fluid loss during exercise as a result of excessive sweating, yet they may not experience thirst and tend to underestimate their fluid needs. Therefore, close attention must be paid to maintenance of adequate fluid and salt intake. Sports drinks can be useful both to replete electrolytes and provide caloric support.

Some outcome measures typically used for COPD, such as the 6-minute walk test, shuttle walk test, and measures of dyspnea, are also appropriate for patients with CF. The choice of health-status measurement tool needs to be tailored to the age and concerns of the patient. Tools that address well-being specifically in relation to having cystic fibrosis include the Quality of Well-Being Scale (37), the Cystic Fibrosis Questionnaire (38), and the Cystic Fibrosis Quality of Life Questionnaire (39). Figure 8.3 summarizes some of the issues relevant in the pulmonary rehabilitation of the CF patient.

## Non–Cystic Fibrosis Bronchiectasis

Non–cystic fibrosis bronchiectasis represents a large number of different diagnoses and thus a highly varying patient population. Causes of non-CF bronchiectasis are many and include congenital disease, common variable immune deficiency, chronic obstructive pulmonary disease, history of childhood or severe adulthood infections, chronic infection with bacteria such as atypical mycobacteria, allergic bronchopulmonary aspergillosis, sarcoidosis, and many more. Published guidelines for the treatment of bronchiectasis recommend including exercise as part of the treatment plan (40). Several trials have reported data strongly supporting the use of outpatient pulmonary rehabilitation for non-CF bronchiectasis with benefits that included significant improvement in exercise tolerance (41–43), reduction in dyspnea (42), and improvements in disease and cough-related quality of life measures (42).

Similar program modifications and special considerations for providing pulmonary rehabilitation apply to patients with non-CF bronchiectasis as apply to patients with CF, with a few exceptions. Patients with non-CF bronchiectasis are not likely to be as adversely affected by specific pathogens, such as *Burkholderia cenocepacia*, though general precautions to avoid transmission of bacteria should be maintained. This population is also more likely to be older and overweight, which may contribute to decreased exercise tolerance and deconditioning differently than in the CF population, and may require a focus on weight loss rather than weight gain or maintenance. Additional modifications may need to be made depending on the underlying cause of the bronchiectasis.

# RESTRICTIVE LUNG DISEASES

A variety of different diseases can lead to restrictive pulmonary physiology. Interstitial lung diseases from many different causes can cause lung volume restriction and diffusion problems. In addition, extrapulmonary factors such as chest wall disorders and neuromuscular weakness can lead to effective restriction of the lungs, as can severe obesity. These different groups of disorders are discussed separately below.

## Figure 8.3   Pulmonary rehabilitation program modifications for patients with cystic fibrosis

**Exercise assessment**

- Cardiopulmonary exercise testing
- Identification of any exercise-induced bronchospasm (EIB)

**Exercise training**

- Warm-up and cool-down periods
- Strength and endurance training: upper and lower extremity
- Sodium chloride and fluid replacement especially when exercising in heat
- Monitoring of oxygen saturation; maintaining $SpO_2$ greater than 90%
- Monitoring of blood sugar values in patients with CF-related diabetes

**Age-appropriate patient and family education topics**

- Basis of symptoms (cough, sputum production, and dyspnea)
- Medical therapy (antibiotics, bronchodilators, corticosteroids, vitamins, pancreatic enzymes, DNase, CFTR modulators based on genotype)

- Secretion clearance techniques
  - Controlled cough
  - Postural drainage
  - Vibration vest and positive end-expiratory devices
  - Bronchodilators
- Pacing and energy conservation techniques
- Pursed-lip breathing
- Strategies to remain active in school, work, and recreational activities
- Benefits of long-term maintenance of regular exercise
- Potential role for lung transplantation in long-term disease management plan

**Nutrition evaluation and counseling**

- Weight monitoring during training
- Age-appropriate outcome measures for exercise tolerance, dyspnea, and health status
- Management of blood glucose levels and appropriate use of insulin in patients with CF-related diabetes

## Interstitial Lung Diseases

Chronic interstitial lung disease is a heterogeneous group of disorders characterized by variable degrees of inflammation, fibrosis, or both, in the interstitial or alveolar compartments of the lung parenchyma. Examples of interstitial lung disease (ILD) and exercise training and education topics are listed in figure 8.4. Symptoms common to ILD include exertional dyspnea, dry cough, exercise intolerance, and fatigue. There is great variation in symptoms and treatment responsiveness, and symptom progression often leads to profound disability. If ILD is secondary to another disease process, such as connective tissue disease, patients may have additional symptoms including arthralgias, myalgias, esophageal reflux, or joint deformity (8). In contrast to COPD, wherein the principal respiratory derangements are airflow obstruction and lung hyperinflation, ILD typically manifests as a restrictive ventilatory defect, with low lung volumes and reduced diffusing capacity. Patients tend to have rapid, shallow breathing as a result of these alterations in respiratory mechanics, and are more likely to require oxygen as their diffusing capacity diminishes, especially during exercise. This often leads to decline in health-related quality of life related to the disease itself or due to treatment side effects (44).

The primary drivers of intolerance are based on two factors. First, impaired gas exchange leads to exertional hypoxemia, which can be very severe even in spite of normal resting oxygenation, a hallmark feature of ILD. This hypoxemia increases pulmonary vascular resistance leading to vasoconstriction and ultimately pulmonary hypertension. This contributes to the second factor, cardiac dysfunction from a combination of diminished venous return and inappropriate heart rate response. The combination of these factors causes

## Figure 8.4    Forms of interstitial lung disease

- Primary—Idiopathic Interstitial Pneumonias
    - Acute interstitial pneumonia (AIP)
    - Cryptogenic organizing pneumonia (COP)
    - Desquamative interstitial pneumonia (DIP)
    - Idiopathic pulmonary fibrosis (IPF)
    - Lymphoid interstitial pneumonia (LIP)
    - Nonspecific interstitial pneumonia (NSIP)
    - Respiratory-bronchiolitis interstitial lung disease (RB-ILD)
- Secondary—Inciting Exposure
    - Acute respiratory distress syndrome (ARDS)
    - Connective tissue disease-related ILD (CTD-ILD)
    - Drug-induced pneumonitis
    - Hypersensitivity pneumonitis
- Sarcoidosis
- Other
    - Langerhans cell histiocytosis
    - Lymphangioleiomyomatosis
    - Neurofibromatosis
    - Vasculitis

impaired oxygen delivery and muscle fatigue. Fibrosis does cause decreased compliance in which the increased dead space ventilation is compensated for by increasing the respiratory rate, resulting in the characteristic rapid and shallow breathing. This was often thought to lead to exercise limitation, but testing has shown that patients with ILD have a large ventilatory reserve after peak exercise. Evaluation of exertional hypoxemia with a 6-minute walk test should be performed prior to initiating an exercise program. Patients should be monitored for dizziness or syncope from impedance of venous return in the setting of pulmonary hypertension.

Another focus of pulmonary rehabilitation should be strength training. As is true of patients with other chronic respiratory conditions, patients with ILD commonly suffer from weight loss, reduction in muscle mass, and deconditioning (45–48). Leg fatigue is often cited as the predominant symptom leading to exercise cessation, which is likely a combination of these factors. ILD patients are at risk for steroid myopathy, which can be reversed with appropriate strength training (8).

Many forms of ILD are progressive over time, with severely disabling symptoms, and are associated with impaired quality of life (49), yet medical treatment options are often limited. In turn, many patients experience anxiety, hopelessness, depression, and embarrassment about their persistent cough. Selected people with advanced disease may be candidates for lung transplantation, yet this too is a major physical and psychological undertaking. Pulmonary rehabilitation is ideally suited to meet several of the needs of patients with ILD, and it is typically mandatory in preparation for lung transplantation (50, 51).

Figure 8.5 summarizes some of the issues relevant in the pulmonary rehabilitation of patients with interstitial lung disease.

Studies have shown that patients with ILD who complete pulmonary rehabilitation can significantly improve their 6-minute walk test distance, subjective degree of dyspnea, and quality of life. It is unclear how results compare to COPD, but studies have shown that these meaningful results do not last as long as those with COPD who complete pulmonary rehabilitation. The duration of benefit may improve with a longer course of rehabilitation, and the goal is to refer early before cardiac dysfunction manifests (8). As always, the exercise program should be tailored to meet the abilities and needs of the individual patient.

Because of the complex, multifactorial basis of exercise limitation in ILD and frequent comorbidity, cardiopulmonary exercise testing is desirable in assessing the patient referred to pulmonary rehabilitation. This assesses exercise capacity, assesses mechanisms underlying exercise limitation, detects the extent of oxygen desaturation, helps in identifying comorbidities, and facilitates formulation of the exercise prescription. The incremental shuttle walk test (ISWT) is felt to better measure gains attained in ILD patients completing pulmonary rehabilitation, rather than the 6-minute walk test, given that it is a symptom-limited maximal exercise capacity test (2, 52).

The patient's oxygen requirements should be assessed by exercise oximetry, performed at the

## Figure 8.5 Pulmonary rehabilitation program modifications for patients with interstitial lung disease

**Exercise assessment**

- CPET when possible
- 6-minute walk or shuttle walk test

**Assessment of oxygen requirements**

- 6-minute walk test
- Exercise oximetry: test at highest intensity level to be performed using the patient's own portable system

**Exercise training**

- Strength and endurance training of the upper and lower extremities
- Strong focus on pacing and energy conservation techniques
- High $FiO_2$ may be required during exercise training

**Age-appropriate patient and family education topics**

- Nature and expected course of disease
- Physiological basis of symptoms and exercise limitation (emphasize that cough is not a contagious condition)

- Expected benefits versus potential adverse effects of medical therapy
- Rationale for and proper use of supplemental oxygen
- Pulmonary airway clearance techniques (especially for persons with bronchiectasis)
- Recognition of symptoms and signs of secondary infection
- Prevention strategies: influenza and pneumococcal vaccines
- Community resources
- Advance directives
- Coping techniques for assistance in managing anxiety and depression
- Training in options for and outcomes of mechanical ventilation

**Nutrition evaluation and counseling**

- Prevention of muscle or weight loss
- Use of disease-appropriate health-status outcomes measurement tools

---

highest intensity of activity, within both rehabilitation and the home environment. Patients must also be tested using the type of portable oxygen system they use in the home setting, since some systems (such as the pulse delivery of oxygen by electronic demand device) often do not maintain adequate oxygen saturation during exercise in this patient population. Oxygen demands may be very high, necessitating the use of high-flow supplemental oxygen or reservoir devices. These requirements may pose as barriers to continuing an exercise regimen at the completion of a rehabilitation program.

General goals of exercise training are to increase strength, endurance, and functional capacity and, in turn, to improve quality of life. Demonstrated benefits of pulmonary rehabilitation among patients with interstitial lung disease or pulmonary fibrosis include the following:

- Improved exercise endurance
- Improved quality of life
- Reduced dyspnea
- Identification of supplemental oxygen requirements, especially during exercise (53–58)

The greatest improvements in exercise endurance have been seen in patients with asbestosis and idiopathic pulmonary fibrosis, and less so in patients with connective tissue disease-associated ILD. Patients with lower baseline 6MWT distances had the greatest degree of improvement (58). Because patients with ILD have restrictive physiology and high oxygen requirements, rehabilitation may not result in reductions in dyspnea for all persons. Patients should be taught pacing and energy conservation strategies as well as paced breathing techniques. An individualized plan should be formulated to enable each patient to continue participation in hobbies and desired activities as long as possible.

Several education topics are recommended for patients with ILD during pulmonary rehabilitation (figure 8.5). Given the magnitude of disabling symptoms and the progressive nature and poor long-term prognosis of some forms of ILD, particular emphasis must be placed on helping patients cope with dyspnea, anxiety, and depression. Pulmonary rehabilitation can also serve as an environment in which patients with ILD can learn about lung transplantation and the potential option for mechanical ventilation. Discussions can and should be held regarding advance directives and end-of-life care.

Although several measures of dyspnea, including the Borg dyspnea scale, Baseline Dyspnea Index, Transition Dyspnea Index, Medical Research Council's dyspnea scale, and visual analog scale, have all been used in patients with ILD, the best means of assessing dyspnea continue to be studied. Likewise, the health-status instruments most able to detect change in health status after pulmonary rehabilitation among patients with ILD are unknown. The SF-36, SGRQ, CRQ, Quality of Well-Being Scale, and World Health Organization QOL Scale have been used to measure health status among patients with ILD, although most were developed for COPD rather than ILD. Recent studies have shown that they may be reliable surrogate tools (59).

## Neuromuscular Disease

The neuromuscular disease umbrella encompasses a large number of different diagnoses, including muscular dystrophies with a variety of disease manifestations, motor neuron disorders such as postpolio syndrome, and diseases such as amyotrophic lateral sclerosis (ALS), spinal cord injury, and other diseases with loss of motor neuron innervation. Chest wall disorders with restrictive physiology are also included here.

Many patients with restrictive chest wall disease or neuromuscular disease with respiratory impairment (with or without underlying lung disease) may benefit from pulmonary rehabilitation. The incidence, severity, and natural history of respiratory impairment in these disorders vary widely, but respiratory complications occur in the majority of people at some point in the illness. Patients with stable disease may present with chronic symptoms. In patients with progressive

> ### Figure 8.6   Examples of conditions wherein pulmonary rehabilitation may be of benefit
>
> - Restrictive chest wall disease (e.g., kyphoscoliosis, pneumoplasty)
> - Neuromuscular disease with respiratory involvement
> - Muscular dystrophy
> - Parkinson's disease
> - Multiple sclerosis
> - Postpolio syndrome
> - Myasthenia gravis
> - Amyotrophic lateral sclerosis
> - Neuromuscular disease (including stroke) and comorbid primary lung disease

disease, symptoms change over time. For example, in patients with muscular dystrophy, those with early diaphragmatic or bulbar involvement are especially vulnerable to developing respiratory symptoms and limitations (60). Others may not develop symptoms until their disease is advanced. Many of these patients have concomitant skeletal muscle or joint dysfunction. Examples of chest wall and neuromuscular disorders are listed in figure 8.6.

People with neuromuscular disease or chest wall disease tend to have a restrictive ventilatory defect on pulmonary function testing. Many have a rapid, shallow breathing pattern, especially during exercise. Other physiological derangements may include respiratory muscle weakness, position-related mechanical disadvantage of the respiratory muscles, chest wall distortion, and reduced chest wall compliance (especially in kyphoscoliosis). Mechanical and physiological abnormalities lead to gas exchange disturbances, often with an elevated $PaCO_2$ (resulting from alveolar hypoventilation) and hypoxemia (related to ventilation–perfusion mismatch or a shuntlike effect at the lung bases). Cardiopulmonary testing in patients with diverse neuromuscular disease may show reduced oxygen uptake, decreased work capacity, and reduced ventilation as well as deconditioning (61).

The previously noted mechanical and physiological respiratory abnormalities plus frequent concomitant peripheral muscle dysfunction lead to exercise intolerance. Respiratory muscle weakness or fatigue and increased oxygen consumption resulting from peripheral muscle weakness or incoordination (62) contribute to exertional dyspnea. Impaired muscle function also results in a weak, impaired cough. Furthermore, secretion clearance may be compromised by poor lung expansion or chest wall distortion. Some patients, especially those with degenerative neuromuscular disorders such as muscular dystrophy, amyotrophic lateral sclerosis (ALS), multiple sclerosis, and Parkinson's disease, develop swallowing dysfunction and therefore are at risk for aspiration. Collectively, these disturbances increase the risk of respiratory infection. Sleep-disordered breathing, including obstructive sleep apnea and the worsening of alveolar hypoventilation during sleep, is very common among people with neuromuscular and restrictive chest wall disorders, especially in the advanced stages of disease.

A large systematic review suggested that there was evidence that strengthening exercises in combination with aerobic exercise are effective for patients with muscle disorders (63). It also found evidence indicating effectiveness of a combination of muscle strengthening and aerobic exercise in patients with diverse disorders, and evidence to support breathing exercises for patients with myasthenia gravis and myotonic muscular dystrophy. Importantly, there was no evidence of adverse effects or harm from exercise.

To date, no clear published guidelines exist regarding optimal exercise strategies for the different forms of neuromuscular disease, and further investigation is needed in this area. Consultation with the patient's neurologist or a physiatrist may be helpful in formulating a safe and appropriate exercise prescription. Aerobic conditioning may be helpful in maintaining mobility and reversing deconditioning. Ambulation and cycle exercise can be performed by patients who have responded to medical therapy or are in an early stage of disease. More frequent exercise sessions of shorter duration (interval training) may be used to avoid overstressing already limited capabilities.

Strength training is usually included, but exercises may vary from resistive training to active range of motion. Those types of strength training that can induce muscle injury should be avoided. Other interventions that may be helpful include orthotics, airway clearance, and inspiratory muscle training (63). Physical therapy or occupational therapy consultation may be necessary to identify the potential needs for adaptive equipment or orthotics necessary to maintain independence with ADLs, work, driving, or higher-order activities such as attending school.

Close attention should be given to training the patient in energy conservation and pacing techniques. Vocational rehabilitation may be useful for selected patients. Family members should be taught the basis of the patient's functional limitations and the optimal ways to provide assistance. Pursed-lips breathing training may not be appropriate for all people with neuromuscular disease. Oxygen saturation should be monitored during exercise and supplemental oxygen titrated to achieve $SaO_2$ equal to or greater than 88%. If appropriate, evaluation for sleep-disordered breathing should be considered.

Patients should also be taught strategies to assist with cough and secretion clearance such as the insufflator-exsufflator device, vibration vest, or positive expiratory pressure device (64). Patients should be taught to identify early signs of respiratory infection and develop a clear process of communication with the health care provider to decide on a treatment strategy. Discussion of advance directives, mechanical ventilation, tracheostomy, home and community resources, and skilled nursing or chronic ventilator facilities helps patients evaluate their options should they no longer be able to remain at home. Pulmonary rehabilitation program modifications to be considered for patients with chest wall and neuromuscular disorders are shown in figure 8.7.

# PULMONARY HYPERTENSION

Pulmonary rehabilitation facilities will be increasingly involved in the care of individuals afflicted with pulmonary artery hypertension (PAH). Issues common to other chronic lung diseases are similarly manifest in patients with PAH, such as the need to improve exercise capacity, manage activities of daily living, and address quality-of-life concerns (65). There is evidence of peripheral muscle dysfunction that is similar to the muscle wasting seen in COPD (66). These patients share many of the clinical needs familiar to others struggling with chronic lung diseases, and pulmonary rehabilitation facilities can have a significant role in the care and management of this significant and compelling illness.

## Figure 8.7   Pulmonary rehabilitation program modifications for patients with chest wall and neuromuscular disorders

**Exercise assessment**

- Disease type and severity
- Individual patient needs and functional limitations
- Consultation with neurologist or physiatrist in formulating exercise prescription (appropriate type and intensity of exercise) if needed

**Exercise training**

- Nature and goals of training program individualized
- Avoidance of excess muscle fatigue
- Aerobic and strength training: ambulation, cycling, water-based exercise
- More frequent, shorter-duration exercise sessions if necessary
- Interval training possibly beneficial
- Inspiratory muscle training for selected patients

**Additional considerations**

- Supplemental oxygen to keep $SpO_2$ greater than 88%
- Potential role for noninvasive assisted ventilation during exercise

- Identification of patients who may be in need of nocturnal noninvasive assisted ventilation (CPAP or BiPAP)
- Assessment of need for assistive or orthotic equipment to maintain independence with ADLs
- Inpatient pulmonary rehabilitation for patients with severe functional limitation or intensive nursing or medical care needs

**Age-appropriate patient and family education topics**

- Respiratory manifestations or complications of neuromuscular or chest wall disease (tailored to the person's condition)
- Secretion clearance and cough techniques
- Recognizing signs of disease destabilization and infection
- Rationale for and benefits of noninvasive assisted ventilation
- Supplemental oxygen
- Tracheostomy and mechanical ventilation
- Advance directives
- Community resources, skilled nursing facilities, chronic ventilator facilities

Much like COPD—which includes chronic bronchitis, emphysema, and asthma—those suffering with PAH have distinct and unique diagnoses that have been lumped under an umbrella term and share PAH as a common defining reality. In fact, patients with COPD may also have elevated pulmonary artery pressure and be unaware of it; as such, they may be actively enrolled in pulmonary rehabilitation (67). It is likely that pulmonary artery pressures vary with exertion at a subclinical level and that the pulmonary vascular bed exhibits adequate capacitance for pressure variation. The various etiologies that can include PAH are diverse, and it is important for the clinician to first understand the disease process the patient presents as these diseases tend to be multisystemic and involve various other clinical realities beyond pulmonary disease. Pulmonary HTN can

arise as a consequence of processes affecting the pulmonary vascular bed directly, or it may occur in conjunction with several respiratory or systemic diseases. Idiopathic primary pulmonary HTN is a disorder wherein the pulmonary vasculature is affected in the absence of identifiable risk factors or coexisting disease. Common causes of secondary pulmonary HTN include advanced parenchymal lung disease such as COPD or interstitial lung disease, chronic thromboembolic disease, left ventricular (LV) failure, HIV infection, certain collagen vascular diseases, drugs or toxins, sleep-disordered breathing, and hepatic cirrhosis with portal hypertension.

It is important to realize that these illnesses, once treated, will have different trajectories with regard to pulmonary artery pressures—for example, chronic pulmonary embolism versus scleroderma. The former diagnosis will likely see some decline in PAH over the many years of anticoagulation therapy, while the latter diagnosis has an inexorable deterioration in PAH which may in fact be the cause of death for these patients. It had been said the most common cause of right-sided heart disease is left-sided heart disease, and given the prevalence of cardiac disease in our society this may well be true. It is thus fortunate that many pulmonary rehabilitation providers are cognizant of cardiac rehabilitation realities as cardiac disease is clearly the most common comorbidity in our pulmonary rehabilitation centers. PAH does have unique and important aspects of the disease state that challenge our centers, and knowledge of these physiologic issues as well as appropriate management skills is paramount to providing proper care.

Perhaps the most challenging aspect of caring for PAH patients is the reality that one does not have a mechanism to easily evaluate the level of pulmonary artery pressures at any given time. Unlike the measurement of systemic blood pressure or the measurements of oxygen saturation, the pulmonary rehabilitation specialist is confronted with a significant physiologic problem and is required to use surrogate measurements and other clinical insights to anticipate evolving pulmonary artery pressure elevation. That other providers are equally confounded about being in the dark about PAH levels at any given time gives little solace to clinicians. It is for this reason that the following bullet points be addressed and acknowledged routinely in the care of patients referred with PAH.

- Patients must be counseled and interrogated as to their compliance with their medication used for the management of PAH each and every time they present for an exercise session. There is little rationale to initiate exercise if a patient has not been compliant or has forgotten to take their medication.

- Resting oxygen levels must be evaluated and an oxygen saturation at or above 90 must be established prior to initiating exercise. Oxygen saturations below 90 are associated with increased pulmonary artery pressures so it behooves the clinician to attempt to address adequate oxygen saturations at the onset of a rehabilitation session. It is fairly common to see $SpO_2$ levels to drop once exercise therapy has begun, so initiating exertional therapy with oxygen levels below 90 is ill conceived.

- Adequate oxygen equipment must be available to offer increasing $FiO_2$ as systemic arterial desaturations will occur and must be addressed in a timely fashion. Saturations that cannot be maintained above 90 should be considered a reason to terminate the exercise session.

- A baseline pulse is important to document, and the rapid evolution of tachycardia, while routinely seen in these patients, is of concern as it speaks to increasing pulmonary vascular resistance. Patients must be encouraged not to Valsalva during exercise, and pulses that reach 130 and above should be considered a cautionary level and decreasing efforts should be considered. Any decrease in BP is a red flag and exercise must be terminated immediately.

- The use of any upper-body exercise is to be kept at a low level and should not routinely include resistance training and range of motion exercises. Stretches should be brief. Weight training of the upper extremity is relatively contraindicated. If there is a specific need for this type of therapy, clearance with the PAH specialist should be obtained.

- As the ability to stop exercise is critical to avoiding hypotension and clinical deterioration, therapists should consider one-on-one patient care in those known to have severe or moderate-to-severe PAH despite therapy. When the pulmonary artery pressure is unclear, a resting tachycardia over 100 warrants close observation during exercise therapy.

- Close communication about patient status during the rehabilitation effort must be made with those primarily caring for the patient.

There are known risk factors for prognosis and survival that the clinician should be aware of as one interacts with these patients. A large study (68) observed that clinical findings such as PAH associated with portal hypertension, modified NYHA/WHO functional class IV, men over 60 years old, and family history of PAH to be independently associated with increased mortality. PAH associated with connective tissue disease, renal insufficiency, modified NYHA/WHO functional class III, resting systolic blood pressure (BP) <110 mmHg, resting heart rate >92 beats/min, 6MWD <165 m, BNP >180 pg/mL, presence of pericardial effusion, % predicted DLCO ≤32%, and mean right atrial pressures >20 mmHg within the year preceding enrollment were also associated with significantly increased risk of death, as were scleroderma and nonscleroderma connective tissue disease categories. On the other hand, modified NYHA/WHO functional class I, 6MWD ≥440 m, BNP <50 pg/mL, and % predicted DLCO ≥80% were associated with improved survival. As many centers may see sporadic cases of PAH it is advisable to review pertinent literature, as novel therapies and changing clinical realities are quickly evolving.

Exertional dyspnea, chest pain, fatigue, palpitations, dizziness, and hemoptysis are characteristic symptoms of pulmonary HTN (69). When severe, pulmonary HTN can lead to exercise-induced syncope or sudden death. The symptom of exercise-induced dizziness or presyncope is generally an ominous sign of severe disease. Decreased exercise capacity, early-onset lactic acidosis, and increased oxygen cost of work result from a combination of cardiocirculatory and gas exchange impairments. Patients with pulmonary HTN often have ventilatory limitation (with low breathing reserve) yet have demand for increased total ventilation to maintain effective alveolar ventilation and gas exchange. Physical deconditioning from relative inactivity will compound these problems. A decreased exercise tolerance is associated with reduced survival in pulmonary hypertension (70).

In the past, pulmonary HTN was erroneously considered a contraindication to exercise testing and training because of concerns of low cardiac output, arrhythmias, pulmonary venous congestion, hypoxemia, and circulatory collapse. However, cautiously administered submaximal exercise testing and training under close supervision by experienced personnel is relatively safe (71). Furthermore, the improved exercise tolerance and increased survival of patients on supplemental oxygen and newer medical therapies (72–74), the recognition that deconditioning is a coexisting factor contributing to exercise intolerance, and the inclusion of selected pulmonary HTN patients in lung transplantation programs have supported the use of pulmonary rehabilitation.

Although exercise training in the setting of pulmonary rehabilitation has not been demonstrated to improve pulmonary artery pressure or cardiac output, it nevertheless can lead to improvement in exercise tolerance by augmenting physical conditioning. In a recently published meta-analysis of PAH and exercise training (106 patients, 53 with exercise and 53 control), exercise training led to an increase in 6-minute walk distance as well as peak oxygen uptake (75). No serious adverse events were reported. It is notable that there was no change in the World Health Organization's functional class status as a result of the pulmonary rehabilitation intervention. Pulmonary rehabilitation is currently undertaken as a routine part of pretransplantation preparation for these patients. There is an accumulating body of evidence supporting the positive outcomes pulmonary rehabilitation provides. Early literature demonstrated benefits with individuals who began with higher levels of initial 6-minute walks (>380 meters), but subsequent studies have also demonstrated significant increases in 6-minute walks in those starting with lower level capacity (79). There is no data on the impact of pulmonary rehabilitation and survival in these patients.

Although cardiopulmonary exercise testing is useful in identifying factors contributing to exercise limitation, an incremental exercise test to maximal capacity should be avoided. A submaximal study is safer, especially in patients with exercise-induced syncope, presyncope, or arrhythmia. The 6-minute walk test is a useful alternative method to assess exercise tolerance of pulmonary HTN patients (70) and provides information on prognosis.

Oxygen saturation should be monitored and oxygen therapy titrated to maintain $SpO_2$ at greater than 90%. Because of the potential for hypoxemia during exercise to further increase pulmonary artery pressures and lead to arrhythmias or circulatory collapse, it is reasonable to adjust the oxygen supplementation to achieve a higher $SpO_2$ than would usually be considered necessary in the context of pulmonary rehabilitation for patients with other conditions.

Special safety precautions are necessary to prevent falls for anticoagulated patients with pulmonary HTN. Monitoring for any dizziness, palpitations or presyncope, systemic HTN, or hypotension is of paramount importance. To this end, high-intensity exercise, or any activities that could lead to increased intrathoracic pressure or decreased RV preload and precipitate circulatory collapse (such as weightlifting without controlled breathing or other resistive exercises that require Valsalva effort), should be rigorously avoided. In general, low-intensity aerobic exercise, such as treadmill or level surface walking, and stretching or active range of motion exercise are the mainstays of therapy (77, 78). Telemetry monitoring

## Figure 8.8 Pulmonary rehabilitation program modifications for patients with pulmonary hypertension

**Exercise assessment**

- 6-minute walk test
- CPET
- Measurement of oxygen saturation during exercise

**Exercise training**

- Low-intensity aerobic exercise (treadmill or level surface walking)
- Pacing and energy conservation
- Avoidance of certain activities
  - High-intensity exercise
  - Activities that may lead to increased intrathoracic pressure such as weightlifting or resistive exercise that requires Valsalva effort
- Telemetry monitoring for patients with known arrhythmia
- Oxygen saturation monitoring
  - Supplemental oxygen to keep $SpO_2$ greater than 90%
  - Confirmation that patient's own portable system provides adequate $SpO_2$
- Close blood pressure and pulse monitoring during exercise
- Exercise cessation if patient develops chest pain, dizziness, light-headedness, or palpitations

- Possible higher-intensity exercise posttransplantation

**Crucial additional considerations**

- Close partnership between pulmonary rehabilitation provider and patient's physicians
- Fall avoidance for anticoagulated patients
- No disruptions in continuous IV vasodilator therapy

**Age-appropriate patient and family education topics**

- Anatomical and physiological basis for symptoms resulting from pulmonary HTN
- Signs of right-heart failure
- Importance and benefits of supplemental oxygen
- Risks and benefits of anticoagulation
- Vasodilator therapy
- Lung transplantation
- Mechanical ventilation
- How to exercise safely to prevent deconditioning
- Nutritional evaluation and counseling (where needed)

may be advisable during exercise for patients with arrhythmias. Patients should be monitored for exercise-induced hypertension or hypotension, and exercise should be stopped if the patient develops chest pain, palpitations, dizziness, light-headedness, or syncope. Extreme caution must be undertaken to ensure that continuous intravenous vasodilator therapy is not interrupted if a patient is still on such therapy.

Pulmonary HTN patients should be taught strategies for pacing and energy conservation, and some may benefit from assistive equipment for ADLs. Each patient must be assessed individually to understand the severity of their disease and the constellation of factors contributing to

their exercise intolerance or functional limitation. Patients should be educated regarding the benefits and risks of pharmacological therapy. Special considerations for patients with pulmonary HTN participating in pulmonary rehabilitation are given in figure 8.8. Representative pulmonary rehabilitation exercise guidelines used by one specialty transplant center are shown in figure 8.9.

# LUNG CANCER

Lung cancer is the leading cause of cancer deaths among men and women in the United States and elsewhere in the developed world. Cigarette

> ## Figure 8.9 Exercise protocol for patients with pulmonary hypertension
>
> - Patients should stop exercising immediately if they become symptomatic.
> - Oxygen saturation and vital signs should be monitored during exercise and should be kept within recommended ranges.
> - Low-resistance exercise (dumbbells, cuff weights, and elastic bands) is recommended; higher-intensity resistance training is not recommended.
> - Lying to sitting position is acceptable after instruction in paced breathing, avoidance of Valsalva, and body mechanics. Forward bending from the waist, with the head in a lowered position, is not recommended as this may exacerbate symptoms of lightheadedness and produce a Valsalva effect.
> - Patients may use the stationary bicycle using arms and legs at low resistance levels.
> - Arm ergometry at low resistance levels is permitted but must have a documented clinical need.
> - Patients may walk on a level surface track or treadmill.
> - Patients may perform stretching exercises.

and health status and can reduce fatigue among cancer patients undergoing chemotherapy (82, 83). Pulmonary rehabilitation has been shown to be a useful adjunct for patients undergoing surgical resection of lung cancer (84, 85, 86).

# PULMONARY REHABILITATION AND THE SURGICAL PATIENT

When considering major surgery for a patient with chronic lung disease, medical personnel must assess whether the patient has adequate respiratory reserve to tolerate surgery and estimate the risk of postoperative complications. Screening spirometry is needed for all patients with chronic respiratory disease before thoracic or upper abdominal surgery.

In general, any patient undergoing thoracic, upper abdominal, or abdominal aortic aneurysm surgery is at risk of developing postoperative pulmonary complications, particularly if the person has smoked within 2 months of surgery or has underlying chronic lung disease or poor general health status.

The following are common postoperative respiratory complications:

- Infection
- Atelectasis
- Worsened gas exchange
- Bronchoconstriction
- Thromboembolic disease
- Respiratory failure requiring prolonged mechanical ventilation

Comprehensive exercise testing may provide useful information in the preoperative assessment of patients whose pulmonary function results are marginal. Low exercise tolerance is associated with poor surgical outcome and reduced survival. Occasionally, pulmonary rehabilitation can lead to such an improvement in exercise capacity that a patient initially considered inoperable may become a candidate for potentially curative surgery (87, 88).

Pulmonary rehabilitation can optimize the respiratory patient's medical and functional status before major surgery, help prevent postoperative complications, and speed up the restoration of functional status. The principles of pre- and postoperative pulmonary rehabilitation (includ-

smoking is the major cause of lung cancer, and women are more susceptible than men to tobacco carcinogens (76). Asbestos and other environmental exposures, including passive smoke exposure, are other etiological factors. Lung cancer contributes substantially to a high-symptom burden, impaired quality of life, high health care costs, and a 5-year survival of only approximately 14%.

Many patients with lung cancer, including those recovering from radiation or chemotherapy, are excellent candidates for pulmonary rehabilitation, especially given that many also have COPD (80). Moreover, deconditioning, cachexia, anxiety, muscle weakness, and fatigue are common contributors to disability among patients with lung cancer, and these conditions can potentially improve after pulmonary rehabilitation (81). Exercise can improve strength, sense of well-being,

ing exercise training) for respiratory patients facing surgery are the same as for rehabilitation in general. However, some specific considerations apply to the patient preparing for or recovering from surgery.

When feasible (i.e., nonemergent surgery), patients should abstain from cigarette smoking for at least 2 months preoperatively (89); a specific smoking cessation program or counseling may be necessary in this regard. Patients should be trained preoperatively in lung expansion and airway clearance techniques, including deep breathing, incentive spirometry, posture, splinting, and assisted coughing. Patients should also be familiarized with the planned surgical procedure and chest tubes as well as trained in pacing, energy conservation, pain management, venous thrombosis prevention, bed mobility, and methods for performing transfers. Nutrition counseling and anxiety management are also important.

Exercise training duration should be based on the time frame for surgery as dictated by medical necessity. Short-duration (2 to 4 weeks) preoperative pulmonary rehabilitation for respiratory patients about to undergo major elective surgery is feasible, although its safety and benefits need confirmation in larger randomized controlled trials. Various types of exercise training programs have been used successfully for these patients (90, 91, 92).

Postoperatively, patients should be mobilized as early as possible. The implementation of pain control and lung expansion strategies learned before surgery is crucial to minimize atelectasis and assist in the clearance of secretions. Gas exchange should be monitored closely, and noninvasive positive pressure ventilation should be used, when necessary. Adequate nutrition should be assured. Stretching, range of motion, and ambulation exercises should begin as soon as is medically feasible (93).

After hospital discharge, exercise training can be continued in a standard outpatient pulmonary rehabilitation program. Uncontrolled clinical studies have demonstrated that postoperative pulmonary rehabilitation (after lung cancer resection surgery) improves walking endurance, increases peak exercise capacity, and reduces dyspnea (94, 95, 96, 97). Further studies are needed to assess the impact of postoperative pulmonary rehabilitation on perioperative complications and survival.

A summary of the program content and components that need to be emphasized or modified for patients undergoing pulmonary resection or other

**Figure 8.10** Pulmonary rehabilitation program modifications for patients with lung cancer or those undergoing thoracic or upper abdominal surgery

- Exercise training to increase muscle strength and endurance
- Pulmonary rehabilitation once chemotherapy or radiation therapy is completed
- Self-management strategies
- Assessment of need for assistive equipment and services
- Psychosocial intervention: coping, stress, and anxiety management techniques
- Education
  - Breathing retraining
  - Pacing
  - Energy conservation
  - Nutrition
  - When to seek health care services

thoracic or upper abdominal surgery is shown in figure 8.10.

## Lung Volume Reduction Surgery

Lung volume reduction surgery (LVRS) is a procedure wherein severely emphysematous lung tissue is resected via open sternotomy or video-assisted thoracoscopy in an effort to improve pulmonary function, respiratory mechanics, and exercise tolerance for highly selected patients with severe emphysema. Those who experience debilitating dyspnea and exercise intolerance despite optimal medical therapy and who are otherwise medically stable may be candidates. The surgical techniques, details of patient selection, and clinical outcomes have been reviewed elsewhere (97, 98, 99). Improvements in $FEV_1$, lung volume, gas exchange, exercise tolerance, dyspnea, quality of life, and survival have been demonstrated after LVRS (100). The noted benefits result at least in part from improved elastic recoil, reduced hyperinflation, improved respiratory muscle function, improved cardiac function, and reduced central respiratory drive.

Pulmonary rehabilitation administered before LVRS is safe and effective (101, 102). In the National Emphysema Treatment Trial (NETT) wherein 1,218 patients underwent outpatient pulmonary rehabilitation before and after randomization to LVRS versus medical care, pulmonary rehabilitation led to significant improvements in peak exercise workload (cycle ergometry), walking endurance (6-minute walk test), dyspnea, and quality of life. Improvements in $VO_2$ max and muscle strength can also result from pulmonary rehabilitation before LVRS. No increased incidence of adverse events has been reported in pulmonary rehabilitation for patients with severe COPD preparing for LVRS as compared with persons with more moderate severity of disease. In addition, exercise training and pulmonary rehabilitation may potentially reduce some of the postoperative complications, and postoperative training may hasten recovery.

The principles of pulmonary rehabilitation for patients considered for LVRS are similar to those for patients with chronic lung disease. Good communication among the patient and family, the pulmonary rehabilitation staff, and the referring pulmonary and surgical physicians is crucial for optimal results. This collaboration will include formulating patients' goals and designing the exercise training regimen, including modes, intensity, and duration. A specific exercise prescription can be formulated based on the results of comprehensive cardiopulmonary exercise testing. After LVRS, pulmonary rehabilitation is helpful in reversing deconditioning, improving mobility, and monitoring oxygenation and the need for medications.

Aspects of pulmonary rehabilitation that require special consideration for patients undergoing LVRS are shown in figure 8.11.

# Lung Transplantation

Pulmonary rehabilitation also plays an essential role in the management of patients who are undergoing lung transplantation. Patients with chronic lung disease who are being considered for transplantation should undergo pulmonary rehabilitation prior to and following transplantation (103).

## Before Transplantation

Pretransplant pulmonary rehabilitation is important for several reasons. Goals include optimizing then maintaining functional status before surgery.

---

**Figure 8.11  Pulmonary rehabilitation program modifications for patients undergoing lung volume reduction surgery**

- Assessment to determine the selection of surgical candidates
- Communication between pulmonary rehabilitation and surgical team
- Formulation of exercise prescription based on CPET
- Preoperative exercise training to reduce postoperative complications
- Education
  - Risks versus benefits of surgery
  - Lung expansion techniques and mobilization postoperatively
  - Pain management
- Nutrition support
- Postoperative exercise training
  - Adjusted training regimen: increased intensity and duration over time
  - Modification of immediate postoperative rehabilitation as a result of the following:
    - » Prolonged air leaks
    - » Extended tube thoracostomy
  - Concurrent medical conditions that precluded transplantation

Even though dyspnea and functional status may improve considerably, this usually does not obviate the need for transplantation, given the progressive nature of the underlying disease. Optimal disease management requires that the patient understand the disease and the benefits as well as potential adverse effects of its treatment regimen, the proper use of supplemental oxygen, how to manage symptoms, and how to recognize and manage acute disease exacerbations. Moreover, lung transplantation is a major surgical procedure with substantial risk of perioperative complications and mortality (104) and the requirement for lifelong medical therapy. Pulmonary rehabilitation allows the patient to learn about the benefits and risks of transplantation, thereby helping with the informed consent process.

Impaired exercise capacity is an important predictor of thoracic surgical outcomes and survival among patients with several forms of advanced lung disease. The increased exercise tolerance achieved after pulmonary rehabilitation may, therefore, improve survival, although this has not been convincingly proven. Pulmonary rehabilitation is an ideal setting in which to identify persons who for various reasons may prove to be suboptimal candidates for surgery. It is possible that pretransplant pulmonary rehabilitation may also decrease the risk of perioperative pulmonary complications and even decrease the duration of hospitalization after transplant. A disease-specific approach to rehabilitation should be undertaken, as emphasized throughout these guidelines.

Patients who are awaiting lung transplantation are typically those with the most severe underlying pulmonary disease. As a result, the intensity of exercise training may need to be reduced. Interval training may be beneficial. Patients should exercise close to the highest workload they can tolerate from the standpoint of dyspnea or leg fatigue. Patients with severe pulmonary hypertension will require lower-intensity exercise, must be closely monitored for hemodynamic stability, and should avoid maneuvers that can increase intrathoracic pressure. Exercise should be supervised to ensure that the prescribed workload can be safely tolerated but is intense enough to have a beneficial effect.

The patient must maintain the intensity of exercise achieved in pulmonary rehabilitation up to the time of surgery, preferably by continuing exercise in a pulmonary rehabilitation center, complemented by home-based exercise. Alternatively, patients may require repeated intermittent admissions to pulmonary rehabilitation and should at least maintain close contact with the pulmonary rehabilitation staff. During the time the patient is waiting for a transplant, the disease can progress, requiring reassessment and modifications to the patient's exercise program, medications, and oxygen prescription. Ongoing attendance in a pulmonary rehabilitation maintenance exercise program and periodic review of the home exercise prescription allow the pulmonary rehabilitation team frequent opportunities for reassessment and may also improve compliance and minimize the severity of pretransplant medical complications (105).

Pulmonary rehabilitation is an ideal setting in which to educate the patient and family regarding the following:

- The surgical procedure
- The perioperative period: controlled coughing, incentive spirometry, pain management
- Wound care, chest tubes, drains, valves
- Potential complications of transplantation
- Benefits and side effects of immunosuppressive agents
- Lung expansion and secretion clearance techniques
- Methods of assisted ventilation
- Strategies to optimize nutrition
- Management of anxiety and depression
- Postdischarge issues and requirements for follow-up

## After Transplantation

Exercise intolerance and functional disability often persist after lung transplantation despite restoration of near-normal lung function and gas exchange. Skeletal muscle dysfunction plays an important role in this exercise impairment. After transplantation, muscle weakness may be present for up to 3 years, and peak exercise capacity may be decreased to 40 to 60% of predicted for up to 2 years. Immunosuppressive medications can aggravate muscle dysfunction. Muscle function can be improved with exercise training in pulmonary rehabilitation (106, 107, 108, 72). Aerobic endurance exercise training can improve exercise capacity of patients after lung transplantation (72).

Postoperative rehabilitation can begin as early as 24 hours after surgery. The goals in this phase include optimizing airway clearance and lung expansion postextubation, decreasing the requirements for supplemental oxygen, and improving stability in the erect posture. Patients may experience tingling or pain in their extremities while the body adjusts to the immunosuppressive medication. Rehabilitation in this early period should include range of motion, basic transfer activities (e.g., sitting to standing), breathing pattern efficiency, upper- and lower-extremity strengthening, functional mobility (e.g., ambulation), and airway clearance techniques. Directed coughing is especially important because of the impairment in the cough reflex that results from denervation of the donor lung.

Resistive exercise of the upper and lower extremities can be performed in addition to simple ambulation. Special walkers can be used to facilitate walking while chest tubes are still in place. Analgesia needs to be adjusted so exercise can be performed without worsening incisional pain. Poor posture can also result from incisional discomfort. Pain may be relieved by medications, heat or ice, massage, and transcutaneous electrical nerve stimulation. When surgery has been performed via a median sternotomy or anterolateral thoracotomy, adequate time (i.e., 4 to 6 weeks) should be allowed before the patient can engage in strenuous upper-extremity exercises such as arm cycling and high-intensity strength training.

Before discharge, it is important to check that the patient's gait is stable and lower-extremity strength is adequate to lessen fall risk. Oxygen saturation levels should be monitored during different levels of exertion so that patients and their families are aware of oxygen requirements during ADLs and exercise at home. Specific assistive medical equipment should be given where necessary.

After hospital discharge, patients may return to the program site to resume pulmonary rehabilitation. Postural awareness, maintenance of good posture, use of back protection measures, avoidance of rotation, and flexion facilitate incisional integrity and reduce the risk of spinal compression fractures due to underlying osteoporosis. A major goal of rehabilitation during this phase is to achieve increased tolerance for activities of daily living.

The 6-minute walk test can usually be performed by the patient before resuming outpatient rehabilitation. Serial repetition of walk tests at regular intervals (e.g., 3, 6, or 12 months after transplant) can be helpful in monitoring progress; a decrease in exercise tolerance may be an early indicator of infection or rejection. On the other hand, some patients may be able to exercise at progressively higher intensity, duration, or both after uncomplicated lung transplantation because they are no longer primarily ventilatory limited. Patients may need reassurance that they can safely perform activities that are more strenuous than those performed before transplant. Pulmonary rehabilitation staff must also be aware that musculoskeletal problems may arise once the patient is exercising at a higher intensity or duration level.

Posttransplantation education should focus on the following:

- Maintenance of regular exercise
- Proper nutrition
- Recognition of symptoms and signs of infection or organ rejection
- Long-term adverse effects of immunosuppression, such as neuropathy, gait disturbances, or osteoporosis

Modifications to pulmonary rehabilitation of particular relevance to patients undergoing lung transplantation are given in figure 8.12.

# Patients with Coexisting Respiratory and Cardiac Disease

The common coexistence of cardiac disease with respiratory disease can pose many challenges to the pulmonary rehabilitation team. Many patients with COPD have concomitant congestive heart failure or coronary artery disease. Special consideration must be given to the educational, psychosocial, and exercise needs of such patients to determine whether pulmonary rehabilitation, cardiac rehabilitation, or both may be appropriate. To this end, the pulmonary rehabilitation provider and pulmonary rehabilitation program medical director should work closely with the patient's referring physician to do the following:

- Identify the multifactorial basis of symptoms and functional limitations.
- Formulate a safe program of exercise training.
- Determine those aspects of a rehabilitation program that may provide the greatest benefit to the patient.

Pulmonary and cardiac rehabilitation share many features, including the combination of exercise training, education, risk factor reduction,

## Figure 8.12 Pulmonary rehabilitation program modifications for patients undergoing lung transplantation

**Pretransplant**

- Disease-specific approach to exercise training
- Exercise intensity as tolerated by dyspnea, leg discomfort, and cardiorespiratory status
- Exercise intensity generally less than post-transplantation training
- Home-based exercise for stable patients
- Periodic review of home exercise program and maintenance of exercise
- Maintenance of $SpO_2$ greater than 90%

**Age-appropriate patient and family education topics**

- Risks versus benefits of transplantation
- Potential complications
- Postoperative care
- Benefits and adverse effects of immunosuppressive medications
- Lung expansion and secretion clearance techniques
- Nutrition
- Methods of assisted ventilation
- Anxiety management, coping, and relaxation techniques
- Patient and family expectations from transplantation

**Immediate posttransplant period**

- Optimized airway clearance and lung expansion
- Monitoring of changing requirements for supplemental oxygen

- Improved stability in erect posture
- Range of motion, basic transfer activities
- Breathing pattern efficiency
- Upper- and lower-extremity strengthening
- Functional mobility and stable gait
- Postural drainage and directed cough techniques
- Analgesia titrated to exercise
- Special walker to facilitate walking with chest tubes

**Postdischarge**

- Exercise training
- Strength and endurance training of lower and upper extremities
- Continued oxygen saturation monitoring
- Emphasis on postural awareness and breathing efficiency
- Intensity and duration of exercise increased over time
- Assessment of need for assistive devices
- Educational topics
  - Back protection
  - Symptoms and signs of infection or rejection (including decreased exercise tolerance)
  - Purpose and potential adverse effects of immunosuppressive therapy
  - Maintenance of proper nutrition
  - Importance of maintaining regular exercise
  - Importance of medication adherence

and psychosocial intervention. The goals of each include improving or maintaining functional independence, enhancing self-efficacy, and initiating behavioral changes that promote positive disease modification. As with a patient who has COPD, skeletal muscle dysfunction and impairment contribute significantly to exercise intolerance in congestive heart failure, and exercise training is beneficial in this disease (73). Improvements in outcomes across several areas have been noted,

including exercise capacity, skeletal muscle function, dyspnea, fatigue, and functional status (74). Current guidelines exist for the use of cardiac rehabilitation (109) and should be used as a guide when dealing with patients who have concomitant pulmonary and cardiac disease.

Many people have symptoms, exercise intolerance, and functional status limitation resulting from both cardiac and pulmonary disease. The choice of cardiac or pulmonary rehabilitation in these patients often depends on the predominant factors identified as contributing to exercise limitation. Other factors affecting program choice include physician or patient preference, insurance reimbursement, and local availability. The healthy lifestyle and exercise training that are promoted in a pulmonary rehabilitation program will likely benefit a patient who has concomitant cardiac disease.

Patients with underlying cardiac disease and pulmonary disease participating in a pulmonary rehabilitation program may require telemetry monitoring. As is the case for respiratory patients, they should stop exercising if they develop chest pain; discomfort; a burning sensation, heaviness, or pressure in the chest, neck, jaw, or arms; dizziness; unusual shortness of breath; palpitations; or extreme fatigue. Such symptoms may prompt the need for further medical testing before resuming exercise training.

# SUMMARY

While most of the experience in the field of pulmonary rehabilitation is in working with patients with COPD, a growing body of literature supports the use of pulmonary rehabilitation in many other populations of patients with chronic respiratory impairment, with improvement in respiratory symptoms, functional status, mood, and tolerance of ADLs. It is important to be mindful of adjustments that need to be made based on specific diagnosis, and working closely with the patient's primary care physician or pulmonologist is critical to designing a disease-specific, effective rehabilitation program.

**VISIT THE WEB RESOURCE** ——————————————————————————————
for links to additional resources and various tools, checklists, and forms.

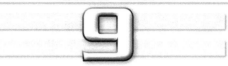

# Program Management and Reimbursement Realities

**Trina Limberg, BS, RRT, MAACVPR**
University of California, San Diego

**June Schulz, RRT, FAACVPR**
Sanford Health, Sioux Falls, SD

**Karen Lui, BSN, MS, MAACVPR**
GRQ Consulting LLC, Washington, DC

This chapter reviews the principles of pulmonary rehabilitation program management, which include the roles and responsibilities of the interdisciplinary team, program delivery models, and the operational and administrative aspects of providing pulmonary rehabilitation services. Access to adequate space and equipment can influence delivery models. Extending community access to populations of patients with diverse needs is increasingly important. Programs require the availability of trained competent staff, medical director oversight, and a structure that is predicated on evidence-based medicine and established clinical practice guidelines.

## INTERDISCIPLINARY TEAM

The interdisciplinary team structure consists of the medical director, program coordinator or director, and other professionals who provide specialized services, as listed in figure 9.1. The structure of the interdisciplinary team depends on a number of factors: the program budget, reimbursement, and the availability of team members and resources.

Because of program and staffing constraints, the program coordinator may also by necessity have to assume the role of the rehabilitation specialist either as a primary role or to provide coverage in the event of staffing absences. Under the supervision of a licensed health care professional, team members may work full time or part time, on call, or as consultants provided competencies have been met and maintained. The Guidelines Committee of the AACVPR recommends that the pulmonary rehabilitation program have an organized team of dedicated pulmonary rehabilitation professionals to ensure optimal outcomes.

## Medical Director

Pulmonary rehabilitation services must be provided under the direction of a licensed physician who has training or experience in the care of patients with chronic respiratory disease. A medical director is the designated licensed physician ultimately responsible for the safety and quality of care provided. This physician is involved in creating the rehabilitative plan of care, provides supervision

## Figure 9.1   The interdisciplinary pulmonary rehabilitation team

### Core Team Members

- Medical director
- Program coordinator or director (physical therapist, nurse, respiratory therapist)
- Rehabilitation specialist (physical therapist, nurse, respiratory therapist)

### Other Resource Professionals Who May Serve as Adjunct Staff

- Physical therapist
- Nurse or nurse practitioner
- Respiratory therapist
- Exercise physiologist
- Clinical psychologist
- Dietitian or nutritionist
- Social worker
- Occupational therapist
- Pharmacist
- Physiatrist
- Physician extender
- Psychiatrist
- Chaplain or pastoral care associate
- Administrative assistant

of the referral, participating in the initial assessment and treatment plan development, and reassessing the patient's progress and goals during the rehabilitation intervention. The medical director identifies factors contributing to the patient's exercise limitation and disability. The medical director should be directly involved with the program director and interdisciplinary team members in formulating an exercise prescription and overall treatment plan. Hosting regular conferences with the team may be an option that supports communication across the team and provides continued education opportunities.

As the program progresses, the medical director, program director, and entire team review the patient's progress at reassessment intervals and whenever changes in the clinical condition warrant review. It is required that a physician personally see the patient sufficiently often to evaluate the patient's progress and, when necessary, make adjustments to the treatment plan. Physician evaluation should occur approximately every 30 days or more frequently if patient needs demand closer scrutiny.

Administrative involvement of the medical director includes working with the program director to review and approve of the mission statement, policies, protocols, and procedures. The medical director and program director should jointly review budgetary matters and attend administrative meetings to help monitor and direct program growth and development.

Educational efforts of the medical director include participating in conferences with patients, staff, and colleagues. Education of health care professionals, especially those in training, should be a prominent role of all members of the pulmonary rehabilitation team, and the medical director should actively participate in this process. In particular, medical students, residents, and pulmonary fellows should be encouraged to take electives in pulmonary rehabilitation, under the direction of the medical director. This will enhance understanding of pulmonary rehabilitation and foster timely referrals from the medical community. Advocacy for pulmonary rehabilitation by the medical director can raise public awareness as well as increase the visibility and understanding of this service in the medical community.

Historically, Medicare and Medicaid guidelines in the United States declare that all reimbursable services in pulmonary rehabilitation are incident to physician services. Although new legislation has changed reimbursement so that pulmonary rehabilitation is no longer reimbursed as an "incident

of the rehabilitation process, and is available for consultation during treatment sessions. Although referrals may come from various health care providers in the community, the medical director is ultimately responsible for determining the appropriateness of the pulmonary rehabilitation plan of care for the patient. The program coordinator and team members should have access to the medical director to review cases that warrant additional consideration for patient safety and to confirm a diagnosis and medical need as being appropriate for pulmonary rehabilitation treatment.

The medical director partners with the program director to carry out a variety of responsibilities, including functioning as a clinician, administrator, educator, and advocate. Clinical responsibilities include providing expertise on the appropriateness to" service, this has not changed the nature of the medical director's responsibility of oversight and care of patients enrolling in these programs.

## Physician Oversight of Pulmonary Rehabilitation Sessions

In addition to medical oversight of pulmonary rehabilitation by the medical director, adequate physician coverage of pulmonary rehabilitation sessions is required. The physician who provides direct supervision and deals with emergency issues does not necessarily have to be the medical director and does not require the continuous physical presence of a physician. Rather, the physician must be in close physical proximity to the rehabilitation area and available for consultation.

The physician in the rehabilitation setting may be needed to assess acute changes that can occur in chronic respiratory patients such as the onset of an exacerbation. The availability of the supervising physician or the medical director can help the responsible team member with assessments and with determining if additional care is needed, especially in the event of acute symptom changes. Physicians also have a unique opportunity to assess patients during exercise training, thus enabling clinical observations not commonly possible in the office setting. Clinical progress and concerns that evolve during rehabilitation can then be communicated to the referring physician.

The specific delineation of responsibility for direct supervision of pulmonary rehabilitation must be established by each program and documented in the rehabilitation protocol manuals. Documentation in the rehabilitation record of physician involvement in rehabilitation program activities is necessary.

## Program Coordinator or Director

The pulmonary rehabilitation program coordinator (sometimes also called the program director) is generally responsible for all program operations. No other member of the team has as much responsibility as the coordinator. This professional also plays a pivotal role in the rehabilitation team, serving as a liaison between the patient, medical director, referring health care providers, administrators, and other rehabilitation staff. The program coordinator oversees patient admission and the initial patient assessment, and ensures that the individualized treatment plan is implemented and coordinated among the interdisciplinary staff. The coordinator has clinical, administrative, educational, and advocacy responsibilities and works in close collaboration with the medical director in all aspects of pulmonary rehabilitation services and management.

The coordinator also oversees clinic and provider schedules, incoming referrals, and training of team members. The coordinator creates and sets the standard for clinical performance of team members. Ideally, the coordinator should work in tandem with the medical director. The medical director assumes responsibility for medical oversight of all clinical team members and the delivery of medical services. The program coordinator is "hands on" for day-to-day operations and acts as clinical resource and backup for the team. The coordinator tracks patient admissions, clinical changes, and patient progress.

In view of these responsibilities, the Guidelines Committee of the AACVPR recommends that the program coordinator have graduated from an accredited school in a field related to cardiopulmonary health (e.g., physical therapy, respiratory therapy, nursing, exercise physiology, occupational therapy) and hold the national certification or licensure for that health care profession. The coordinator must have special training and experience in treating patients with pulmonary diseases and in the delivery of pulmonary rehabilitation services. Appendix C details the competencies required. The Guidelines Committee recommends that the program coordinator have a minimum of 3 years of clinical pulmonary rehabilitation experience after a bachelor's degree or higher, or at least 5 years of pulmonary rehabilitation experience after an associate's degree.

The program coordinator must be familiar with payer coverage requirements and rules, for optimizing reimbursement. Establishing and maintaining documentation that supports admission and ongoing care of patients who can benefit from pulmonary rehabilitation treatment is crucial. Program coordinators will want to develop a strategic plan to engage potential internal and external referral sources such as community physicians and health care plans, while informing about clinical practice guidelines. These efforts can lead to more appropriate referrals and establish community relationships that foster increased patient access. Figure 9.2 provides an overview of program coordinator duties.

## Figure 9.2 Program coordinator duties

**Leadership Responsibilities**

- Oversees the department budget
- Prepares and submits requests for capital equipment
- Advocates for department computer and software needs
- Works with human resources to develop job descriptions and hiring criteria, conducts interviews, and spearheads the hiring and orientation process
- Performs annual performance reviews for team members
- Provides coaching for improved performance of team members and works with labor relations staff to process disciplinary measures when warranted
- Supervises clinic staff and front office receptionist or program assistant
- Prepares a master program schedule and defines maximum program appointment capabilities
- Works with the information system department to develop provider templates and clinic calendars in the hospital electronic system
- Learns the hospital electronic record system and becomes a skilled resource for the department
- Participates in ambulatory care licensed clinic meetings to stay abreast of regulatory requirements and changes in hospital policy
- Plans in-service training for the team
- Develops department specific protocols
- Develops leader goals, department quality improvement efforts and measures patient satisfaction
- Oversees purchasing needs for medical and office supplies

- Tracks program metrics and reports for referral volume, clinic visits, and financial reports
- Maintains membership to professional organizations to keep abreast of reimbursement and clinical practice changes
- Maintains knowledge of Medicare coverage rules and area commercial health plans
- Prepares department and recruits team members to achieve program certification
- Reviews (annually) and maintains charge data for the hospital system charge master
- Advocates for clinic needs, such as additional space, facility repairs, equipment replacements, audiovisual needs, cleaning services, and medical equipment upgrades
- Oversees payer authorizations and charge entry to ensure accurate coding
- Tracks department untoward events and reviews outcomes with the medical and clinical team at regular staff meetings
- Uses untoward event data to develop training for clinical staff
- Advocates for funding to support education and professional development of team members
- Engages in community and professional organization activities in support of patient population

**Clinical Duties**

- Maintains clinical skills and professional licensure
- Conducts assessments and delivers pulmonary rehabilitation services
- Conducts regular team meetings to review patient admissions and progress
- Organizes conferences with the medical director and team to review incoming patient cases

# Rehabilitation Specialist

The rehabilitation specialist may come from diverse academic backgrounds and clinical experiences. This professional must have formal education in a cardiopulmonary health care specialty (e.g., physical therapy, respiratory therapy, nursing, exercise physiology, occupational therapy, psychology, nutrition) and possess special training and experience that supports him or her to meet the competencies described in appendix C. The rehabilitation specialist participates in the skilled, discipline-specific evaluations and ongoing treatment (e.g., exercise training, education, and psychosocial support) of the patient, under the direction of the program coordinator and medical director.

## Staffing Requirements

Patients with chronic respiratory disease need close monitoring during exercise training because of changing medical concerns, such as hypoxemia, bronchospasm, dyspnea, chest pain, dysrhythmias, weakness, and comorbidities.

There are no recommended staffing ratios or supportive literature for pulmonary rehabilitation supervised exercise or education sessions. Therefore, staffing should be based on patient need, disease severity, and acuity. Patient safety is the single most important concern when assessing and delivering care. The input of interdisciplinary team members is essential to developing staffing coverage for sessions. Access to space and equipment may also play a role in determining class size and duration.

## Staff Competencies

Staff competencies must be maintained and documented in accordance with usual requirements for respective disciplines. All team members should meet and maintain competencies, including licensure renewals, CPR certification, required continuing education units (CEUs), and required JCAHO and HIPAA training sessions. In some instances, age-appropriate competencies may have to be demonstrated. Continuing education is necessary in the practice of pulmonary rehabilitation to maintain a high level of expertise. Attendance of annual national and state AACVPR meetings will meet many continuing education requirements. The Guidelines Committee recommends joining state or regional chapters of the AACVPR (if available) and participating in meetings and education events.

Training interdisciplinary team members to become rehabilitation specialists will require an orientation program and precepting with experienced team members. Training should be ongoing to include the review and inclusion of new evidenced-based guidelines and study findings. Program certification requirements for professional competency and emergency training should be reviewed and met annually.

Pulmonary rehabilitation staff competencies are provided in appendix C.

## Figure 9.3 Staff responsibilities

- Conduct comprehensive patient assessments
- Communicate findings to referring physicians that warrant discussion or medical follow-up
- Develop an individualized treatment plan with collaborative patient goals
- Establish medical necessity for a skilled level of care and services
- Ensure patient safety
- Provide interactive education and skills training sessions for patients and their families
- Engage family members whenever possible
- Monitor, reassess, and modify treatment to support patient progress
- Participate in pulmonary rehabilitation team conferences, staff meetings, and in-services, as appropriate
- Collect and review patient and program outcomes
- Develop a home program plan to promote long-term adherence to recommended lifestyle changes
- Maintain communication with referring providers
- Initiate departmental emergency procedures as necessary
- Recommend pulmonary rehabilitation to potential patients

## Staff Responsibilities

The pulmonary rehabilitation team must have the competency to provide comprehensive pulmonary rehabilitation. These responsibilities are listed in figure 9.3.

# PROGRAM CONTENT AND STRUCTURE

The specific program configuration depends on staff and space availability and budgetary considerations. Medicare currently allows 36 1-hour outpatient pulmonary rehabilitation sessions, up to two 1-hour sessions per day. At the discretion of the Medicare administrative contractor, up to 36 additional hours of pulmonary rehabilitation may be allowed on a case-by-case basis. Exercise training must be included and documented as a component of each hour. In general, most program durations range from 6 to 12 weeks. The program configuration often depends on resource and space availability; the program duration for each patient ideally depends on the initial assessment findings and progress toward individual treatment plan goals.

On occasion, certain medical circumstances may necessitate readmission to a pulmonary rehabilitation program. Patients with chronic lung disease are susceptible to periodic exacerbations or other complications that may significantly reduce their health status. For example, frequent exacerbations or hospitalizations, new or worsening comorbid conditions and surgical interventions such lung resection for lung cancer, transplantation, or lung volume reduction surgery may be valid reasons for readmission to a pulmonary rehabilitation program. Such reenrollment requires appropriate evaluation and documentation of medical necessity. Coverage for further pulmonary rehabilitation sessions should be determined through the patient's insurer.

## Assessment and Goal Setting

The initial pulmonary rehabilitation assessment sets the foundation for all services provided during pulmonary rehabilitation. This assessment is performed by the program coordinator or rehabilitation specialist. The evaluation includes a review of the patient's medical history, current medical regimen, and comorbid conditions. The purpose of the assessment is to identify problems, establish short- and long-term goals in collaboration with the patient, and develop a comprehensive individualized plan of care. The plan of care must be approved by either the referring physician or the medical director. This assessment is described in chapter 2.

## Oxygenation Assessment

The patient's oxygenation status should be assessed at the initial evaluation prior to starting the program, during supervised exercise sessions, and with the discharge assessment. In addition to the assessment, a review of prescribed equipment and home use should be done at the initial assess-

ment and monitored throughout the treatment duration. Assessments may reveal that hypoxemia is inadequately treated, warranting changes in flow setting or delivery equipment or both. Patients should be educated on how and when to use their prescribed oxygen systems.

## Exercise Training

An individualized physical conditioning and exercise program using proper breathing techniques is essential for strength and endurance training to improve functional capabilities. To ensure the safety of patients with pulmonary disease, clinicians should address appropriate bronchodilation, adequate oxygenation, and optimal dyspnea management. Safety assessment also involves addressing musculoskeletal issues, such as joint and muscle problems and osteoporosis, and neurological issues, such as balance problems and fall risk. Breathing retraining, energy conservation, and relaxation techniques are often taught in conjunction with exercise. Supervised exercise training is facilitated by the use of various types of equipment. The goal should also include the development of an exercise program that can be translated into the home environment and incorporated into the patient's activities of daily living (ADLs). Many pulmonary rehabilitation programs also offer ongoing or maintenance exercise classes for patients to continue participation after completing the program. Typically, these services are self-pay, although some commercial plans may extend coverage. Disease-specific approaches to exercise training are detailed in chapters 3 and 8.

## Self-Management Education

The educational component of pulmonary rehabilitation includes group lectures, small-group demonstrations, interactive sessions, and one-on-one sessions for specifically identified patient needs. Educational needs are determined during the initial evaluation and should be reassessed during the program. The objective is to promote patient self-efficacy and healthy behavior changes through learning self-management skills. Acute exacerbations can lead to deteriorating lung function; for this reason, clinical guidelines recommend provider and patient collaboration in the development of action plans to help patients identify symptom changes and act swiftly to modify treatments or seek medical attention. All members of the pulmonary rehabilitation team participate in this process. The rationale, process, and content of self-management education are detailed in chapter 4.

## Psychosocial Assessment and Intervention

Recognizing and addressing psychosocial issues and challenges are necessary for optimal outcomes in pulmonary rehabilitation. Problems such as depression, anxiety, and cognitive impairment are common in patients with chronic respiratory disease. These comorbidities contribute to functional limitation and may blunt potential gains made in pulmonary rehabilitation. An assessment of anxiety, depression, cognitive impairment, and other psychosocial issues is therefore an integral component of pulmonary rehabilitation. Assessment findings should be reported to the referring physician when follow-up is warranted, especially if patients are experiencing substantial impairments. Some psychosocial issues improve with pulmonary rehabilitation. Reassessment of psychological status and refinement of interventions are essential components of discharge planning. The psychosocial component of pulmonary rehabilitation is detailed in chapter 5.

# ADMINISTRATIVE ASPECTS OF PROGRAM MANAGEMENT

The pulmonary rehabilitation staff must be familiar with the policies and procedures of their department and facility. These usually include the items in figure 9.4.

## Facilities and Equipment

The facilities and equipment used for the pulmonary rehabilitation program should meet state, federal, and JCAHO safety code standards. Sufficient space should be available for the multiple services provided. The equipment budget should address equipment expenses in relation to purchase, maintenance, and depreciation. The physical area can vary greatly depending on program structure, patient population, needs, and resources. Because the program is often the first contact patients and the general public have with the health care facility that houses it, the program plays an important role in public relations for the entire organization.

### Figure 9.4  Policies and procedures

- Mission statement
- Scope of care, including location of services, hours of operation, content, description, schedule, patient selection criteria, and emergency procedures
- Staff requirements, including job descriptions, responsibilities, in-service attendance, evaluations, and dress code
- Medical record documentation
- Continual quality improvement
- Patients' rights
- Administrative policies, including organizational ethics and management of information as mandated by HIPPA (privacy, confidentiality, security, record retention, availability of medical records)
- Infection surveillance and control
- Safety
- Facility orientation, including confidentiality, payroll, security, employee benefits, and risk management

An organized, clean, and well-maintained facility provides patients with a sense of involvement and enhances patient satisfaction and safety. Figure 9.5 lists considerations for pulmonary rehabilitation space and equipment.

## Emergency Procedures and Equipment

Appropriate emergency procedures and supplies must be available in the pulmonary rehabilitation exercise testing and training areas. The staff must be certified at least in basic life support and ongoing clinical competency demonstrations, including mock drills. All staff members should be familiar with the program's emergency policies and procedures. Minimum emergency equipment is listed in figure 9.6.

## Location of Services

Pulmonary rehabilitation can be conducted in outpatient, home-based, or community-based

## Figure 9.5   Considerations for space and equipment

- Adequate and convenient parking, including handicapped parking spaces
- Waiting or reception area
- Access to the building for people with disabilities
- Easily accessible water or drinking source
- Restrooms with handicap access
- Sufficient space for conducting initial evaluations, conducting administrative activities, hosting education sessions, exercise facilities, and space for clinical staff
- Exercise training equipment such as level surface track, motorized treadmills, stationary bikes, rowing or elliptical machines, arm ergometer, stair stepper, mats, weights, and chairs
- Unobstructed course for conducting field tests such as the 6-minute walk or shuttle walk test
- Blood pressure and oximetry monitoring equipment
- Oral thermometer
- Oxygen source (e.g., piped in, liquid, concentrators, compressed gas cylinders) and delivery systems
- Oxygen therapy interfaces such as nasal cannulas, reservoir cannulas, and nonrebreathing masks
- Various oxygen conservation and delivery devices such pulsed-dose systems, standard regulators

- Optional: Flam cabinets for full oxygen cylinder storage and not full (labeled)
- Regulatory safety rules limit storage; using freestanding flam cabinets can increase storage capacity while maintaining regulatory compliance
- Optimal light, temperature, ventilation, and humidity
- Strict avoidance of perfumes, scented deodorants, hair sprays, etc., by staff and patients
- Storage space for equipment (oxygen, wheelchairs, walkers, respiratory therapy equipment) and locked medical records
- Hand-washing facilities with antibacterial soap and waterless disinfectant
- Absence of chemical odors from cleaning agents, new paint, or whiteboard markers
- A copy of the Patient's Bill of Rights displayed in the department
- Confidentiality of patient records and patient privacy
- First-aid supplies
- Emergency equipment
- Optional: ADL facilities such as a teaching kitchen, bed, washer and dryer, and tool bench to help train patients in their specific ADLs needs

settings. Delivering patient education and some concepts of pulmonary rehabilitation may be initiated during the inpatient stay. These guidelines focus on the outpatient setting, which is by far the most common in the United States. Although many outpatient programs are located within the four walls of the traditional acute care hospital, some are located in satellite facilities not in immediate proximity to the hospital. A number of comprehensive outpatient rehabilitation facilities (CORFs) may provide respiratory therapy services. Additionally, a limited number of physicians' offices provide pulmonary rehabilitation. The consideration regarding the physical location of a rehabilitation program is secondary to the absolute requirement that the program meet all the necessary standards

regarding accessibility for the patient, safety, provision of services, adequate physical space, and availability of staff and physician resources.

More diverse delivery models of pulmonary rehabilitation are needed to expand access to those who are unable to get to centers and for models that may support rehabilitation gains posttreatment in the patient's community.

## Program Performance Measures

Outcome assessment in pulmonary rehabilitation includes patient-centered clinical outcomes (see chapter 7) and program performance measures. Both are necessary for pulmonary rehabilitation and essential for certification from AACVPR.

> **Figure 9.6    Minimum emergency equipment**
>
> - Dedicated oxygen source, regulator, and interfaces (i.e., nasal cannula, nonrebreathing mask, etc.)
> - Bag-valve mask device with various mask sizes
> - Oral airways in various sizes
> - Pulse oximeter
> - First-aid supplies
> - Standard defibrillator or automatic external defibrillator (AED) with pads

Program performance measures determine how effective the program is in meeting its quality improvement goals. In 2009, the National Quality Forum approved two measures submitted by AACVPR: improvement in *health-related quality of life* and *functional capacity* in COPD patients before and after pulmonary rehabilitation. In 2015, an additional program measure, improvement in *dyspnea*, was developed. When calculated using the number of patients who meet the outcome (numerator) compared to all patients (denominator), these measures provide a percentage of patients who reflect improvement in the outcome. All three described performance measures reflect pulmonary rehabilitation program impact based on improvement based on the minimally clinical important difference for the instrument used. Denominator exclusions are also described to ensure that only patients where the outcome could be measured reliably are included. See chapter 8 and the AACVPR Pulmonary Rehabilitation Outcome Resource Guide (available on the AACVPR website) for the three AACVPR-required program performance measure descriptions and algorithms to calculate program measures:

- Improvement in Dyspnea at Completion of Pulmonary Rehabilitation (PR)
- Improvement in Functional Capacity at Completion of Pulmonary Rehabilitation (PR)
- Improvement in Health-Related Quality of Life at Completion of Pulmonary Rehabilitation (PR)

Examples of other program performance outcomes include the following:

- Smoking cessation intervention for all smokers and smoking cessation rates
- Nutrition intervention for all patients who need it
- Tracking BMI in those with weight gain or loss goals
- Oxygen therapy use for those who have a demonstrated medical need
- Activity promotion, pedometers, patient diary
- Education, before and after by use of knowledge and skills assessments
- Patient satisfaction
- Adherence, sessions attended, dropout rate
- Referrals made to other disciplines
- Level of adherence with care plan
- Monitoring for psychological problems

Performance measures must be incorporated into every pulmonary rehabilitation program and documented in the medical record.

## Documentation

Accurate and thorough documentation facilitates effective communication among the team, the referring physician, and third-party payers. Documentation is also a necessary precursor to reimbursement. It must reflect the need for professional supervision of the treatment, the level of skilled care, and progress toward rehabilitation goals. The physician's order for pulmonary rehabilitation must be present before the initiation of services. This must include the pulmonary diagnosis and reason for referral.

Within the pulmonary rehabilitation program, documentation is used to delineate the functional abnormalities of the patient, define the clinical rationale for treatment, note patient progress, and demonstrate outcomes. Each pulmonary rehabilitation session must be documented to reflect the services provided. Detailed discussions of the necessary documentation are given in the preceding chapters in this book. A brief summary of elements to be documented is shown in figure 9.7.

## Team Conferences

Collaboration and communication in an interdisciplinary team enhance quality of care. Team conference information is useful to document the patient's progress toward the established goals and outcomes. Staff team conferences and staff–patient team conferences should be held as necessary to

## Figure 9.7 Documentation

### Initial

- Physician's evaluation of the history of the respiratory illness and significant comorbidity
- Diagnostic tests relevant to the patient's specific pulmonary problems
- Symptom assessment, including levels of dyspnea, cough, and fatigue
- Secretion clearance abilities
- Sleep quality
- Prescribed respiratory therapy treatments and equipment use such as nebulizer or oxygen therapy and secretion clearance device use
- ROM limitations and the presence of any pain that may impact exercise and activity abilities
- Patient's perception of diagnosis, treatments, and current level of function
- Habits including smoking history; if actively smoking include quit history, quit methods, and interest to quit
- Secretion clearance abilities
- Specific problems and functional deficits in areas of exercise, upper-extremity range of motion, gait, and balance
- Fall risk
- ADL performance, nutrition status, knowledge base
- Psychosocial status, specifically the availability of good social support
- Employment status: working, disabled, or retired
- Rehabilitation potential: poor, fair, good, or excellent

- Individualized short- and long-term goals
- Written physician acceptance of the specific plan of care

### Continuing

- Date of service, treatment time, procedure or modality, signature
- Notes describing the patient's progress toward treatment goals
- Notes that match billing codes
- Pain scale and location of pain
- Vital signs
- Oxygen delivery system, interface, and flow setting
- Adverse or untoward events
- Rationale for continued need for rehabilitation services
- Notes from team conferences held at the beginning and at the end of a patient's participation in the program
- Documentation of continuing physician involvement and direction during the course of the program

### At Discharge

- Postprogram evaluation
- Recommendations for a home program plan for collaborative self-management
- Discharge summary and communication to the referring health care provider, which may include the progress made during pulmonary rehabilitation, recommendations for self-care maintenance, symptom management techniques, and a home exercise program

meet the needs of the rehabilitation patient and to optimize outcomes.

# POSTREHABILITATION MAINTENANCE

An important goal of pulmonary rehabilitation is to promote long-term maintenance of gains made during the formal pulmonary rehabilitation program. This is best achieved through health behavior change, including long-term adherence to exercise recommendations. Many programs provide postrehabilitation maintenance sessions, although these are not formal components of pulmonary rehabilitation.

Exercise maintenance programs might also be appropriate formats to support returning to exercise after recovering from a milder exacerbation of respiratory disease. Patients with less severe functional impairment or comorbidity may be candidates for joining a community gymnasium or exercise program. Structured patient support groups, such as better breathing clubs, are also useful adjuncts to postrehabilitation, but they do not substitute for exercise maintenance programs.

Although there are no current guidelines for operating postrehabilitation maintenance exercise services, program leaders may consider requiring a physician referral and acknowledgment of enrollment from the primary care or referring provider. Given that patients often have polypharmacy situations and multiple comorbid conditions, obtaining an updated medical history and medication list at regular intervals can be very useful as patients often attend sessions for many years and medical status can change. It may also be prudent to have documents that provide patients with the scope and criteria for participating in maintenance services such as safety and attendance requirements. If patients are required to be independent with exercise equipment use, this should be monitored over time and reassessed if physical status changes. In those patients whose medical condition causes a prolonged absence, such as with a serious acute exacerbation, suspending services and requesting a referral for reassessment may be indicated. There are occasions where patients meet medical necessity and require return to regular rehabilitation sessions to restore function; in many instances these patients are able to return to maintenance at a later time. The Guidelines Committee suggests that the program coordinator, medical directors, and team members meet to review operating practices and discuss the best practice that supports patient safety and quality aftercare.

# REIMBURSEMENT REALITIES

The rules for reimbursement are constantly changing, and it is critical that billing and documentation requirements for all third-party payers be followed carefully to ensure appropriate reimbursement. Program coordinators, the medical director, and other members of the team should be familiar with current reimbursement guidelines of Centers for Medicare and Medicaid Services (CMS) and other third-party payers.

The Omnibus Act of 2003 created legislation that was enacted in 2006 to create Medicare Administrative Contractors (MACs). These MACs are responsible for Medicare beneficiaries in specific geographic regions, including claims processing, payment, audits, and enforcement of Medicare regulations. The intent of this legislation was to improve communication and reimbursement strategies, thus providing improved service to Medicare recipients. Under the auspices of the AACVPR, MAC committees have been established. Each pulmonary rehabilitation program should be aware of these committees and their interactions with the local Medicare administrative contractor in the region to ensure a correct understanding of new or specific policy issues.

In 2008, new legislation was passed allowing reimbursement of specific pulmonary rehabilitation sessions. This became federal law in January 2010. There is now a single code (G0424) that specifically bundles all pulmonary rehabilitation services into comprehensive 1-hour sessions for COPD diagnosis. Separate billing cannot be made for the individual components such as 6-minute walk assessment, exercise training, education, smoking cessation counseling, or psychosocial intervention. Up to 2 hours per day may be provided per patient; a component of each hour must include exercise training. Medicare allows 36 of these sessions, with provisions for an additional 36 if medically necessary.

Medicare will cover pulmonary rehabilitation for patients with moderate, severe, and very severe COPD. These levels of severity are based on existing Global Initiative for Chronic Obstructive Lung Disease (GOLD) criteria, which can be accessed at www.goldcopd.com. Currently, Medicare has established pulmonary rehabilitation reimbursement rates for the hospital and the office settings. These rates are subject to change.

Reimbursement for pulmonary rehabilitation for patients with non-COPD diagnoses is handled differently. At the time of the writing of these guidelines, reimbursement follows local coverage determination (LCD) policies. Knowledge of local coverage policy is mandatory for non-COPD diagnosis reimbursement. The AACVPR website (www.AACVPR.org) is a source for updates in coverage.

Although many third-party payers follow Medicare practices, many do not. Differences thus exist throughout the United States in how reimbursement guidelines are applied by various third-party payers that are not Medicare based. Some services may not be covered, such as nonindividualized education or training, maintenance care, documentation time, duplication of clinical services, films or videos, and treatment that lacks documented medical necessity.

> ### Figure 9.8   Strategies to improve success
>
> - Identify the need for services in the area (competition in the community)
> - Tailor services to patient and community demographics (e.g., set up a posttransplantation program in a tertiary care center)
> - Engage patients and families for their input to the rehab experience and use the information to improve the patient experience
> - Assess the opportunities and challenges of the infrastructure (e.g., parking, accessibility)
> - Define the scope of service and develop a charge master with adequate pricing
> - Identify and cultivate a physician referral base
> - Promote the program (e.g., feedback to physicians, patient testimonials) and patient satisfaction scores
> - Provide patients with a contact list of health care system leaders
> - Work to engage health care system public relations officers to help with community public service announcements, web page and brochure development
> - Build a competent, compassionate interdisciplinary team that exudes professionalism and quality
> - Use the AACVPR media kit, and observe National Pulmonary Rehabilitation Week

The program coordinator must be familiar with the process of obtaining prior authorization for the pulmonary rehabilitation program by the insurance companies because coverage varies depending on the patient's policy. Networking with other program coordinators is critical in providing the awareness, knowledge, and support needed to obtain appropriate reimbursement. A close liaison between the coordinator and the facility's business office is necessary to ensure that billing information is complete and accurate. Reimbursement problems that occur must be addressed promptly and effectively.

# STRATEGIES FOR PROGRAM SUCCESS

Program success depends in part on physician and consumer awareness, which is accomplished through organized strategies. An optimal strategy should address both referring physicians and patients. Strategies that may improve the success of the program are summarized in figure 9.8.

The ultimate success of pulmonary rehabilitation services depends on satisfied patients and enthusiastic interdisciplinary team members. Pulmonary rehabilitation must be viewed and marketed from a global perspective, remembering that prevention is integrated into every component of the program.

# SUMMARY

Successful pulmonary rehabilitation programs need the efforts of a dedicated and skilled interdisciplinary team, a supportive environment, and a well-organized infrastructure. Staff share the common goal of enhancing the lives of a challenging and unique group of patients suffering from chronic respiratory disease. Careful attention to all the aspects of program management provided in these guidelines will foster the development and implementation of a successful program.

**VISIT THE WEB RESOURCE** ———————————————
for links to additional resources and various tools, checklists, and forms.

# Putting It All Together

## Performance Measures, Outcomes, Valid and Reliable Tools, and Program Certification

**Anne M. Gavic, MPA, RCEP, MAACVPR**
Northwest Community Hospital, Arlington Heights, IL

**Steven W. Lichtman, EdD, MAACVPR**
Helen Hayes Hospital, West Haverstraw, NY

Measurement of quality has gained a prominent role in health care through the years. In particular, since publication of *Crossing the Quality Chasm* in 2001 (1), health care organizations have been directed to systematically measure and assess quality-related data, identify gaps in care, and identify opportunities for improvement. Quality measurement allows health care professionals and services to assess how we are doing as compared to best clinical practice and known evidence and identify gaps in care. Careful assessment of quality data leads to identification of opportunities for improvement and ultimately to enhanced program quality and patient care.

In addition to improving patient care, quality measurement has become increasingly important from a health care payment and regulatory perspective. The Centers for Medicare and Medicaid Services (CMS) and other payers continue to move away from traditional payment models and toward models that include performance and quality measurement. Health care organizations are required to show evidence of quality in order to recuperate optimal payment for that service. Under this model, hospitals and physician-led services may increase or decrease their reimbursement for services based on selected performance measures or standards.

Various regulatory bodies, including the Joint Commission (www.jointcommission.org), determine the quality of a program or health care organization based, in part, on measurement of program results or outcomes, and how they relate to national standards.

Each service within a health care organization contributes to the overall level of quality in the system. In this light, pulmonary rehabilitation programs have a responsibility to continuously assess their program's success related to patient outcomes, program processes, financial stability, and patient satisfaction.

Pulmonary rehabilitation includes provision of multifaceted care toward specific expected results or outcomes. Patients are assessed for physical, psychosocial, and behavioral factors to determine their individual needs and to create a treatment plan that will most likely move that patient to the most positive outcome.

Recognizing the importance of quality measurement, AACVPR has created tools and resources to increase awareness and knowledge of measuring quality, to collect, analyze and benchmark data, and to report data relative to program quality. These tools are available on the AACVPR website. Each of these resources is rooted in the same evidence base, each of these tools intersects with the others, and success in one area will likely lead to success in another.

# MEASURING THE QUALITY OF PATIENT CARE

Measuring the quality of care allows the care provider to determine:

- If there is a gap in patient care
- If there are variations in the quality of care
  - Across providers
  - Among patients
  - Among regions

Through the measurement of these aspects of patient care, performance measures drive program improvement. Teams of health care providers who review their performance measures are able to make adjustments in care, share successes, and probe for causes when progress comes up short— all on the road to improved patient outcomes. As a growing number of measures are publicly reported, consumers are better able to assess quality for themselves, and then use the results to make choices, ask questions, and advocate for good health care.

Increasingly, private and public payers use measures as preconditions for payment and targets for bonuses, whether it is paying providers for performance or instituting nonpayment. Therefore the aim of implementing performance measure processes is to improve program processes leading to improved patient outcomes.

## Performance Measures

Performance measures allow an organization to monitor important aspects of its program systems and processes. In a health care setting, performance measures are derived from practice guidelines. Performance measures are developed based on data from specific measured outcomes for which there is strong evidence and goals or benchmarks have been established. In developing performance measures, the following considerations are taken into account:

- Is the measure related to a meaningful patient outcome?
- Can the outcome be reliably measured?
- Can the measure be clearly defined?
- Is the person or program held accountable for this performance measure able to change practices to improve the outcome?
- Can the measure be determined without undue cost or effort?
- Will it produce unintended negative consequences?
- Can it be used to distinguish high from low program quality?

AACVPR has established three performance measures for pulmonary rehabilitation: improvement in perception of dyspnea, improvement in functional capacity, and improvement in health-related quality of life. AACVPR pulmonary rehabilitation–specific performance measures are discussed in detail in chapter 7.

Ultimately, performance measures give providers a way to assess health care against recognized standards.

- How do patients know if their health care is good care?
- How do providers pinpoint the steps that need to be improved for better patient care?
- How do insurers and employers determine whether they are paying for the best care that science, skill, and compassion can provide?

## Performance Measurement

Performance measurement is a process by which an organization monitors important aspects of its programs, systems, and processes. Performance measurement specifically involves measuring the number of patients who meet an established goal against all patients completing the pulmonary rehabilitation program within a given time. In this way, a percentage of patients meeting the goal or performance measure can be determined.

## Performance Management

Performance management is a process used to set goals and regularly check progress toward goal achievement. This involves goal setting, examining data, and acting on the results to improve performance toward the specified goals. Performance management involves utilizing the performance measure data to identify gaps in care or opportunities for improvement and ultimately to improve program processes and patient care.

## Outcomes

An outcome represents a specific result a program is intended to achieve regarding patient care. Outcome measurements quantify the health status of a patient, or the change in health status resulting from health care intervention as defined by the National Quality Forum (NQF). Patient-reported outcome measures should be based on validated and reliable tools, relevant to the objectives of care. Measurement of outcomes should result in findings that are actionable—that is, the health care provider can implement quality improvement processes to improve relevant patient outcomes.

## AACVPR Pulmonary Rehabilitation Performance Measures

Performance measures, and their associated outcome measures, need to be based on strong published scientific evidence. The three AACVPR patient-related performance measures (functional capacity, decreased perception of shortness of breath, and improved quality of life) related to pulmonary rehabilitation participation have a strong foundation in research. Additional benefits of pulmonary rehabilitation participation have also been reported and may be observed in selected patients.

Assessment data measured at program initiation and again at program completion provide the patient outcomes. Measuring and evaluating individual patient outcomes provides information about that patient's progress toward his or her goals. Aggregate data from all patients completing the program within a given time period provides a snapshot of the interventions that have been most successful (or least successful) in moving patients toward their goals. This can be valuable in highlighting areas for improvement.

Chapter 7 provides a detailed overview of patient-centered outcomes in pulmonary rehabilitation. In addition, a comprehensive Pulmonary Rehabilitation Outcomes Toolkit is available at www.aacvpr.org.

# AACVPR OUTPATIENT PULMONARY REHABILITATION REGISTRY

In order to collect and analyze meaningful data, it is important to have a systematic method of data collection. To encourage uniform data collection and assist with basic data analysis and outcomes evaluation, AACVPR created a pulmonary rehabilitation registry. The registry allows for collection of various data sets, including patient demographics, relevant medical information, and clinical and behavioral information, that can be used to determine patient and program outcomes.

Only valid and reliable tools were included in the registry in an effort to maintain standardization of data collected. All instruments or methods recommended for measurement of the pulmonary rehabilitation performance measures, as outlined in chapter 7, are included in the registry. Data can also be recorded for other patient clinical measures, such as changes in anthropometric data, oxygen use, and pulmonary function test results, as well as behavioral factors such as changes in nutrition, physical activity, or smoking behaviors. The pulmonary rehabilitation registry data collection form can be found on the AACVPR website and provides a detailed outline of all data fields.

# PULMONARY REHABILITATION PROFESSIONAL CERTIFICATE

AACVPR offers formal certification for health care providers who practice in pulmonary rehabilitation programs. Staffing for pulmonary rehabilitation is, by design, multidisciplinary. Health care professionals working in pulmonary rehabilitation may include but are not limited to nurses, respiratory therapists, exercise physiologists, and physical therapists. Each discipline brings a strength to the team, and the patient will benefit from collaboration between these disciplines. AACVPR recognizes that in order to provide the very best care, each pulmonary rehabilitation professional, regardless of discipline, must possess a set of core competencies that ensure foundational knowledge and skills to provide that care. The AACVPR Clinical Competency Guidelines for Pulmonary Rehabilitation Professionals outline those competencies necessary to provide high-quality care (2) (see appendix C). However, no specific training on these competencies or method of assessing an individual's understanding of these competencies previously existed.

To meet this need, AACVPR partnered with the American Association of Respiratory Care (AARC) to create a certificate in pulmonary rehabilitation. To receive this certificate, the candidate must review 12 modules related to essential elements of pulmonary rehabilitation and successfully complete an exam at the conclusion. Modules in the Pulmonary Rehabilitation Certificate include:

- Pulmonary Rehabilitation
- Pathophysiology and Assessment of COPD
- Assessment and Management of Patients other than COPD
- Pharmacologic Interventions
- Supplemental Oxygen Administration
- Exercise Assessment, Prescription, and Training in PR
- Pulmonary Function Testing
- Tobacco Cessation
- Nutrition for the Patient with Pulmonary Disease
- Psychosocial Assessment and Intervention in Pulmonary Rehabilitation
- Patient Self-Management and Collaboration
- Outcomes Measurement in PR
- Palliative Care

# PULMONARY REHABILITATION PROGRAM CERTIFICATION

The remaining questions are: How do I know if my program is meeting a high level of quality? Is my program meeting established guidelines and standards? How does it measure up against other programs in the nation?

AACVPR program certification was developed in 1998 to recognize programs that demonstrate high standards within key components in program management, clinical care, and outcome measurement safety as outlined in this book.

In addition, program certification recognizes programs that report patient and program outcomes and demonstrate efforts to foster optimal outcomes in the care of persons with chronic lung disease.

The intent of program certification is to:

- Recognize programs that meet important quality standards and that provide high quality care as evidenced by reported processes and outcomes
- Provide patients and their families a way to identify those programs that meet a high level of quality, as evidenced by achievement of national certification
- Inform and educate regulatory bodies of the criteria for and value of national certification
- Urge payers to recognize the value of a program's achievement of national program certification

Eligible programs must be in operation for a minimum of 12 months at the time of completing the certification application. Program certification is awarded for a 3-year period, at which time programs are eligible to apply for recertification.

## Resources for Certification

The most current certification and recertification applications are available on the AACVPR website. Resources for certification include the following:

- AACVPR clinical competency guidelines for pulmonary rehabilitation professionals. *J Cardiopulm Rehabil Prev.* 2014;34:291–302
- *ACSM Guidelines for Exercise Testing and Prescription, Tenth Edition*, 2017
- *ACSM Resource Manual for Guidelines for Exercise Testing and Prescription, Seventh Edition*; 2013
- American Thoracic Society/European Respiratory Society statement on pulmonary rehabilitation. *Am J Respir Crit Care Med.* 2013;188(8):e13-e64
- Pulmonary rehabilitation: joint ACCP/AACVPR evidence-based clinical practice guidelines. *Chest.* 2007;131(5 Suppl):4S-42S

Resources and training that support achievement of certification and recertification are offered at the AACVPR national meeting, teleconferences, webinars, and state affiliate meetings. Best-practice models for program documentation are available online for AACVPR members.

# Key Components of Certification

The pulmonary rehabilitation program certification application includes eight focus areas or pages that must be completed and submitted in order for AACVPR program certification to be awarded. Those areas include:

- Program staff and competencies
- Individualized treatment plan
- Medical emergencies
- Emergency preparedness
- Exercise prescription policy
- Performance measures
  - Improvement in functional capacity
  - Improvement in dyspnea
  - Improvement in health-related quality of life

## Program Staff and Competencies

AACVPR believes that all health care professionals working in pulmonary rehabilitation must have a level of knowledge, skills, and competencies that allow them to provide best care to their patients. Essential competencies for pulmonary rehabilitation are described in the AACVPR Clinical Competency Guidelines for Pulmonary Rehabilitation Professionals document cited previously. Program certification requires evidence of competency for each health care professional working in the pulmonary rehabilitation program. Evidence of assessment of competency in four separate areas must be provided, and must be in line with the published core competencies.

The AARC/AACVPR Pulmonary Rehabilitation Certificate may be used in place of evidence of four competencies for any pulmonary rehabilitation professional who has successfully completed the certificate. An individual may submit their pulmonary rehabilitation certificate document instead of competencies for one certification or recertification application only.

## Individualized Treatment Plan (ITP)

In the Institute of Medicine's landmark report *Crossing the Quality Chasm* (1), six aims to improve health care quality were outlined. The list describes health care that is

- Safe
- Effective
- Patient-centered
- Timely
- Efficient
- Equitable

Safety is the first of the six aims to improve health care quality noted in the Institute of Medicine's report. It states that health care should be safe—avoiding injuries to patients from the care that is intended to help them (1).

## Medical Emergencies and Emergency Preparedness

The key to providing safe care in pulmonary rehabilitation is having processes in place that address care of patients in the event of a medical emergency. In addition, staff training to ensure rapid and appropriate response to an emergency and provision of care within their scope of practice is essential.

To address this and ensure procedures are in place to care for patients in an emergency, the program certification application requires submission of emergency procedures that address the most common emergencies. In addition, evidence of pulmonary rehabilitation staff training related to emergency response completed at least four times per year must be provided.

## Exercise Prescription Policy

Pulmonary rehabilitation includes essential components of exercise training, education, counseling, and support designed to move patients toward optimal health and self-management within any constraints of their disease.

Routine participation in exercise training will likely result in improved functional capacity, but may also affect other factors such as weight, body composition, and psychosocial indices. To be most effective, patients must be guided to participate in exercise at a level that is both safe and effective. For this reason, program certification requires demonstration of a standardized but individualized process for prescribing exercise. See chapter 3 for exercise prescription details.

The ITP is the roadmap or guide to providing a patient's care in pulmonary rehabilitation. Without this guide, there is risk of care being provided ineffectively, or in the same way to all patients without regard for their individual needs. The ITP includes a baseline description of the patient's disease or disability, initial assessments and measurements, as well as outlining elements (or goals) to be accomplished during the program, based on best evidence and research and what the patient has agreed is important to them. It should be clear enough that any staff member caring for a patient understands the individual patient needs, the goals for care, interventions that have been provided, and what still remains to be done.

Elements of the ITP include

- Initial patient assessment
- Plan; goals, interventions, education
- Reassessment
- Discharge and follow-up

The initial assessment and measurements, taken when a patient begins the program, provide a baseline from which to evaluate the patient's individual needs, determine necessary interventions, and measure progress by comparing the baseline to subsequent measurements.

The plan is designed to educate, counsel, and guide the caregiver and patient toward the established goals. The plan specific to pulmonary rehabilitation includes supervised exercise, as well as individual and group education, counseling for behavior change, and both formal and informal support. Periodic reassessment throughout the program will determine the patient's progress toward—or movement away from—agreed-upon goals.

The value of the ITP from a quality perspective is that imbedded within the ITP are all measurements and data necessary for evaluating outcomes and reporting on performance measures.

The final or discharge assessment is the opportunity to repeat measurements done at program initiation. A comparison of this final measurement to the initial measurements allows for assessment of change in health indices and determination of individual patient outcomes.

Aggregate measurements of functional capacity, perceived shortness of breath, and health-related quality of life for all patients over a given period of time can be used to report and evaluate the program's performance measure data.

The ITP is at the core of care provision in pulmonary rehabilitation. It guides patient care, ensures it is individualized to the needs of each patient and that the care is provided in a systematic way that ensures optimal outcomes. An example of a well-designed ITP is also provided in appendix A.

## Performance Measures

As noted earlier, the final portion of the program certification application focuses on the three performance measures for pulmonary rehabilitation:

- Improvement in functional capacity
- Improvement in dyspnea
- Improvement in health-related quality of life

To complete the application, data must be provided on both the total number of patients completing the program and the percentage of patients who met each performance measure. Importantly, each of the three performance measure sections concludes with this question:

> What is ONE change that you can make in your rehab process to help you increase your percentage, or if you achieved 100%, how do you plan to maintain your percentage as you continue to work to improve your patient outcomes?

Quality is about more than measurement. It is about identifying any gaps in care and considering what might be done differently to close those gaps and to maintain the very highest level of care.

# SUMMARY

The importance of quality in health care cannot be overstated. It has assumed an ever-increasing role in regulatory standards, credentialing, and payment for health care services. More importantly, health care professionals are urged to position quality squarely at the center of patient care—providing the very best care, in the right way, all of the time. Pulmonary rehabilitation programs must strive to provide the highest level of care to patients who put their lives in our hands expecting optimal outcomes.

For this to happen, our focus must consistently be on identification of gaps in care and how those gaps can be narrowed. Gaps are identified through data collection, measurement, and analysis. Outcome and performance measure data from pulmonary rehabilitation programs will help to identify areas of strength and areas where there are opportunities for improvement. Staff education and credentialing, such as completion of the pulmonary rehabilitation certificate, contribute to pulmonary rehabilitation professionals having a high level of knowledge and competency to provide care. Weighing a pulmonary rehabilitation program against established standards, such as with program certification, provides a way to maintain program excellence and strive for continuous quality improvement.

Compliance with evidence-based guidelines and standards of care, as delineated in this book, needs to be seen as the "right thing to do for our patients" by all health care providers, rather than just another regulatory step that is "required" to do.

**VISIT THE WEB RESOURCE**
for links to additional resources and various tools, checklists, and forms.

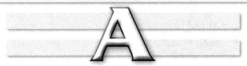

# Forms, Questionnaires, Assessments, and Individualized Treatment Plan Example

**T**his appendix contains tools to help practitioners gather information and assess rehabilitation patients, as well as questionnaires for participants to evaluate a rehabilitation program. Practitioners or patients should fill out each form as necessary. Included are an initial interview form, a participant questionnaire, a physician referral form, a program evaluation form, and a participant nutritional assessment form.

## Initial Interview Form

Name: _____ Date: _____

Address: _____ Phone: _____

Emergency contact: _____ Phone: _____

Age: _____ Sex: _____ Occupation: _____

Height: _____ Weight: _____ Highest level of education: _____

Marital status: _____ Advance directives: _____

Diagnosis: _____ Insurance provider: _____

Referring physician: _____

Primary care physician: _____

Referral source: _____

Chief complaint: _____

### History

How many times have you been hospitalized in the last year as a result of lung problems? _____

How many days were you in the hospital in the last year as a result of lung disease? _____

How many E.R. visits have you had in the past year as a result of breathing difficulty? _____

Last hospital admission: _____ Release: _____

Previous hospitalizations: _____

Have you ever attended a pulmonary rehabilitation program? _____

Have you ever had any chest injuries or surgeries?   Yes   No

   Type _____

Do you have any upcoming surgeries?   Yes   No   _____

Do you have any physical limitations that may affect your ability to exercise (sensory loss, amputation, stroke, surgeries,

   fractures, etc.)? _____

Do you have any other medical problems?

Cardiovascular disease _____

Hypertension _____

Diabetes _____

G-I problems _____

Reflux/hiatal hernia _____

Osteoporosis _____

Sinusitis _____

Vision or hearing problems _____

Other _____

Have you ever had or do you have:

| | | | |
|---|---|---|---|
| Emphysema | _____ | Valley fever | _____ |
| Asthma | _____ | Tuberculosis | _____ |
| Bronchitis | _____ | Pleurisy | _____ |
| Pneumonia | _____ | Lung cancer | _____ |
| Bronchiectasis | _____ | Sinus trouble | _____ |
| Blood clot in lung | _____ | Other | _____ |
| High pressure in lungs | _____ | | |

*(continued)*

**A.1** Pulmonary rehabilitation initial interview form.

Reprinted courtesy of the Pulmonary Rehabilitation Program at St. Joseph's Hospital and Medical Center, Phoenix, AZ.

Do you have a family history of respiratory disease? _____

Have you ever used tobacco? _____ What form?   Chew   Smoke _____

Do you chew/smoke now? _____ How long did you use or have you used tobacco? _____

When did you stop chewing/smoking?_____

If you are still smoking, do you plan to quit? _____

Do you live with any smokers?_____

Other substance abuse? _____

Have you ever been exposed to:

| Asbestos dust | Yes | No | Paint fumes | Yes | No |
|---|---|---|---|---|---|
| Cotton dust | Yes | No | Plastic fumes | Yes | No |
| Mining dust | Yes | No | Solvent fumes | Yes | No |
| Other dust | Yes | No | Other fumes | Yes | No |

Do you consume alcohol? _____ How much? _____

Do you have any allergies (food, pollen, drugs, etc.)? _____

How many colds do you get per year?_____

Vaccines:        Flu     Yes    No        Pneumonia     Yes    No

Do you ever have chest pain? _____ Location _____

Type of pain _____ Frequency _____

Have you ever had a heart attack?_____ When? _____

## Major Symptomatology

What are your symptoms today? _____

What were your symptoms last year?_____

What were your symptoms 5 years ago? _____

When did you realize that you had lung problems?_____

## Disease Impact

Do you sleep flat or with your head elevated? _____

If elevated, how high? _____

Do you awaken during the night? _____ How often? _____

Why?_____

Do your ankles ever swell up? _____ When?_____

Do you cough?_____ What part of the day?_____

Do you cough up sputum?_____ When? _____

Describe _____

Have you ever coughed up blood? _____

## MRC Dyspnea Scale

[0] _____ Breathless with strenuous exercise

[1] _____ Shortness of breath when hurrying on the level or walking up a slight hill

[2] _____ Walks slower than people of the same age on the level because of breathlessness, or has to stop for breath when walking at own pace on the level

[3] _____ Stops for breath after walking about 100 yards or after a few minutes on the level

[4] _____ Too breathless to leave the house or when dressing or undressing

**A.1** (continued)

Do you use oxygen?_____ How often?_____ Liters per minute_____

Type of oxygen delivery system _____ Supplier_____

Are you on any home respiratory therapy?_____ Type_____

How do you clean the equipment? _____

Do you have trouble eating? _____ Why?_____

Do you have trouble gaining or losing weight? _____

Have you experienced a recent weight change?_____

Do you have a special diet?_____

Are you able to care for yourself?_____

Are you able to take care of your home? _____

Do you exercise? _____ If yes, how?_____ How often? _____

Do you have exercise equipment? _____ Type _____

Has your physician limited your activities?_____

Do you have any special interests or hobbies?_____

What activities does your breathing difficulty prevent you from doing that you would like to do? _____

Does your breathing interfere with your ability to have sexual relations? _____

Are others close to you affected by your health?_____

If yes, how? _____

Are you affected by trying to live up to others' expectations? _____

How? _____

Do you find yourself worrying daily? _____ occasionally?_____ almost never? _____

Does your income cover your expenses and needs? _____

Do you live alone?_____

Do you have transportation? _____ What form?_____

How do you heat and cool your home? _____

Do you have any pets?_____

**Medications**

| Type | Amount | Frequency |
| --- | --- | --- |
| | | |
| | | |
| | | |
| | | |
| | | |
| | | |
| | | |
| | | |
| | | |
| | | |
| | | |

Medication compliance:   Yes   No

M.D.I. technique: _____

Spacer:  Yes   No     Type:_____     Needs training:  Yes   No     *(continued)*

**A.1**   *(continued)*

**Observations**

Color _____ Skin turgor _____

Mentation _____ Energy level _____

Nutritional status _____

Blood pressure _____ Pulse _____ Edema _____

Respirations (rate, rhythm, depth) _____

Accessory breather? _____ Pursed lips? _____

Abdominal breathing? _____ Other _____

Auscultation _____

**Data From Patient's Records**

FEV$_1$ _____ FEV$_1$/FVC _____ ABGs _____ Hb/Hct _____

Alb _____ EKG _____ Other _____

**Client's Stated Goals**

Please state your goals or what you expect to achieve from this rehabilitation program.

_____

_____

Patient's signature _____

**Estimated Learning Ability**

_____ No baseline, slow learner          _____ Some baseline, slow learner

_____ No baseline, good learner          _____ Some baseline, good learner

_____ Needs only comprehensive review and reinforcement

Degree of motivation _____

Candidacy:   Accept _____ Reject _____

Evaluator's signature _____

**A.1** *(continued)*

## Participant Questionnaire

Date: _____  Physician: _____

Name: _____

Address: _____

City/state: _____  Zip: _____  Phone: _____

Age: _____  Birth date: _____  Marital status:  M   S   W   D

Spouse's name: _____

Social Security #: _____  Medicare #: _____

Insurance: _____

_____

Diagnosis: _____

**Living Situation**  _____ House  _____ Apartment  _____Mobile home  _____ Condo

Level:  _____ Single  _____ Multi

Entrance:  _____ Incline  _____ Stair(s) # _____

Household members: _____

(Relationships & names) _____

Household pets: _____

(Types & names) _____

Usual household duties I perform:  _____ Cooking  _____ Cleaning  _____ Finances  _____ Laundry

_____ Transportation  _____ Yard work  _____ Grocery shopping

My major source(s) of support: (names and relationships) _____

**Transportation**  _____ Currently drive  _____ Rely on family  _____ Rely on friends

_____ Use public transportation  _____ Is a real problem for me

**Occupational History**

Current or former occupation: _____

Retirement/disability date: _____

Occupational exposure:  _____ Welding  _____ Pottery  _____ Asbestos  _____ Mines/foundry

_____ Gas/fumes  _____ Quarry  _____ Sandblasting  _____ Chemicals  _____ Dust

**Educational History**

The last grade I completed was: _____

I learn information best by:  _____ Explanation  _____ Reading  _____ Video/TV  _____ Computer  _____ Demonstration

**Medical History**

(Please check those that apply; mark with F if family history exists)

| | | |
|---|---|---|
| _____ Asthma | _____ Tuberculosis | _____ Fractures (specify) _____ |
| _____ Chronic bronchitis | _____ Diabetes | _____ Cancer |
| _____ Emphysema | _____ Sinus problems | _____ Pneumonia |
| _____ Bronchiectasis | _____ High blood pressure | _____ Heart disease |
| _____ Osteoporosis | _____ Arthritis | _____ Sarcoidosis |
| _____ Cystic fibrosis | _____ Pulmonary fibrosis | _____ Collapsed lung |

*(continued)*

**A.2**  Pulmonary rehabilitation participant questionnaire.

Adapted from Pulmonary Rehabilitation Programs at Long Beach Memorial Medical Center, Long Beach, CA, Mt. Diablo Medical Center, Concord, CA, and Union Hospital, Dover, OH.

## Allergy History

I have seen an allergist. ____ Yes ____ No

Was skin testing performed? ____ Yes ____ No

I am allergic to the following:

    Food(s): _____

    Medications: _____

    Environmental: ____ Dust ____ Mold ____ Pollens ____ Grass Other:_____

I have difficulty when exposed to the following environmental irritants:

    ____ Dust ____ Smog ____ Solvents ____ Humidity ____ Perfumes/colognes

    ____ Rapid changes in temperature ____ Tobacco smoke ____ Wind ____ Other: _____

## Vaccine History

I receive the flu vaccine annually. ____ Yes ____ No

    If no, why not? _____

I have received the pneumonia vaccine. ____ Yes ____ No

    Year received: _____

## Smoking History

____ I have never smoked.

____ I have smoked in the past but do not smoke now.

    Year started: _____ Year quit: _____

    Number of packs smoked per day:_____

____ I am currently a smoker.

    Number of packs smoked per day:_____

Exposure to secondhand smoke: ____ None ____ Home ____ Work ____ Social situations

## Pulmonary Health History

Cough: ____ Yes ____ No

    ____ A.M. ____ P.M. ____ Nighttime ____ Around the clock

Mucus: Normal color:_____ ____ Thick ____ Thin ____ Moderate

    Amount/day: ___ 1 tsp. ___1-2 tsp. ___ 1 Tbsp. ___1/4 cup ___ 1/2 cup ___ 1 cup ___ >1 cup

    When: ___ A.M. ___ P.M. ___ Around the clock

I use the following to help me raise my mucus:

    ____ Drink warm liquids    ____ Inhalers

    ____ Aerosol treatments    ____ Chest percussion

    ____ Postural drainage    ____ Increase my fluids

I have coughed up blood. ____ Yes ____ No When: _____

I have taken steroid pills (e.g., prednisone). ____ Yes ____ No

    Length of time: _____ Last date:_____ Highest dose: _____

I experience the following:

    ____ Chest pain    ____ Dizziness/unsteadiness    ____ Hoarseness

    ____ Fatigue    ____ Ankle swelling    ____ Weight change

    ____ Wheezing

    Known trigger factors:_____

**A.2** *(continued)*

I have been on a ventilator (respirator) in an intensive care unit. _____ Yes _____ No  Last date: _____

What I remember most about that experience is: _____

_____

I see my lung doctor every (please give a time frame): _____

## Pulmonary Infections

Number/year: _____

Antibiotic usually taken: _____

I know I have an infection when: _____

## Pulmonary Hospitalizations

Number in past year: _____     Number in previous year: _____

## Emergency Room Visits for Pulmonary Reasons

Number in past year: _____     Number in previous year: _____

## Shortness of Breath

I have experienced shortness of breath since: _____

My breathing is most difficult: _____ Early A.M. _____ A.M. _____ P.M. _____ Bedtime

I do the following to decrease or avoid being short of breath:

_____ Stop and rest                        _____ Use aerosol machine

_____ Use inhalers                         _____ Use belly or diaphragm breathing

_____ Use a fan or air conditioner         _____ Open windows

_____ Remove myself from the irritant      _____ Limit my activity

_____ Practice a relaxation technique      _____ Avoid exposure to irritants

_____ Check the air pollution forecast     _____ Check my peak flow

_____ Use pursed-lip breathing             _____ Avoid tobacco smoke exposure

## Dietary History

Current height: _____     Current weight: _____

I have recently had a change in my weight. _____ Yes _____ No

Gained _____ pounds     Lost _____ pounds

Over this period of time: _____

I can attribute this weight change to: _____

I would like to weigh: _____ pounds

I follow the following type of diet:

_____ No special diet          _____ Low saturated fat        _____ Ulcer

_____ Low sodium (salt)        _____ Caloric restriction      _____ Hiatal hernia

_____ Low cholesterol          _____ Diabetic                 _____ Other _____

My appetite is: _____ Good _____ Fair _____ Poor

I drink this amount of each of these a day:

Water _____     Sodas _____     Coffee _____

Tea _____       Wine _____      Hard liquor _____

Milk _____      Juice _____     Beer _____  (continued)

**A.2** *(continued)*

I have difficulty with:   chewing         ____ Yes   ____ No

swallowing      ____ Yes   ____ No

digestion       ____ Yes   ____ No

I take vitamins.   ____ Yes   ____ No

If yes, please list: _____

**Sleeping History**

Usual bedtime _____   Usual time of waking up _____

Naps taken during the day:   Number: _____   Length: _____

Number of pillows used when sleeping: _____

Medications/strategies used to help me sleep: _____

| Medication name/strength | Amount and frequency on a daily basis | Time(s) of the day medication taken | Purpose of medication | Comments that you have |
|---|---|---|---|---|
| Example: 1. Albuterol | 2 puffs 4 times a day | 6 A.M., 2 P.M., 6 P.M., 11 P.M. | improve breathing | works well |
| Example: 2. Lasix 40 mg | 1 tablet once a day | in the morning usually 6 A.M. | blood pressure | |
| | | | | |
| | | | | |
| | | | | |
| | | | | |
| | | | | |

**Activities of Daily Living**

Use this shortness of breath scale to answer the following questions:

Scale:   0 = None;   1 = Minimal;   2 = Moderate;   3 = Great;   4 = Unable

To what degree do you get short of breath at rest? ____

To what degree do you get short of breath when climbing stairs? ____

How many stairs? ____

To what degree do you get short of breath during the following activities:

____ Eating

____ Simple personal care (washing face, combing hair, etc.)

____ Taking full bath or shower

____ Dressing

____ Picking up or straightening up

____ Sweeping or vacuuming

____ Shopping

____ Laundry

____ Cooking and doing dishes

____ Walking around your house

____ Walking your own pace on level surface

____ Walking one block

____ Walking with others your age

____ Walking up a slight hill

**A.2**   (continued)

**Activity/Exercise History**

_____ Yes _____ No     I currently do purposeful walking _____ days a week for _____ minutes.

_____ Yes _____ No     I do calisthenics _____ days/week.

_____ Yes _____ No     I do purposeful exercise programs.

The following things limit my ability to remain active:

_____ Shortness of breath          _____ Lightheadedness

_____ Fatigue                      _____ Joint problems (specify): _____

I have the following exercise equipment available:

_____ None

_____ Stationary bike        _____ Treadmill          _____ Stair stepper

_____ Pool                   _____ Weights            _____ Other: _____

**Equipment/Assistive Device History**

I use the following items:

_____ Walker                 _____ Eyeglasses

_____ Wheelchair             _____ Electric cart

_____ Cane                   _____ Hearing aid

_____ Four-point quad cane   _____ Other: _____

**Respiratory Home Care Equipment History**

I use the following items:                               Frequency used:

_____ Peak flow meter                                    _____

_____ Aerosol machine (e.g., Pulmoaide)                  _____

_____ Suction machine                                    _____

_____ Ventilator                                         _____

_____ Mechanical chest percussor                         _____

_____ PEP valve                                          _____

_____ Oxygen: _____ Flow rate    System: _____ Concentrator

                                         _____ Tank

                                         _____ Liquid

                                         _____ Pulse

Oxygen used:   _____ Continuously   _____ Only when I need it   _____ With sleep only   _____ With exercise only

              _____ With sleep and exercise

I change my oxygen tubing every:

_____ Week   _____ 2 weeks   _____ 3-4 weeks   _____ 1-2 months   _____ Oops! I didn't know I needed to change it.

My home care equipment vendor is: _____

**Day-to-Day Living**

I am sexually active   _____ Yes   _____ No

My present interests and hobbies are: _____

Former interests and hobbies in which I can no longer participate are: _____

This is what I do for fun: _____

I would describe my present temperament (mood) as: _____
(examples: worried, sad, impatient, frustrated, depressed, anxious, contented, cheerful, etc.)          _(continued)_

**A.2**  _(continued)_

This is what makes me feel this way: _____

I use the following to relax:

| | | |
|---|---|---|
| ____ Read | ____ Alcohol | ____ Other: _____ |
| ____ Deep breathing | ____ Yoga | |
| ____ Smoke | ____ Pursed-lip breathing | |
| ____ TV | ____ Tranquilizer | |

This has been the most difficult adjustment for me because of my lung disease:

_____

This is how my lung disease has affected how I feel about myself:

_____

My goals for completing pulmonary rehabilitation are: _____

_____

**A.2** *(continued)*

---

## Outpatient Pulmonary Rehabilitation Program

### Physician Referral Form

Name: _____ DOB: _____

Diagnosis: _____

1. I agree to have my patient participate in the _____ Outpatient Pulmonary Rehabilitation Program.

2. I am aware that certain diagnostic data (such as PFTs, 6-minute walk test, CXR, EKG, cardiopulmonary exercise test) may be required and will be requested by the program director if not already available.

3. I agree to have my patient counseled in all areas related to pulmonary rehabilitation.

4. I agree to continue the regular care of my patient throughout his/her participation in the program.

Physician signature: _____

Phone: _____    Special considerations:

Fax: _____    _____

Date: _____    _____

_____

_____

**A.3** Outpatient pulmonary rehabilitation physician referral form.

Used by permission from St. Francis Hospital and Medical Center, Hartford, CT.

## Pulmonary Rehabilitation Physical Therapy Evaluation

Patient name: _____

MRN: _____

MD: _____

Today's date: _____ Time in: _____ Time out: _____ Age: _____ ☐ F ☐ M

Diagnosis: _____ Onset: _____

_____ Onset: _____

_____ Onset: _____

**PMH:** ☐ Hypertension ☐ Diabetes ☐ Cancer ☐ Osteoporosis ☐ Cardiac ☐ Fracture ☐ Surgery
☐ H/O falls ☐ Signs of abuse/neglect

Other: _____

_____

Current medications: _____

_____

☐ Bone density test: _____ Exercise test complete: ☐ Yes, max watts: _____ ☐ No, scheduled: _____

Pulmonary rehabilitation history: _____

_____

Home exercise: _____

Mental status: _____

Social/Family status: _____

Three greatest difficulties: _____ , _____ , _____

Patient goals: _____ , _____ , _____

Cough: _____

Oxygen use: *At rest:* _____ by _____ *Exercise:* _____ by _____ *Sleep:* _____ by _____

Smoking history: _____

**Pain**

Location: _____ Duration: _____ Character: _____

Current: _____/10 Best: _____/10 Worst: _____/10 Increases with: _____ Decreases with: _____

Edema: ☐ No ☐ Yes Location: _____ Exacerbated by: _____

**Examination**

Auscultation: _____

Breathing pattern: ☐ Diaphragmatic: _____ ☐ Accessory muscle use: _____ ☐ Pursed Lips: _____

Range of motion: UE: _____ LE: _____

Strength: UE: _____ LE: _____

Posture/Skin/Physical Characteristics/Other: _____

Gait: _____

Foot evaluation: ☐ Overpronator ☐ Normal pronator ☐ Supinator Given shoe list: ☐ Yes ☐ No

Other: _____

*(continued)*

**A.4** Pulmonary rehabilitation physical therapy evaluation form.

Patient name:_____ MRN:_____

**Precautions**

- ❑ Aspiration
- ❑ Incisional
- ❑ Osteoporosis
- ❑ Hypertension
- ❑ Hernia
- ❑ Musculoskeletal
- ❑ Cardiac
- ❑ Diabetes
- ❑ Risk of falls
- ❑ Other:_____

**Problems**

- ❑ Retained secretions
- ❑ Ineffective breathing pattern
- ❑ Limited range of motion
- ❑ Postural deviations
- ❑ Decrease mobility
- ❑ Pain
- ❑ Oxygen desaturation
- ❑ Decreased strength
- ❑ Altered mental status
- ❑ Altered nutritional status
- ❑ Smoking
- ❑ Decreased functional level (ADLs, self care)
- ❑ Other:_____

**Treatment/Plan**

- ❑ Cough techniques
- ❑ Flutter/Acapella/Vest
- ❑ PD and percussion
- ❑ 3-day trial pulmonary hygiene
- ❑ Breathing retraining
- ❑ Postural exercises
- ❑ Chair exercises
- ❑ Ice
- ❑ Hot packs
- ❑ TENS
- ❑ Nutritional consult
- ❑ Smoking cessation consult
- ❑ General conditioning
- ❑ Progressive ambulation
- ❑ Strengthening
- ❑ Stretching
- ❑ Home exercise program
- ❑ Footwear education
- ❑ Referral to outpatient physical therapy

**Special Considerations**

- ❑ Use pillows/wedge for floor exercise
- ❑ Incisional precautions until _____
- ❑ No upper body flexion or rotation
- ❑ Give osteoporosis handout
- ❑ BP daily
- ❑ Monitor blood glucose
- ❑ Preexercise          ❑ Postexercise
- ❑ Other: _____

**Goals Developed Collaboratively With Patient:**

*Short-Term Goal: In* _____ *weeks patient will:*

1. Ambulate _____ feet in 6 min. with _____ rests and _____ assist with _____ assistive device

2. _____

3. _____

4. _____

*Long-Term Goal: In* _____ *weeks patient will:*

1. Ambulate _____ feet in _____ min. with _____ rests and _____ assist with _____ assistive device

2. _____

3. _____

4. _____

Patient's rehab potential: ❑ Poor   ❑ Fair   ❑ Good   ❑ Excellent

Frequency of treatment: _____   Duration of program: _____

Physical therapist: _____   Date: _____

Physician's Medicare Certification: I certify that this patient is under my care. The above treatment plan of care has been reviewed by me and I authorize it to be implemented for the next 30 days.

Physician's signature: _____   Date: _____

**A.4**   *(continued)*

**1.5–2 METs**

Walking 1 mph

Standing

Driving automobile

Sitting at desk or typing

**2–3 METs**

Walking 2.5–3 mph

Dusting furniture, light housework

Preparing a meal

**3–4 METs**

Sweeping

Vacuuming

Ironing

Walking 3 mph

Golfing (power cart)

Pushing light lawnmower

**4–5 METs**

Calisthenics

Cycling outdoors 6 mph

Painting

Golfing (carrying clubs)

Playing tennis (doubles)

**5–6 METs**

Walking 4 mph

Digging in garden

Ice or roller skating 9 mph

Doing carpentry

**6–7 METs**

Stationary cycling (vigorous)

Playing tennis (singles)

Shoveling snow

Mowing lawn (nonpowered)

**A.5** Representative levels of energy expenditure (in METs).

*Note:* One MET is the level of energy expenditure at rest, or approximately 3.5 ml/kg/min of oxygen consumption.

# Nutritional Assessment

Name: _____ Date: _____

Height: _____ Weight: _____

What is your "usual" adult weight? _____

Have you gained or lost any weight recently?    No    Yes    How much? _____

Over what period of time? _____

What do you attribute it to? _____

Have you noticed any changes in your eating habits since your pulmonary problems began? _____

If so, describe them: _____

Do you follow any of these dietary restrictions?

   Low salt    Diabetic    Gout    Ulcer    Low fat/cholesterol    Hiatal hernia    Other:_____

Caloric intake: _____

How would you describe your appetite?_____

Is this usual for you?    No    Yes

Do you take vitamin or mineral supplements?    No    Yes    Specify name, strength, and frequency.

_____

_____

Do you have any food allergies?    No    Yes    What are they?

_____

_____

Describe any problems you have with:

   Dental: _____

   Chewing: _____

   Swallowing: _____

   Digestion: _____

   Constipation or diarrhea: _____

   Bloating: _____

   Nausea: _____

   Fatigue: _____

   Shortness of breath: _____

How many ounces of the following fluids do you drink:

| | Daily | Weekly | Rarely |
|---|---|---|---|
| Water | _____ | _____ | _____ |
| Soft drinks* | _____ | _____ | _____ |
| Juice | _____ | _____ | _____ |
| Milk | _____ | _____ | _____ |
| Coffee* | _____ | _____ | _____ |
| Tea* | _____ | _____ | _____ |
| Beer | _____ | _____ | _____ |
| Wine | _____ | _____ | _____ |
| Hard liquor | _____ | _____ | _____ |

*Caffeine/decaffeinated

**A.6**  Nutritional assessment form.

Reprinted courtesy of the Pulmonary Rehabilitation Program at Mt. Diablo Medical Center, Concord, CA.

FOR STAFF USE ONLY:

%IBW: _____     BMI: _____

Weight change:     Mild     Moderate     Severe

Supplements?_____

Available labs:     Albumin _____     Cholesterol _____     Other _____

Possible drug or nutrient interactions?

_____

_____

Comments:

_____

_____

Assessment and recommendations:

_____

_____

_____

_____

Date: _____     Dietitian: _____ , RD

**A.6**  *(continued)*

Reprinted courtesy of the Pulmonary Rehabilitation Program at Mt. Diablo Medical Center, Concord, CA.

| | True | False | Not Sure |
|---|---|---|---|
| 1. The diaphragm is a muscle that does most of the work of breathing. | 1 | 2 | 3 |
| 2. Emphysema is a disease that primarily affects air sacs (alveoli). | 1 | 2 | 3 |
| 3. "Pursed-lip breathing" helps prevent small airways from collapsing. | 1 | 2 | 3 |
| 4. People with chronic lung disease can abruptly stop taking a steroid medication such as prednisone at any time without ill effects. | 1 | 2 | 3 |
| 5. Changing the flow rate on oxygen equipment can be dangerous for a person with chronic lung disease. | 1 | 2 | 3 |
| 6. For a person with chronic lung disease, eating six small meals a day rather than three large meals can help to reduce shortness of breath during and after meals. | 1 | 2 | 3 |
| 7. For a person with chronic lung disease, foods that are high in protein, such as fish, are an important part of the diet. | 1 | 2 | 3 |
| 8. Drinking water has no effect on the mucus in the lungs. | 1 | 2 | 3 |
| 9. A person with chronic lung disease should rinse out the mouth after using a steroid metered-dose inhaler. | 1 | 2 | 3 |
| 10. When climbing stairs, a person with chronic lung disease should hold his or her breath briefly while taking a step. | 1 | 2 | 3 |
| 11. For people with chronic lung disease, the most efficient method of completing a task is to work quickly in short bursts and to take frequent rests. | 1 | 2 | 3 |
| 12. During activity, people with chronic lung disease should exhale when they exert themselves. | 1 | 2 | 3 |
| 13. If someone with chronic lung disease is taking antibiotics, it is fine for that person to stop taking them when he or she feels better. | 1 | 2 | 3 |
| 14. During diaphragmatic breathing, it is important for a person with chronic lung disease to pull in the abdomen during inhalation. | 1 | 2 | 3 |
| 15. It is important for a person with chronic lung disease to keep the shoulder muscles relaxed to decrease the amount of oxygen used for breathing. | 1 | 2 | 3 |
| 16. A bronchodilator, such as Albuterol, gets rid of infection. | 1 | 2 | 3 |

**A.7** Sample quiz for patients with chronic lung disease.

Adapted, by permission, from Y. Schere, L. Schmeider, and S. Shimmell. 1995. "Outpatient instruction for individuals with COPD," *Perspectives in Respiratory Nursing* 6 (3):3.

## Pulmonary Rehabilitation Perioperative Education Sessions and Support Group

Name: _____

Patient ID#: _____

**Education Sessions**

**Date**

_____ Spacers/MDIs

_____ Pulmonary issues

_____ ABG/PFTs

_____ Nutrition

_____ Home equipment

_____ Exercise responses

_____ Urinary incontinence

_____ Medications

_____ Charting/Inhalers

_____ Lung disease pathology

_____ Anatomy and physiology I

_____ Anatomy and physiology II

_____ Preoperative aspects (pre only)

_____ Transplant medications (post)

_____ Transplant issues (1st Monday of each month, 11:30 A.M.)

_____ Transplant medications (pre-op participants only, 3rd Monday of each month, 11:30 A.M.)

**Date**

_____ Oxygen

_____ Chest PT

_____ Carolina Organ Procurement Association

_____ Doctor's day

_____ Osteoporosis

_____ Graduate program

_____ Home program

_____ Graduation

_____ Travel issues

_____ Topic of choice

_____ Progress review

_____ _____

_____ _____

_____ _____

**Support Group**
(List dates)

_____   _____   _____   _____

_____   _____   _____   _____

Monday/Wednesday lectures: 3:45-4:30

Tuesday support group: Intensive 2:45-3:30

Perioperative 3:45-4:30

Thursday lectures: 2:45-3:30

Friday lectures: 2:15

All lectures will be held in the Meltzer room of the fitness building.

*If it has been three months since you last heard a lecture, it may need to be repeated.

**A.8** Pulmonary rehabilitation perioperative education sessions and support group.

Used by permission of the Duke University Pulmonary Rehabilitation Program.

# INDIVIDUALIZED TREATMENT PLAN: Pulmonary Rehabilitation / RC SERVICES

**EXERCISE: See MD orders.**
Exercise workloads will be progressed gradually within limits of patient's ability.
Progression based on Borg dyspnea of 3-5 and absence of untoward symptoms during exercise.

**INDIVIDUAL COUNSELING:** Education on disease self management strategies including:
☐ Dyspnea control techniques at rest, activity and ADLs ☐ Inhaled and respiratory medications
☐ Exacerbation prevention & management ☐ O2 Rx, system, safety ☐ ADL management and pacing
☐ Panic & depression management ☐ Nutrition & weight management ☐ Smoking cessation
☐ Home exercise plan & guidelines ☐ Intimacy ☐ Safe travel ☐ Advanced directives

**PATIENT GOALS**
☐ Breathe better ☐ Take medications correctly
☐ Increase endurance/stamina ☐ Improve Cholesterol Results
☐ Improve weight ☐ Symptom management
☐ Control panic / anxiety ☐ Stop smoking / maintain cessation
☐ Return to Work ☐ Weight loss _____ lbs
☐ Return to recreation/hobby ☐ Other: _____

**Admitting Diagnosis:**

Name: _____ Date: _____
☐ history of pneumonia ☐ hospitalized for resp. exacerbation
☐ CHF ☐ HTN Cardiac other: _____
☐ Ortho _____ ☐ Osteoporosis _____
☐ Neurological _____
☐ GERD GI disorder: _____
☐ Diabetes ☐ glucometer ☐ Rx _____
☐ Depression ☐ Anxiety ☐ Rx _____ ☐ counselor
☐ OSA ☐ CPAP / BiPAP ☐ Insomnia ☐ Rx _____
☐ Surgeries _____
Clinical Note: _____

| Problems / Goals | Plan | Initial Assessment Session # 1 <br> Date/Initial : _____ | Reassessment Session # _____ <br> Date/Initials: _____ | Reassessment Session # _____ <br> Date/Initial: _____ | Final Assessment Session # _____ <br> Date/Initial: _____ |
|---|---|---|---|---|---|
| **Education by RN or RCP** ☐__ sessions <br> **Problem:** <br> ☐ Knowledge deficit self management <br> ☐ Ineffective control of dyspnea <br> **Goal:** <br> ☐ Effectively partners with MD / team to prevent and manage disease-related impairments | Education topics: training by RN or RCP <br> ☐ Disease overview <br> ☐ Breathing strategies, dyspnea control at rest, with panic, exercise, ADLS <br> ☐ Respiratory medication <br> ☐ Exacerbation prevention, management <br> ☐ Panic control <br> ☐ Secretion clearance <br> ☐ travel ☐ intimacy <br> ☐ Home exercise program <br> ☐ Advance directives | ☐ Knowledge deficit of disease self management strategies <br> ☐ Poor control of dyspnea <br> Barriers to learning: <br> ☐ speech ☐ hearing <br> ☐ vision ☐ literacy <br> ☐ cognitive <br> ☐ <br> ☐ ready to learn | ☐ Demonstrates disease self-management strategies <br> ☐ Dyspnea control during rest, ADLS and exercise <br> ☐ Using Rxs as directed <br> ☐ Mobilizes secretions effectively <br> ☐ Demonstrates strategies for anxiety and depression management | ☐ Demonstrates disease self-management strategies <br> ☐ Dyspnea control at rest / with activity <br> ☐ Using Rxs as directed <br> ☐ Mobilizes secretions effectively <br> ☐ Demonstrates strategies for anxiety and depression management | ☐ Demonstrates disease self-management strategies <br> ☐ Dyspnea control at rest / with activity <br> ☐ Using Rxs as directed <br> ☐ Mobilizes secretions effectively <br> ☐ Demonstrates strategies for anxiety and depression management |
| **Hypoxemia** <br> **Problem:** <br> ☐ Hypoxemia <br> ☐ No home O2 <br> ☐ No port. O2 <br> ☐ Needs O2 Rx recommendation <br> ☐ poor knowledge O2 use/safety <br> **Goal** <br> ☐ Hypoxemia managed <br> ☐ Port system <br> ☐ Using O2 as Rx'd / safely | ☐ Monitor SpO2 at rest and with exercise <br> ☐ Recommend appropriate FiO2 to patient and physician <br> ☐ Assist pt to contact DME for home O2 ☐ portable O2 <br> ☐ Train in appropriate use of O2 at rest and with exercise <br> ☐ Train in O2 safety <br> ☐ Train in O2 systems | Initial SpO2: _____ <br> FiO2 _____ <br> Port O2 _____ <br> Stationary O2 _____ <br> DME _____ | ☐ Demonstrates knowledge of O2 Rx at rest and with exercise <br> ☐ Demonstrates knowledge of O2 safety <br> ☐ Using O2 as Rx'd <br> ☐ Has home O2 as Rx'd <br> ☐ Uses port. O2 as Rx'd | ☐ Demonstrates knowledge of O2 Rx at rest and with exercise <br> ☐ Demonstrates knowledge of O2 safety <br> ☐ Using O2 as Rx'd <br> ☐ Has home O2 as Rx'd <br> ☐ Uses port. O2 as Rx'd | ☐ Demonstrates knowledge of O2 Rx at rest and with exercise <br> ☐ Demonstrates knowledge of O2 safety <br> ☐ Using O2 as Rx'd <br> ☐ Has home O2 as Rx'd <br> ☐ Uses port. O2 as Rx'd |

160

| Problem / Goal | Assessment | Instruction | Outcome | Outcome | Outcome |
|---|---|---|---|---|---|
| **Psychosocial Assess-ment: Problem:**<br>☐ Depression<br>☐ Anxiety<br>☐ Panic<br>☐ Ineffective coping<br>☐ Impaired quality of life (QOL)<br>**Goal:**<br>☐ Improved psychosocial coping strategies<br>☐ Verbalizes coping mechanisms<br>☐ Adequate treatment of depression<br>Improved QOL | Depression:<br>☐ self report<br>☐ depression screening test<br>score: _____<br>☐ Anger ☐ Anxiety<br>☐ Stress ☐ Panic<br>☐ Impaired QOL<br>☐ QOL score _____<br>Medications _____<br>☐ Referred for MD counseling | Instruction:<br>☐ Review screening results<br>☐ Benefits of exercise<br>☐ Relaxation techniques<br>☐ Stress management<br>  ☐ On meds currently<br>  ☐ Receiving counseling<br>  ☐ Recommend counseling<br>  ☐ Recommended follow-up with MD for consideration of Rx<br>☐ Train in coping strategies | ☐ Management of stress and depression<br>☐ Practicing Interventions<br>☐ Counseling referral<br>☐ Demonstrates coping strategies | ☐ Management of stress and depression<br>☐ Practicing Interventions<br>☐ Met<br>☐ Progressing<br>☐ Not progressing<br>☐<br>☐ Counseling referral | ☐ Management of stress and depression<br>☐ Practicing Interventions<br>☐ Met<br>☐ Progressing<br>☐ Not progressing<br>☐<br>☐ Counseling referral |
| **Activities of Daily Living Problem:**<br>☐ Impaired ADL management<br>**Goal:** ☐ ADL management with control of dyspnea | ☐ Impaired ADL management<br>☐ Fear +/or severe dyspnea with stairs<br>☐ Need for OT eval<br>☐ Need for assistive devices | Instruction:<br>☐ ADL performance with pacing, dyspnea control<br>☐ OT evaluation<br>☐ Assistive device evaluation recommendations and resources<br>☐ Train in dyspnea control / pacing with stairs | ☐ Management of ADLs with control of dyspnea<br>☐ Following OT recommendations<br>☐ Has ordered assistive devices<br>☐ Appropriate stair climbing<br>☐ Met<br>☐ Progressing<br>☐ Not progressing<br>_____ | ☐ Management of ADLs with control of dyspnea<br>☐ Following OT recommendations<br>☐ Has ordered assistive devices<br>☐ Appropriate stair climbing<br>☐ Met<br>☐ Progressing<br>☐ Not progressing<br>_____ | ☐ Management of ADLs with control of dyspnea<br>☐ Following OT recommendations<br>☐ Has ordered assistive devices<br>☐ Met<br>☐ Progressing<br>☐ Not progressing<br>_____ |
| **Nutrition & Weight Management Problem:**<br>☐ Overweight<br>☐ Cachexia<br>**Goal:**<br>☐ BMI 21 to 25<br>☐ Wt loss 1-2 lb per week<br>☐ prevent further weight loss<br>☐ Waist Circumference<br>< 35 in female<br>< 40 in male | Knowledge deficit management of<br>☐ Overweight:<br>☐ Cachexia<br>☐ Osteoporosis<br>☐ lack of Vit D / Ca++ sup Poor understanding of:<br>☐ role of exercise in weight control<br>☐ wt control with Prednisone<br>Admit Weight _____<br>Admit Ht _____<br>Admit BMI _____<br>Admit WC _____ | ☐ RD consult<br>☐ Review BMI or WC and identify target weight and strategies for weight control<br>☐ Education class (nutrition strategies, role of supplements, Prednisone and weight control strategies)<br>☐ Education re: need for ongoing weight monitoring<br>☐ Food diary<br>☐ Physical activity log<br>Weight: _____<br>BMI: _____<br>WC: _____ | ☐ BMI 21 to 25<br>☐ wt loss 1-2 lb/ week<br>☐ weight stable<br>☐ WC < 35 female<br>WC < 40 male<br>Weight: _____<br>BMI: _____<br>WC: _____<br>☐ Goal met<br>☐ Progressing<br>☐ Not progressing<br>☐ Referral to structured weight management program _____ | ☐ BMI 21 to 25<br>☐ wt loss 1-2 lb/ week<br>☐ weight stable<br>☐ WC < 35 female<br>WC < 40 male<br>Weight: _____<br>BMI: _____<br>WC: _____<br>☐ Goal met<br>☐ Progressing<br>☐ Not progressing<br>☐ Referral to structured weight management program _____ | ☐ BMI 21 to 25<br>☐ wt loss 1-2 lb/ week<br>☐ weight stable<br>☐ WC < 35 female<br>WC < 40 male<br>Weight: _____<br>BMI: _____<br>WC: _____<br>☐ Goal met<br>☐ Progressing<br>☐ Not progressing<br>☐ Referral to structured weight management program _____ |

# PATIENT CARE PLAN: Pulmonary Rehabilitation

| Problems / Goals | Initial Assessment Session # ___ Date/Initial : ___ | Plan | Reassessment 30 days/Date: ___ Session # ___ Date/Initials: ___ | Reassessment 60 days/Date: ___ Session # ___ Date/Initial: ___ | Final Assessment 90 days/Date ___ Session # ___ Date/Initial: ___ |
|---|---|---|---|---|---|
| **Medications** Problem: □ Medication Non-adherence Goal: □ Adherence to prescribed medications | □ Patient reports taking medications as prescribed ___ % of the time. | □ Review prescribed medications' purpose, schedule, side-effects and importance of compliance | □ Medication list reviewed □ Taking medications 100% of the time □ Met □ Approx ___ % □ Not progressing | □ Medication list reviewed □ Taking medications 100% of the time □ Met □ Approx ___ % □ Not progressing | □ Medication list reviewed □ Taking medications 100% of the time □ Met □ Approx ___ % □ Not progressing, see DC Summary |
| **Inhaled medications** Problem: □ Incorrect inhaled Rx use, technique Goal: □ Correct technique/ timing & care MDI, DPI, nebulizer | Pt demo correct technique: MDI: □ Yes □ No □ NA DPI: □ Yes □ No □ NA Neb: □ Yes □ No □ NA □ When to replace MDI | Instruct correct technique/ timing & care: □ MDI □ DPI □ Nebulizer □ Return demo use of inhaler | Pt demo correct technique/timing: MDI: □ Yes □ No □ Reinstructed DPI: □ Yes □ No □ Reinstructed Neb: □ Yes □ No □ Reinstructed | Pt demo correct technique/timing: MDI: □ Yes □ No □ Reinstructed DPI: □ Yes □ No □ Reinstructed Neb: □ Yes □ No □ Reinstructed | Pt demo correct technique/timing: MDI: □ Yes □ No □ See DC summary DPI: □ Yes □ No □ see DC summary Neb: □ Yes □ No □ See DC summary |
| **Secretion clearance** Problem: □ Ineffective secretion clearance Goal: □ pt demonstrates effective cough, effective secretion clearance | Pt reports: □ No cough □ Non-prod cough □ Prod cough w/ infections □ Prod cough daily <1 Tbsp. □ Prod cough daily > 1 Tbsp. □ Nasal congestion | Instruct: □ Controlled cough □ CPT □ Vibratory PEP device □ VEST □ Role of exercise in secretion clearance □ NS nasal spray ___ | Pt demo correct: Effective cough: □ Yes □ No □ Reinstructed CPT: □ Yes □ No □ Reinstructed Device: □ Yes □ No □ Reinstructed □ NS nasal spray Sputum management: □ Improved □ No Change ___ | Pt demo correct: Effective cough: □ Yes □ No □ Reinstructed CPT: □ Yes □ No □ Reinstructed Device: □ Yes □ No □ Reinstructed □ NS nasal spray Sputum management: □ Improved □ No Change ___ | Pt demo correct: Effective cough: □ Yes □ No □ Reinstructed CPT: □ Yes □ No □ Reinstructed Device: □ Yes □ No □ Reinstructed □ NS nasal spray Sputum management: □ Improved □ No Change ___ |
| **Knowledge deficit** Problem: □ Respiratory Infection Prevention / Management Goal: □ pt describes signs/ symptoms of infection, methods to identify and prevent | Pt reports: □ Rare respiratory infection □ 0-1/yr respiratory infection □ >1/yr respiratory infection □ Hospitalized in past 12 mo x ___ □ Inadequate cleaning of respiratory equipment | Instruct: □ Hydration □ Hand hygiene □ Evaluate sputum □ When to call MD □ s/sx to report: purulent sputum, > dyspnea, > fatigue □ influenza vaccine pneumovax □ cleaning of respiratory equipment | Pt demo: Improved hydration: □ Yes □ No □ Reinstructed Hand hygiene: □ Yes □ No □ Reinstructed Eval sputum: □ Yes □ No □ Reinstructed Verbalize when to call MD: □ Yes □ No □ Reinstructed □ Cleaning of respiratory equipment | Pt demo: Improved hydration: □ Yes □ No □ Reinstructed Hand washing: □ Yes □ No □ Reinstructed Eval sputum: □ Yes □ No □ Reinstructed Verbalize when to call MD: □ Yes □ No □ Reinstructed □ cleaning of respiratory equipment | Pt demo: Improved hydration: □ Yes □ No □ See DC Summary Hand washing: □ Yes □ No □ See DC Summary Eval sputum: □ Yes □ No □ See DC Summary Verbalize when to call MD: □ Yes □ No □ See DC Summary |

## Exercise & Fitness
**Problem:**
- ☐ Deconditioning
- ☐ No regular exercise
- ☐ Knowledge deficit exercise guidelines and safety

**Goal:**
- ☐ Aerobic Exercise 30-60 mins x 9 weeks
- ☐ PR: 2-3/wk
- ☐ Resistance: 2-3 times weekly
- ☐ _____

## Diabetes Management
**Problem:**
- ☐ non-fasting BG
- ☐ < 80
- ☐ >240
- ☐ Poor knowledge of DM management

**Goal:**
- ☐ non-fasting BG 80-240
- ☐ HbA1C <7%
- ☐ self-mngt of DM

---

Current Exercise level:
Type: _____
Frequency: _____
Duration: _____
- ☐ Sedentary or < 3x/week for 20 mins
- ☐ barriers to exercise
_____ Initial MET
Level _____
THR: _____

Diabetic: ☐ Yes ☐ No
Type: _____
- ☐ BG (blood glucose) levels:
- ☐ Self Monitors BG at home:
  - ☐ Yes ☐ No
  Frequency _____
- ☐ HbA1C <7
- ☐ HbA1C _____

---

- ☐ Review with patient benefits and core components of exercise program
- ☐ Review how to measure and monitor dyspnea level
- ☐ Review exercise intensity
- ☐ Review exercise safety guidelines

Home Exercise:
- ☐ Review home exercise guidelines
- ☐ Borg: 3-4/10

- ☐ Obtain glucometer
- ☐ Schedule DM program
- ☐ Non-fasting BG 80-240
- ☐ Review signs/symptoms of hyper/hypoglycemia
- ☐ RD consult/coaching appt
- ☐ Patient to take BG pre & or post exercise.

---

Aerobic Exercise 30-60 mins 3-7x/wk
THR: _____
- ☐ Met
- ☐ Progressing
- ☐ Not progressing
- ☐ Borg _____
MET Level _____
Time: _____ minutes
Home Exercise:
Mode: _____
Freq: _____ times/wk
Time: _____ minutes
N/A
- ☐ non-fasting BG 80-240
- ☐ HbA1C <7% HbA1C _____
- ☐ Met
- ☐ Progressing
- ☐ Not progressing _____

---

Aerobic Exercise 30-60 mins 3-7x/wk
THR: _____
- ☐ Met
- ☐ Progressing
- ☐ Not progressing
- ☐ Borg _____
MET Level _____
Time: _____ minutes
Home Exercise:
Mode: _____
Freq: _____ times/wk
Time: _____ minutes
N/A
- ☐ non-fasting BG 80-240
- ☐ HbA1C <7% HbA1C _____
- ☐ Met
- ☐ Progressing
- ☐ Not progressing _____

---

Aerobic Exercise 30-60 mins 3-7x/wk
THR: _____
- ☐ Met
- ☐ Progressing
- ☐ Further f/u –see DC summary
- ☐ Borg _____
MET Level _____
Time: _____ minutes
Home Exercise:
Mode: _____
Freq: _____ times/wk
Time: _____ minutes
N/A
- ☐ non-fasting BG 80-240
- ☐ HbA1C <7%
- ☐ HbA1C _____
- ☐ Met
- ☐ Progressing
- ☐ Further f/u –see DC summary
- ☐ _____

---

## Staff Signatures/credentials:
_____

_____

**Stamper Plate:**
..............................

---

## Medical Director:

**MD Initial Review**
- ☐ Outcome assessment reviewed
- ☐ Exercise plan approved as documented
- ☐ Exercise plan approved with the following modifications:
- ☐ Treatment plan and goals support patient needs/ abilities
- ☐ Special precautions concerning this patient:

MD Signature _____
Date _____ Time _____

**MD f/u Review**
- ☐ Continue with current program
- ☐ Continue program with the following changes:

MD Signature _____
Date _____ Time _____

**Final Review**
- ☐ Outcome Assessment Reviewed

MD Signature _____

**MD Review**
- ☐ Continue with current program
- ☐ Continue program with the following changes:

MD Signature _____
Date _____ Time _____

_____ is a _____ y/o female who presents to Pulmonary Rehabilitation program with a physician order for monitored exercise and education to optimize physical and social performance and autonomy, increase strength and endurance and control dyspnea. Principle Diagnoses: COPD (496)    Onset Date:

The following information was gathered from the patient:

Smoking Hx: smoked, Number of Pack Years = _____ Quit_____

PMH:   CV    GI       DM      ortho    psychiatric
PSH:

Pulmonary Hosp past 12 months: N/A ED visits for Pulmo past 12 months: N/A
Pulmonary Infections past 12 months: N/A
Knows signs of infections: N/A       Prevention Y/N    Management Y/N

## Current Inhaled Medications
Short-Acting Beta2-agonist: N/A
Long-Acting Beta2-agonist: N/A
Short-Acting Anticholinergic: N/A
Long-Acting  Anticholinergic: N/A
Inhaled Corticosteroid: N/A
Combined Inhaled Corticosteroid & Long Acting Beta2-agonist: N/A
Spacer: N/A            Hx of Thrush: N/A

## Current Oral Pulmonary Medications: N/A

## Respiratory Equipment
Hand Held Nebulizer: N/A       Medication Solution: N/A       Cleans: N/A
Peak Flow Meter: N/A    ❒ Flutter N/A  ❒ Acapella N/A  ❒ Vest N/A
Oxygen: N/A via N/A L/pm: N/A delivery system: Concentrator
Home vendor: N/A

Advance Directive: N/A Gave info: N/A Who has copies: N/A, N/A and N/A
Allergy History:
   Medications:
   Environmental: N/A     pets at home_____
   Food:

Vaccine Hx: Annual flu vaccine annually Yes/yr: pneumovax vaccine Yes/yr:

Coughing Hx: N/A  nasal congestion Y/N  PND Y/N  sinus pain Y/N
Mucus: Color: N/A          Consistency: N/A          Amount/day: N/A
Needs training on secretion clearance Y/N Management of nasal congestion Y/N

Current height:          Current weight:          Wt one year ago_____

Sleep abnormalities: N/A    Total Hrs: N/A   Wake up in the middle of night: N/A for: N/A   Pillows: N/A   Bipap or CPAP: N/A   Home vendor: N/A

Mobility Assistive Device: none    Falls: N/A   Balance: N/A   Stairs at home:

Activities of Daily Living:

| | | | |
|---|---|---|---|
| Bathing: | No barrier 0/10 | Vacuuming: | No barrier 0/10 |
| Toileting: | No barrier 0/10 | Carrying objects | No barrier 0/10 |
| Dressing: | No barrier 0/10 | Laundry: | No barrier 0/10 |
| Cooking: | No barrier 0/10 | Sexual activity: | No barrier 0/10 |
| Eating: | No barrier 0/10 | Shopping: | No barrier 0/10 |
| Washing Dishes: | No barrier 0/10 | Sports/ N/A: | No barrier 0/10 |
| Bending: | No barrier 0/10 | Hobbies/ | No barrier 0/10 |
| Sweeping: | No barrier 0/10 | Pushing/Pulling: | No barrier 0/10 |
| Steps/Stairs: | No barrier 0/10 | | |

Home exercise program: N/A    Equipment available: N/A

Living Situation: House with no incline or stairs
Transportation: Currently drives
Occupational history: Work related exposures    N/A    N/A
Went out on regular retirement.
Education History: grade school
Learning style: ❒ Visual ❒ Auditory and ❒ Kinesthetic
Barriers to learning: N/A
Medical History: N/A, N/A, N/A, N/A and N/A
Language barriers: N/A    Primary language: N/A    Secondary language: N/A
Cultural Barriers:
Impairment: ❒ Hearing ❒ Vision ❒ Cognitive
Aspects of family and home that affect rehabilitation treatment:

Evidence of physician / emotional or financial abuse or neglect N/A
Eligible for Handicap placard N/A    Has placard N/A    Given application N/A

Panic Control: No barrier needs training on control of panic, relaxation techniques, dyspnea control with panic

**Pain Assessment:** Pain: 0/10        Intensity:        Quality:
Location:        Management:

Pulmonary Function Test results on_____showed a N/A
❒ obstruction or ❒ restrictive and N/A reduction in diffusion.

**Physical Exam V/s: see exercise record**
_____; SaO2 _____ % on room air and when using
O2 at_____ L/pm was SaO2_____%; N/A Edema;
Respirations required the use of accessory muscles No barrier; Breath sounds

**Patient Goals:**

❒ Breathe better
❒ Increase my physical endurance
❒ Have energy to enjoy my family and friends
❒ Rely less on others
❒ Ease with daily activities and walking
❒ Feel less anxious about my condition and not panic

❒ Understand and use my medication correctly
❒ Control my cough
❒ Make fewer visits to the hospital or emergency room
❒ Quit smoking
❒ Lose weight
❒ Others goals:

RN Signature: _____

Date: _____Time:_____ Minutes:_____

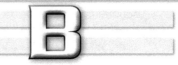

# American Thoracic Society/ European Respiratory Society Statement: Key Concepts and Advances in Pulmonary Rehabilitation

The following is a portion of an American Thoracic Society/European Respiratory Society statement of key concepts and advances in pulmonary rehabilitation. For the complete references cited in this appendix, see the source listed in the credit line at the end of the document. A link to the full article online is provided in the web resource.

This official statement of the American Thoracic Society (ATS) and the European Respiratory Society (ERS) was approved by the ATS Board of Directors, in June 2013 and the ERS Scientific and Executive Committees in January 2013 and February 2013, respectively.

## ABSTRACT

*Background*: Pulmonary rehabilitation is recognized as a core component of the management of individuals with chronic respiratory disease. Since the 2006 American Thoracic Society (ATS)/ European Respiratory Society (ERS) Statement on Pulmonary Rehabilitation, there has been considerable growth in our knowledge of its efficacy and scope.

*Purpose*: The purpose of this Statement is to update the 2006 document, including a new defini-

tion of pulmonary rehabilitation and highlighting key concepts and major advances in the field.

*Methods*: A multidisciplinary committee of experts representing the ATS Pulmonary Rehabilitation Assembly and the ERS Scientific Group 01.02, "Rehabilitation and Chronic Care," determined the overall scope of this update through group consensus. Focused literature reviews in key topic areas were conducted by committee members with relevant clinical and scientific expertise. The final content of this Statement was agreed on by all members.

*Results*: An updated definition of pulmonary rehabilitation is proposed. New data are presented on the science and application of pulmonary rehabilitation, including its effectiveness in acutely ill individuals with chronic obstructive pulmonary disease, and in individuals with other chronic respiratory diseases. The important role of pulmonary rehabilitation in chronic disease management is highlighted. In addition, the role of health behavior change in optimizing and maintaining benefits is discussed.

*Conclusions*: The considerable growth in the science and application of pulmonary rehabilitation since 2006 adds further support for its efficacy in a wide range of individuals with chronic respiratory disease.

# OVERVIEW

Pulmonary rehabilitation has been clearly demonstrated to reduce dyspnea, increase exercise capacity, and improve quality of life in individuals with chronic obstructive pulmonary disease (COPD) (1). This Statement provides a detailed review of progress in the science and evolution of the concept of pulmonary rehabilitation since the 2006 Statement. It represents the consensus of 46 international experts in the field of pulmonary rehabilitation.

On the basis of current insights, the American Thoracic Society (ATS) and the European Respiratory Society (ERS) have adopted the following new definition of pulmonary rehabilitation: "*Pulmonary rehabilitation is a comprehensive intervention based on a thorough patient assessment followed by patient-tailored therapies that include, but are not limited to, exercise training, education, and behavior change, designed to improve the physical and psychological condition of people with chronic respiratory disease and to promote the long-term adherence to health-enhancing behaviors.*"

Since the previous Statement, we now more fully understand the complex nature of COPD, its multisystem manifestations, and frequent comorbidities. Therefore, integrated care principles are being adopted to optimize the management of these complex patients (2). Pulmonary rehabilitation is now recognized as a core component of this process (figure 1) (3). Health behavior change is vital to optimization and maintenance of benefits from any intervention in chronic care, and pulmonary rehabilitation has taken a lead in implementing strategies to achieve this goal.

Noteworthy advances in pulmonary rehabilitation that are discussed in this Statement include the following:

- There is increased evidence for use and efficacy of a variety of forms of exercise training as part of pulmonary rehabilitation; these include interval training, strength training, upper-limb training, and transcutaneous neuromuscular electrical stimulation.
- Pulmonary rehabilitation provided to individuals with chronic respiratory diseases other than COPD (i.e., interstitial lung disease, bronchiectasis, cystic fibrosis, asthma, pulmonary hypertension, lung cancer, lung volume reduction surgery, and lung transplantation) has demonstrated improvements in symptoms, exercise tolerance, and quality of life.

- Symptomatic individuals with COPD who have lesser degrees of airflow limitation who participate in pulmonary rehabilitation derive similar improvements in symptoms, exercise tolerance, and quality of life as do those with more severe disease.
- Pulmonary rehabilitation initiated shortly after a hospitalization for a COPD exacerbation is clinically effective, safe, and associated with a reduction in subsequent hospital admissions.
- Exercise rehabilitation commenced during acute or critical illness reduces the extent of functional decline and hastens recovery.
- Appropriately resourced home-based exercise training has proven effective in reducing dyspnea and increasing exercise performance in individuals with COPD.
- Technologies are currently being adapted and tested to support exercise training, education, exacerbation management, and physical activity in the context of pulmonary rehabilitation.
- The scope of outcomes assessment has broadened, allowing for the evaluation of COPD-related knowledge and self-efficacy, lower- and upper-limb muscle function, balance, and physical activity.
- Symptoms of anxiety and depression are prevalent in individuals referred to pulmonary rehabilitation, may affect outcomes, and can be ameliorated by this intervention.

In the future, we see the need to increase the applicability and accessibility of pulmonary rehabilitation; to effect behavior change to optimize and maintain outcomes; and to refine this intervention so that it targets the unique needs of the complex patient.

# INTRODUCTION

Since the American Thoracic Society (ATS)/European Respiratory Society (ERS) Statement on Pulmonary Rehabilitation was published in 2006 (1), this intervention has advanced in several ways. First, our understanding of the pathophysiology underlying chronic respiratory disease such as chronic obstructive pulmonary disease (COPD) has grown. We now more fully appreciate the complex nature of COPD, its multisystem manifestations, and frequent comorbidities. Second, the science

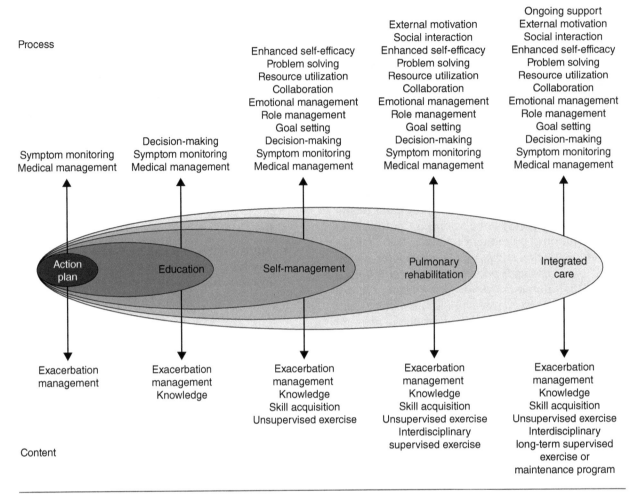

Process

Symptom monitoring
Medical management

Decision-making
Symptom monitoring
Medical management

Enhanced self-efficacy
Problem solving
Resource utilization
Collaboration
Emotional management
Role management
Goal setting
Decision-making
Symptom monitoring
Medical management

External motivation
Social interaction
Enhanced self-efficacy
Problem solving
Resource utilization
Collaboration
Emotional management
Role management
Goal setting
Decision-making
Symptom monitoring
Medical management

Ongoing support
External motivation
Social interaction
Enhanced self-efficacy
Problem solving
Resource utilization
Collaboration
Emotional management
Role management
Goal setting
Decision-making
Symptom monitoring
Medical management

Action plan    Education    Self-management    Pulmonary rehabilitation    Integrated care

Exacerbation
management

Exacerbation
management
Knowledge

Exacerbation
management
Knowledge
Skill acquisition
Unsupervised exercise

Exacerbation
management
Knowledge
Skill acquisition
Unsupervised exercise
Interdisciplinary
supervised exercise

Exacerbation
management
Knowledge
Skill acquisition
Unsupervised exercise
Interdisciplinary
long-term supervised
exercise or
maintenance program

Content

**Figure 1**    A spectrum of support for chronic obstructive pulmonary disease.

and application of pulmonary rehabilitation have evolved. For example, evidence now indicates that pulmonary rehabilitation is effective when started at the time or shortly after a hospitalization for COPD exacerbation. Third, as integrated care has risen to be regarded as the optimal approach toward managing chronic respiratory disease, pulmonary rehabilitation has established itself as an important component of this model. Finally, with the recognition that health behavior change is vital to optimization and maintenance of benefits from any intervention in chronic care, pulmonary rehabilitation has taken a lead in developing strategies to promote self-efficacy and thus the adoption of a healthy lifestyle to reduce the impact of the disease.

Our purpose in updating this ATS/ERS Statement on Pulmonary Rehabilitation is to present the latest developments and concepts in this field. By doing so, we hope to demonstrate its efficacy and applicability in individuals with chronic respiratory disease. By necessity, this Statement focuses primarily on COPD, because individuals with COPD represent the largest proportion of referrals to pulmonary rehabilitation (4), and much of the existing science is in this area. However, effects of exercise-based pulmonary rehabilitation in people with chronic respiratory disease other than COPD are discussed in detail. We hope to underscore the pivotal role of pulmonary rehabilitation in the integrated care of the patient with chronic respiratory disease.

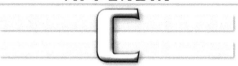

# Clinical Competency Guidelines for Pulmonary Rehabilitation Professionals

**T**able 2 from the Position Statement of the American Association of Cardiovascular and Pulmonary Rehabilitation. A link to the full position statement online is available on the web resource.

| Competency | Knowledge | Skill/Ability |
|---|---|---|
| Patient assessment and management | • Pulmonary anatomy, physiology, and pathophysiology<br>• Pulmonary disease risk factors<br>• Pulmonary assessments, diagnostic tests, and procedures, including pulmonary function testing, multidimensional staging of COPD (i.e., BODE index)<br>• Common comorbidities<br>• Exacerbation risks<br>• Individual patient's needs, expectations of treatment, and cultural framework<br>• Patient readiness to initiate behavior change<br>• The recommendation that pulmonary rehabilitation should be considered for all patients with chronic respiratory disease who have persistent symptoms, limited activity, or are unable to adjust to illness despite otherwise optimal medical management<br>• Current reimbursement criteria for pulmonary rehabilitation<br>• Impact of conditions or processes that might be considered contraindications to pulmonary rehabilitation such as severe bone and joint conditions, unstable cardiac conditions, and significant cognitive impairment<br>• Exercise and treatment protocols should be appropriate across the age, size, and physical development spectrum<br>• Tailoring rehabilitation interventions to meet the needs of the specific patient with regard to the underlying respiratory disease, physical limitations, and comorbidities<br>• Common comorbidities that limit or otherwise influence physical activity, symptom management, and quality of life, which may include metabolic disorders, musculoskeletal conditions, cardiovascular conditions, neuromuscular conditions, psychiatric and mood disorders, or other conditions<br>• Smoking cessation assessment<br>• Nutrition assessment | • Obtain a medical history, review medical records (including comorbidities), laboratory/radiologic data, pulmonary function data, smoking history, and data from questionnaires<br>• A focused symptom history centering on dyspnea—its severity, what brings it on, what relieves it<br>• Physical examination, including vital signs and respiratory and cardiac systems<br>• Critical appraisal of pulmonary function testing, arterial blood gas findings, and other pertinent laboratory/radiologic data<br>• Document patient preferences and goals<br>• Develop an ITP, in conjunction with the patient, with development of reasonable, important, and measurable patient goals<br>• Interactively communicate and counsel the patient/family on the treatment plan through shared decision making<br>• Document and communicate ITP and progress reports to the referring health care provider and other members of the interdisciplinary team<br>• Quantify patient outcomes through pre- and postprogram assessment of preestablished outcomes<br>• Modify therapy goals when clinical findings warrant change<br>• Identification and application of inclusion and exclusion criteria in current pulmonary rehabilitation guidelines<br>• Communicate potential inclusion/exclusion criteria issues with the medical director of the program and/or referring physician<br>• Review reimbursement criteria for pulmonary rehabilitation, including specific third-party payers, and be able to convey this information to the patient<br>• Use of age-appropriate teaching and treatment protocols<br>• Assessment of patients with obstructive, restrictive, and vascular lung disease, lung transplant, and other surgical lung interventions<br>• Accurately classify individuals with obstructive lung disease using spirometric data<br>• Identify limitations to exercise in the individual patient (including respiratory, symptomatic, musculoskeletal, cardiovascular, and psychological)<br>• Take appropriate actions to reduce fall risk in patients at risk for falls (e.g., patients with musculoskeletal or neurological issues or pulmonary hypertension)<br>• Take appropriate actions to intervene with high-flow oxygen in patients who are at risk for exercise-induced hypoxia (e.g., patients with ILD)<br>• Effectively communicate with the medical director and other health care providers on impediments and potential risks to the patient |

| Competency | Knowledge | Skill/Ability |
|---|---|---|
| Dyspnea assessment and management | • Domains of dyspnea measurement (e.g., sensory-perceptual experience, affective distress, symptom impact, or burden)<br>• Measurement tools (e.g., Modified Medical Research Council Dyspnea Scale, modified Borg, University of California San Diego Shortness of Breath Questionnaire, Baseline Dyspnea Index/ Transition Dyspnea Index, Chronic Respiratory Disease Questionnaire Dyspnea domain)<br>• Common descriptors of dyspnea quality (e.g., work/effort, tightness, and air hunger/unsatisfied inspiration)<br>• Breathing strategies<br>• Pharmacological/psychological treatment of dyspnea<br>• Dyspnea treatment options that include:<br> - Pulmonary rehabilitation<br> - Supplemental oxygen<br> - Pharmacologic therapy (e.g., bronchodilators and opioids)<br> - Nonpharmacologic approaches (e.g., breathing retraining, pursed lip breathing, cool air movement on face, and noninvasive ventilation)<br> - Cognitive behavioral therapy<br> - Causes and physiology of dyspnea in patients with lung disease: neurophysiologic mechanisms, cerebral processing of dyspnea, ventilatory constraints, pulmonary gas exchange abnormalities, peripheral muscle dysfunction, cardiac dysfunction, or any combination of the above | • Assessment of dyspnea through the appropriate use of a valid and reliable instrument<br>• Assessment of dyspnea onset/progress during exercise using the modified Borg scale<br>• Critically appraise the patient experience of subjective dyspnea using the common descriptors of dyspnea quality<br>• Instruct the patient through demonstration of effective breathing strategies (e.g., pursed-lip breathing, prolonged expiration, and diaphragmatic breathing)<br>• Facilitate patient mastery of techniques during exercise<br>• Assessment and patient instruction of the pathogenesis of dyspnea for the individual on the basis of the known physiologic mechanisms and pathophysiologic impact of the specific disease process |
| Oxygen assessment, management, and titration | • Limitations and uses of pulse oximetry<br>• Arterial blood gas interpretation<br>• Exercise and activity-induced hypoxemia<br>• Criteria for prescribing LTOT<br>• Oxygen interface devices<br>• Oxygen therapy patient education | • Pulse oximetry<br>• Use appropriate sensor placement to provide stable readings<br>• Communicate potential need for alternate testing (i.e., ABG) when unable to obtain accurate readings or if more thorough information is required (i.e., presence of hypercapnia)<br>• Develop a long-term oxygen therapy prescription<br>• Apply oxygen therapy flow to achieve SpO2 above 88%–90% or per physician recommendation<br>• Titrate flow settings and modify delivery devices when needed as exercise modality changes and intensity increases or decreases<br>• Perform oxygen assessments |

*(continued)*

| Competency | Knowledge | Skill/Ability |
|---|---|---|
| Oxygen assessment, management, and titration *(continued)* | | • Seek recommendations for sleep oxygen prescription (from the referring physician)<br>• Collaborate with the health provider and vendor to select the optimal oxygen delivery system to support adequate oxygenation and lessen the overall impact on patient's personal freedom and quality of life<br>• Assess delivery systems to confirm adequate oxygen prescription with home activity and exercise<br>• Provide the patient with a written oxygen prescription and training for oxygen use with daily activities and exercise<br>• When appropriate, instruct patients in self-monitoring oximetry use<br>• Promote patient understanding of the use, benefits, and risks of oxygen therapy<br>• Emotionally support the patient when implementing lifestyle-altering therapy |
| Collaborative self-management | • Behavior change<br>• Self-efficacy<br>• COPD exacerbation<br>• The importance of regular exercise and activity and potential barriers to regular exercise and activity<br>• Medication adherence, including inhaler technique<br>• End-of-life discussions and advanced directives, including palliative and hospice care | • Practice techniques to promote self-efficacy and health behavior change (i.e., increasing patient knowledge, goal setting, problem solving, and shared decision making)<br>• Practice strategies aimed at the prevention, early recognition, and treatment of the COPD exacerbation (i.e., the action plan)<br>• Address motivational issues<br>• Stress the need to promote physical activity in the home and community settings<br>• Adjust teaching to accommodate individual needs and limitations |
| Adherence | • Exercise/physical activity<br>• Nutrition counseling<br>• Medication and oxygen use<br>• Tobacco cessation | • Identify impairments to learning<br>• Emphasize why exercise is important, barriers to exercise, and how to overcome them<br>• Reinforce medication/oxygen regimens and practice inhaler technique<br>• Tobacco cessation counseling and provide resources<br>• Weight-loss strategies<br>• Weight-gain strategies |
| Medication/therapeutics | • The types of medications used for treatment of patients with COPD/other airway diseases including beta-agonists (short- and long-acting), anticholinergics (short- and long-acting), corticosteroids (e.g., oral and inhaled), phosphodiesterase 4 inhibitors, antibiotics, and combination therapies | • Demonstrate the correct use of devices used for medication delivery (e.g., aerosol, metered dose inhalers, and dry powder inhalers), secretion clearance techniques (e.g., postural drainage, chest physiotherapy, controlled cough technique, and ambulatory and stationary mechanical device use), and breathing techniques (e.g., pursed-lip breathing and diaphragmatic breathing) |

| Competency | Knowledge | Skill/Ability |
|---|---|---|
| Medication/ therapeutics *(continued)* | • The types of medications used for the treatment of patients with other chronic lung diseases (e.g., interstitial lung disease, vascular lung disease, and posttransplantation), including anti-inflammatory agents, immunosuppressive agents, and pulmonary artery vasodilators<br>• Indications/contraindications/side effects of each medication type<br>• The various types of secretion clearance techniques available (e.g., postural drainage, chest physiotherapy, coughing, and mechanical device use), and indications/contraindications/side effects of various techniques<br>• Types of breathing techniques (e.g., pursed-lip breathing and diaphragmatic breathing) and indications/ contraindications/side effects of these techniques<br>• Energy conservation techniques<br>• Demonstrate an understanding of the need for alterations/changes in the therapeutic plan | |
| Diseases not related to COPD | • Asthma, airway hyperresponsiveness, and exercise-induced bronchospasm<br>• Fear and anxiety associated with exercise<br>• Importance of a preexercise warm-up and postexercise cool-down<br>• Importance of peak flow monitoring<br>• Cystic fibrosis/bronchiectasis<br>• Importance of secretion clearance<br>• Cross-infection of patients/infection control<br>• Salt and fluid loss when sweating during exercise<br>• Lung transplantation<br>• Differences of pretransplant vs. posttransplant pulmonary rehabilitation<br>• Different types of ILD including idiopathic pulmonary fibrosis, sarcoidosis, asbestosis, silicosis, pneumoconiosis, pneumonitis, drug-induced lung disease, connective tissue disease, hypersensitivity pneumonitis, ARDS, and bronchiolitis obliterans<br>• Pulmonary hypertension | • Premedication, warm-up before exercise<br>• Good hand washing<br>• Maintains at least 3-ft (1-m) distance between patients when exercising<br>• NaCl and fluid replacement<br>• Secretion clearance techniques, including controlled cough, postural drainage, percussion, vibration, vibration vest and positive end-expiratory devices, flutter and oscillatory airway devices to facilitate airway clearance, respiratory muscle training devices and techniques, and bronchodilators<br>• Administer appropriate levels of supplemental oxygen<br>• Energy conservation<br>• Administer appropriate levels of supplemental oxygen to maintain SpO2 > 90%<br>• Instruct patients with pulmonary hypertension to avoid Valsalva maneuver with activity and exercise |

*(continued)*

| Competency | Knowledge | Skill/Ability |
|---|---|---|
| Diseases not related to COPD *(continued)* | • Anatomical and physiologic basis for symptoms resulting from pulmonary hypertension<br>• Importance of stopping exercise if the patient becomes symptomatic<br>• Rationale for avoiding isometric exercise and heavy weight lifting, Valsalva maneuver in surgical pulmonary patient<br>• Lung cancer treatment (surgery, chemotherapy, radiation therapy) | |
| Exercise testing | • Use of field testing (6MWT, shuttle walk) as outcome measure<br>• Importance of using standardized, consistent course/protocol and encouragement<br>• Published protocol guidelines<br>• Cardiopulmonary exercise testing<br>• Application of exercise testing results into exercise prescription | • Complete 6MWT using American Thoracic Society criteria<br>• Complete shuttle walk using published standards<br>• Complete symptom-limited cardiopulmonary exercise testing on selected patients as appropriate<br>• Appropriately monitor heart rate, blood pressure, perceived exertion, dyspnea, and SpO2<br>• Develop exercise prescription on the basis of exercise testing results when appropriate |
| Exercise training | • Normal and abnormal physiologic responses to exercise<br>• Specific pathophysiologic factors limiting exercise tolerance in pulmonary disease<br>• Physiologic basis of exercise training with pulmonary disease<br>• Exercise prescription on the basis of testing, comorbidities, and pulmonary disease-specific principles<br>• Safety and precautions of exercise training<br>• Function and activities of daily living<br>• Monitoring tools and oxygen administration with exercise training | • Recognition of signs and symptoms of exercise intolerance<br>• Identify exercise limitations of specific comorbidities, including systemic and pulmonary hypertension, diabetes, congestive heart failure, obesity, osteoporosis, and musculoskeletal abnormalities<br>• Develop an individualized and effective exercise prescription, including endurance, strengthening, and flexibility components (use interval training when appropriate)<br>• Accurately interpret and incorporate ongoing data into exercise prescription as individual responses change<br>• Appropriately modify exercise plan for patients with pain<br>• Take appropriate actions to modify exercise plan for patients with potential limitations resulting from patient parameters such as precautions on the basis of blood gas<br>• Utilize results of functional tests for balance and gait assistance to ensure ambulation safety<br>• Proficient use of monitoring tools and interpretation of data during exercise training |
| Psychosocial management | • Influence of pulmonary disease processes on emotional functioning, especially depression and anxiety<br>• Influence of pulmonary disease on social relationships (including family and friends) and quality of life<br>• Influence of pulmonary disease and emotional distress on cognitive functioning, especially memory and problem-solving skills | • Screen for psychological symptom burden (especially depression and anxiety), substance abuse, and poor quality of life<br>• Assessment of cognitive capacity for adequate participation in the rehabilitation program and adherence to medical recommendations<br>• Individual and group education/therapy to address stress management and effective coping strategies |

| Competency | Knowledge | Skill/Ability |
|---|---|---|
| Psychosocial management *(continued)* | • Influence of socioeconomic factors (i.e., work status, income level, educational attainment, and access to health care) on patient functioning<br>• Influence of psychosocial factors on adherence to health behaviors (i.e., smoking, diet, and exercise)<br>• Pharmacologic agents that are commonly used to treat psychological distress<br>• Available institutional/community resources (e.g., psychologist, social worker, and clergy) to address psychosocial needs<br>• Long-term planning needs of some patients, including advance directives, palliative care, and hospice information | • Referral to institutional/community resources to address psychosocial distress or cognitive concerns that are not otherwise addressed<br>• Referral to the mental health specialist should screening suggest significant psychiatric disease<br>• Measure and report outcomes of psychosocial functioning at the conclusion of the program |
| Tobacco cessation | • Psychological and physiologic behaviors of tobacco addiction<br>• Effects of smoking on chronic respiratory disease<br>• Established guidelines for treating tobacco use and tobacco prevention/cessation objectives<br>• Effects of secondhand smoke as a risk factor for chronic respiratory disease<br>• Influence of behavior change strategies on smoking cessation<br>• Available institutional/community resources (e.g., psychologist, social worker, and community smoking cessation programs) to support smoking cessation<br>• Effects, risks, and benefits of pharmacologic agents used to aid in tobacco cessation | • Behavioral interventions to promote tobacco cessation and long-term tobacco-free adherence<br>• Measure and report outcomes of tobacco cessation at the conclusion of the pulmonary rehabilitation program |
| Emergency responses for patients and program personnel | • How to identify and treat life-threatening situations or urgent/adverse and untoward events<br>• Appropriate emergency responses to changing signs and symptoms<br>• Changes in perceived dyspnea at rest or with exercise<br>• Participant comments/complaints<br>• Unexpected events, falls<br>• Sprains and fractures<br>• Abrasions | • Be familiar with the medical emergency policies and procedures on how to treat patients from onset of symptoms until resolution of emergency<br>• All staff should be BLS certified<br>• Use AED, bag-valve-mask, and oxygen correctly<br>• Appropriate emergency procedures in response to changing signs and symptoms such as chest pain<br>• Describe, for emergency personnel, the location of the incident, how to get there, and exits or room numbers<br>• Identify the location of all emergency equipment and supplies |

*(continued)*

| Competency | Knowledge | Skill/Ability |
|---|---|---|
| Emergency responses for patients and program personnel *(continued)* | • Peripheral neuropathy<br>• Muscle weakness<br>• Poor balance<br>• Lack of or inappropriate use of ambulatory assistive device<br>• Possible neck/head injury | • Participate in mock emergency in-service/practice<br>• Have the patient stop activity and assume a comfortable breathing position<br>• Lung auscultation and obtain RR<br>• Encourage the patient to use pursed-lip breathing and panic control techniques<br>• Have the patient use fast-acting bronchodilator medication<br>• Administer oxygen if required<br>• Monitor heart rate, blood pressure, and dyspnea rating<br>• Terminate patient exercise when appropriate<br>• Assess symptoms after terminating exercise and resting<br>• Use fall prevention, including standard screening tools with admission, train the patient in fall prevention techniques and strategies to enhance balance<br>• Practice fall prevention by close monitoring of high-risk patients (e.g., 1:1 monitoring with treadmill walking and use of seated exercises to promote safety)<br>• Recognize the need for assistive ambulatory devices to improve safety<br>• Refer to the appropriate provider for specific balance and/or fall prevention therapy<br>• Assess why fall occurred (i.e., equipment malfunction or participant accident when getting on or off equipment)<br>• Evaluate seriousness of events and then act accordingly |
| Universal standard precautions | • Importance of hand washing and universal precautions<br>• Appropriate actions to prevent spread of methicillin-resistant *Staphylococcus aureus, Clostridium difficile*<br>• Appropriate precautions for patients with varicella zoster (shingles)<br>• Importance of staff immunizations for influenza and varicella zoster<br>• Special precautions taken for patients in the rehabilitation setting with cystic fibrosis (i.e., antibiotic-resistant *Pseudomonas cepacia*)<br>• Signs and symptoms of tuberculosis and appropriate actions for evaluation and isolation | • Demonstrate proper hand washing technique<br>• Wipe down (or instruct patients to wipe down) exercise equipment before use<br>• Take appropriate actions with varicella zoster, instructing patients that lesions should be covered and patients should not attend rehabilitation until lesions have crusted over<br>• Patients with cystic fibrosis should exercise >3 ft away from other patients and contain secretions |

Abbreviations: ABG, arterial blood gases; AED, automated external defibrillator; ARDS, adult respiratory distress syndrome; BLS, basic life support; BODE, body mass index, airflow obstruction, dyspnea, and exercise capacity; COPD, chronic obstructive pulmonary disease; ILD, interstitial lung disease; ITP, individual treatment plan; LTOT, long-term oxygen therapy; NaCl, sodium chloride; PR, pulmonary rehabilitation; RR, respiratory rate; SpO2, pulse oximeter-measured oxygen saturation; 6MWT, 6-minute walk test.

Reprinted by permission from E.G. Collins et al., "Clinical Competency Guidelines for Pulmonary Rehabilitation Professionals: Position Statement of The American Association of Cardiovascular and Pulmonary Rehabilitation," *Journal of Cardiopulmonary Rehabilitation and Prevention* 34, no. 5 (2014): 291–302.

# D

# Example of a Typical Pulmonary Rehabilitation Facility and Examples of Pulmonary Rehabilitation Programs That Meet 2, 3, and 5 Days a Week

This appendix provides one example of a pulmonary rehabilitation facility, including descriptions of the various areas possible and detailed examples of activities that could be included in pulmonary rehabilitation programs.

## EXAMPLE PULMONARY REHABILITATION FACILITY

### Facility Areas

- Waiting or reception area
- Pulmonary rehabilitation administrative assistant's office
- Pulmonary rehabilitation program coordinator's office
- Storage room
- Classroom

### Description of Areas

- Pulmonary rehabilitation waiting or reception area and office
  - Equipment includes desks, computer, chairs for patients, staff equipment and supplies, and public telephone.
- Pulmonary rehabilitation classroom
  - Equipment includes patient notebooks and supplies appropriate for pulmonary rehabilitation training, tables, chairs, whiteboard, and VCR.
- Gymnasium
  - Equipment includes exercise equipment appropriate for pulmonary rehabilitation exercise sessions (e.g., indoor level-surface track, treadmills, stationary bikes, rowing machines, stair stepper, treadmills, floor exercise space, and weights) as well as blood pressure cuffs, stethoscopes, supplemental oxygen sources, pulse oximeters, and emergency equipment.

# EXAMPLES OF PULMONARY REHABILITATION PROGRAMS THAT MEET 2, 3, AND 5 DAYS A WEEK

Practitioners can use these examples to create unique programs.

## Typical twice-weekly, 8-week program outpatient pulmonary rehabilitation schedule*

| Week 1: Nutritional and Respiratory Assessments | |
|---|---|
| Appointment date: _____ Appointment time: _____ | |

| Week 2: Tuesday 01/22/19 1:30 P.M. | Thursday 01/24/19 1:30 P.M. |
|---|---|
| 1:30–2:30 Orientation to program; education session on lung disease<br>2:30–4:00 Supervised exercise | 1:30–2:30 Breathing retraining and inhaler use<br>2:30–4:00 Supervised exercise |

| Week 3: Tuesday 01/29/19 1:30 P.M. | Thursday 01/31/19 1:30 P.M. |
|---|---|
| 1:30–2:30 Lung medications<br>2:30–4:00 Supervised exercise | 1:30–2:30 Medications part 2 or review<br>2:30–4:00 Supervised exercise |

| Week 4: Tuesday 02/05/19 1:30 P.M. | Thursday 02/07/19 1:30 P.M. |
|---|---|
| 1:30–2:30 Food, lungs, and their relationship<br>2:30–4:00 Supervised exercise | 1:30–2:30 What are these tests for?<br>2:30–4:00 Supervised exercise |

| Week 5: Tuesday 02/12/19 1:30 P.M. | Thursday 02/14/19 1:30 P.M. |
|---|---|
| 1:30–2:30 Energy conservation<br>2:30–4:00 Supervised exercise and stairs | 1:30–2:30 Preventing infection<br>2:30–4:00 Supervised exercise and stairs |

| Week 6: Tuesday 02/19/19 1:30 P.M. | Thursday 02/21/19 1:30 P.M. |
|---|---|
| 1:30–2:30 Improving the immune system and relaxation techniques<br>2:30–4:00 Supervised exercise and stairs | 1:30–2:00 Relaxation and panic control<br>2:00–2:45 Living with lung disease<br>2:45–4:00 Supervised exercise |

| Week 7: Tuesday 02/26/19 1:30 P.M. | Thursday 02/28/19 1:30 P.M. |
|---|---|
| 1:30–2:30 Community resources<br>2:30–4:00 Supervised exercise | Individually scheduled 6-minute walk tests*<br>1:30–2:30 Benefits of exercise<br>2:30–4:00 Supervised exercise |

| Week 8: Tuesday 03/05/19 1:30 P.M. | Thursday 03/07/19 1:30 P.M. |
|---|---|
| 1:30–2:00 Taking pulmonary rehabilitation home<br>2:00–3:30 Supervised exercise | 1:30–2:00 Program evaluation and graduation<br>2:00–3:30 Supervised exercise |

*Make sure there is a 5–10 minute rest break between each activity

### Three-Day Pulmonary Rehabilitation Program

- Monday, Wednesday, Friday; 2-hour format
- Check-in: 10 minutes
- Warm-up and breathing retraining: 10 minutes
- Weight training and stretching: 20 minutes
- Aerobic training (ambulation on treadmill or level surface): 20 minutes
- Biking aerobic training (bike ergometer with arms and legs, legs only, or arm ergometry—patient may do one of the bike choices or a combination that would total 20 minutes): 20 minutes
- Cool-down: 10 minutes
- Education: 30 minutes
- Make sure there is a 5–10 minute rest break between each activity

### Five-Day Pulmonary Rehabilitation Program

- Monday through Friday, 4-hour format
- Check-in: 10 minutes
- Circuit weight training: 20 minutes
- Pulmonary hygiene (may include chest physical therapy, nebulizer, instruction in inhaler use, or breathing retraining): 30 minutes
- Floor exercise (breathing retraining, muscle toning, stretching): 60 minutes
- Aerobic training (ambulation on treadmill or level surface): 30 minutes
- Biking aerobic training (bike ergometer with arms and legs, legs only, or arm ergometry—patient may do one of the bike choices or a combination that would total 30 minutes): 30 minutes
- Education: 60 minutes
- Make sure there is a 5–10 minute rest break between each activity.

# Summary of Additional Recommended Guidelines for Pulmonary Rehabilitation

## Canadian Thoracic Society recommended guidelines

1. There are no differences in major patient-related outcomes of pulmonary rehabilitation between nonhospital-based sites (community or home) or hospital-based sites. It is strongly recommended that all COPD patients have access to pulmonary rehabilitation programs regardless of program. *Grade of recommendation: 1A*

2. Aerobic and resistance training offered together is better than aerobic training alone in improving endurance and functional ability. While aerobic training is the foundation of pulmonary rehabilitation, it is recommended that both aerobic and resistance training be prescribed to COPD patients. *Grade of recommendation: 2B*

3. It is recommended that longer pulmonary rehabilitation programs, beyond six to eight weeks duration, be provided for COPD patients. *Grade of recommendation: 2B*

4. It is strongly recommended that patients with moderate, severe, and very severe COPD participate in pulmonary rehabilitation. *Grade of recommendation: 1C*

5. The benefits of pulmonary rehabilitation are realized by both women and men. It is strongly recommended that both women and men be referred for pulmonary rehabilitation. *Grade of recommendation: 1C*

6. It is strongly recommended that COPD patients undergo pulmonary rehabilitation within one month following an AECOPD due to evidence supporting improved dyspnea, exercise tolerance, and health-related quality of life compared with usual care. *Grade of recommendation: 1B*

7. Pulmonary rehabilitation within one month following an AECOPD is also recommended due to evidence supporting reduced hospital admissions and mortality compared with usual care. *Grade of recommendation: 2C*

Reprinted by permission from D.D. Marciniuk et al., "Optimizing Pulmonary Rehabilitation in Chronic Obstructive Pulmonary Disease-Practical Issues: A Canadian Thoracic Society Clinical Practice Guideline," *Canadian Respiratory Journal* 17, no. 4 (2010): 159-168.

# British Thoracic Society recommended guidelines

1. Patients with COPD should be referred for pulmonary rehabilitation regardless of their smoking status. *Grade of recommendation: D*

2. People with chronic respiratory disease should be referred to pulmonary rehabilitation irrespective of coexistent stable cardiovascular disease. *Grade of recommendation: D*

3. Patients with an MRC dyspnea score of 5 who are housebound should not routinely be offered supervised pulmonary rehabilitation in their home. *Grade of recommendation: D*

4. Pulmonary rehabilitation programs should be a minimum of twice-weekly supervised sessions. *Grade of recommendation: D*

5. Pulmonary rehabilitation programs of 6–12 weeks are recommended. *Grade of recommendation: A*

6. A supervised pulmonary rehabilitation program is recommended for patients with COPD. *Grade of recommendation: A*

7. If considering a structured home-based rehabilitation program for patients with COPD, the following important factors need careful consideration: mechanisms to offer remote support and supervision, provision of home exercise equipment and patient selection. *Grade of recommendation: B*

8. Patients hospitalized for acute exacerbation of COPD should be offered pulmonary rehabilitation at hospital discharge to commence within 1 month of discharge. *Grade of recommendation: A*

9. Inspiratory muscle training (IMT) is not recommended as a routine adjunct to pulmonary rehabilitation. *Grade of recommendation: B*

10. No specific hormonal or nutritional supplement can currently be recommended as a routine adjunct to pulmonary rehabilitation. *Grade of recommendation: B*

11. Patients with non-cystic fibrosis (CF) bronchiectasis who have breathlessness affecting their activities of daily living (ADL) should have access to and be considered for pulmonary rehabilitation. *Grade of recommendation: D*

12. The routine referral of patients with asthma to pulmonary rehabilitation is not recommended. *Grade of recommendation: D*

13. Repeat pulmonary rehabilitation should be considered in patients who have completed a course of pulmonary rehabilitation more than 1 year previously. The likely benefits should be discussed and willing patients referred. *Grade of recommendation: B*

14. Earlier repeat pulmonary rehabilitation should be considered in individuals with accelerated physiological decline or if additional benefits on a shorter timescale would be clinically valuable. *Grade of recommendation: D*

15. All patients completing pulmonary rehabilitation should be encouraged to continue to exercise beyond the program. *Grade of recommendation: A*

Reprinted by permission from C.E. Bolton et al., "British Thoracic Society Guideline on Pulmonary Rehabilitation in Adults," *Thorax* 68 (2013): ii1–ii30.

## American Thoracic Society and European Respiratory Society recommended guidelines

1. There is increased evidence for use and efficacy of a variety of forms of exercise training as part of pulmonary rehabilitation; these include interval training, strength training, upper-limb training, and transcutaneous neuromuscular electrical stimulation.

2. Pulmonary rehabilitation provided to individuals with chronic respiratory diseases other than COPD (e.g., interstitial lung disease, bronchiectasis, cystic fibrosis, asthma, pulmonary hypertension, lung cancer, lung volume reduction surgery, or lung transplantation) has demonstrated improvements in symptoms, exercise tolerance, and quality of life.

3. Symptomatic individuals with COPD who have lesser degrees of airflow limitation who participate in pulmonary rehabilitation derive similar improvements in symptoms, exercise tolerance, and quality of life as do those with more severe disease.

4. Pulmonary rehabilitation initiated shortly after a hospitalization for a COPD exacerbation is clinically effective, safe, and associated with a reduction in subsequent hospital admissions.

5. Exercise rehabilitation commenced during acute or critical illness reduces the extent of functional decline and hastens recovery.

6. Appropriately resourced home-based exercise training has proven effective in reducing dyspnea and increasing exercise performance in individuals with COPD.

7. Technologies are currently being adapted and tested to support exercise training, education, exacerbation management, and physical activity in the context of pulmonary rehabilitation.

8. The scope of outcomes assessment has broadened, allowing for the evaluation of COPD-related knowledge and self-efficacy, lower- and upper-limb muscle function, balance, and physical activity.

9. Symptoms of anxiety and depression are prevalent in individuals referred to pulmonary rehabilitation, may affect outcomes, and can be ameliorated by psychological intervention.

Reprinted from M.A. Spruit et al., "An Official American Thoracic Society/European Respiratory Society Statement: Key Concepts and Advances in Pulmonary Rehabilitation," *American Journal of Respiratory Critical Care Medicine* Vol 188, no. 8 (2013): 1011–1027. Available: www.thoracic.org/statements/resources/copd/PRExecutive_Summary2013.pdf

## Australian/New Zealand recommended guidelines

1a. Patients with COPD should undergo pulmonary rehabilitation (strong recommendation, moderate quality evidence).

1b. Pulmonary rehabilitation is provided after an exacerbation of COPD, within 2 weeks of hospital discharge (weak recommendation, moderate quality evidence).

2. Patients with moderate-to-severe COPD (stable or following discharge from hospital for an exacerbation of COPD) should undergo pulmonary rehabilitation to decrease hospitalizations for exacerbations (strong recommendation, moderate-to-low quality evidence).

3a. Home-based pulmonary rehabilitation should be offered to patients with COPD as an alternative to usual care (weak recommendation, moderate-to-low quality evidence).

3b. Home-based pulmonary rehabilitation, including regular contact to facilitate exercise participation and progression, should be offered to patients with COPD as an alternative to hospital-based pulmonary rehabilitation (weak recommendation, moderate-to-low quality evidence).

3c. Community-based pulmonary rehabilitation, of equivalent frequency and intensity as hospital-based programmes, should be offered to patients with COPD as an alternative to usual care (weak recommendation, moderate quality evidence).

4. Patients with mild COPD (based on symptoms) undergo pulmonary rehabilitation (weak recommendation, moderate-to-low quality evidence).

5. The panel is unable to make a recommendation due to lack of evidence evaluating whether programmes of longer duration are more effective than the standard 8-week programmes.

6a. More research is needed to determine the optimal model of maintenance exercise programmes ("in-research" recommendation).

6b. Supervised maintenance programmes monthly or less frequently are insufficient to maintain the gains of pulmonary rehabilitation and should not be offered (weak recommendation, low quality evidence).

7. Pulmonary rehabilitation should be offered to all patients with COPD, irrespective of the availability of a structured multidisciplinary group education programme (weak recommendation, moderate-to-low quality evidence).

8. Further research of oxygen supplementation during training is required in patients with COPD who have exercise-induced desaturation to reduce the uncertainty around its lack of effect to date ("in research" recommendation).

9a. Patients with bronchiectasis undergo pulmonary rehabilitation (weak recommendation, moderate quality evidence).

9b. Patients with interstitial lung disease undergo pulmonary rehabilitation (weak recommendation, low quality evidence).

9c. Patients with pulmonary hypertension undergo pulmonary rehabilitation (weak recommendation, low quality evidence).

Reprinted by permission from J.A. Alison et al., "Australian and New Zealand Pulmonary Rehabilitation Guidelines," *Respirology* 22, no. 4 (2017); 800–819.

# References

## Chapter 1

1. Spruit MA, Singh SJ, Garvey C, ZuWallack R, Nici L, Rochester C, Hill K, Holland AE, Lareau SC, Man WDC, Pitta F, Sewell L, Raskin J, Bourbeau J, Crouch R, Franssen FME, Casaburi R, Vercoulen JH, Vogiatzis I, Gosselink R, Clini EM, Effing TW, Maltais F, Van der Palen J, Troosters T, Janssen DJA, Collins E, Garcia-Aymerich J, Brooks D, Fahy BF, Puhan MA, Hoogendoorn M, Garrod R, Schols AMJ, Carlin B, Benzo R, Meek P, Morgan M, Rutten-van Mölken MPMH, Ries AL, Make B, Goldstein RS, Dowson CA, Brozek JL, Donner CF, and Wouters EFM; on behalf of the ATS/ERS Task Force on Pulmonary Rehabilitation. An Official American Thoracic Society/European Respiratory Society Statement: Key Concepts and Advances in Pulmonary Rehabilitation. *Am J Respir Crit Care Med.* 2013;188(8):e13-e64.

2. Ries AL, et al. Pulmonary rehabilitation: joint ACCP/AACVPR evidence-based clinical practice guidelines. *Chest.* 2007;131(5 suppl):4S-42S.

3. Global Initiative for Chronic Obstructive Lung Disease. https://goldcopd.org.

4. Grone O, Garcia-Barbero M. Integrated care. A position paper of the WHO European office for integrated health care services. *Internat J Integrated Care.* 2001;1:1–15.

5. Sin DD, Anthonisen NR, Soriano JB, Agusti AG. Mortality in COPD: role of comorbidities. *Eur Resp J.* 2006;28:1245–1257.

6. Casas A, Troosters T, Garcia-Aymerich J, Roca J, Hernández C, Alonso C, del Pozo F, de Toledo P, Antó JM, Rodríguez-Roisín R, Decramer M. Integrated care prevents hospitalisations for exacerbations in COPD patients. *Eur Respir J.* 2006;28:123–130.

7. Puhan MA, Gimeno-Santos E, Cates CJ, Troosters T. Pulmonary rehabilitation following exacerbations of chronic obstructive pulmonary disease. *Cochrane DB Syst Rev.* 2009;21(1):CD005305.

8. Hodgkin JE, Balchum OJ, Kass I, et al. Chronic obstructive pulmonary diseases: current concepts in diagnosis and comprehensive care. *JAMA.* 1975;232:1243–1260.

9. Sahn SA, Nett LM, Petty TL. Ten year follow-up of a comprehensive rehabilitation program for severe COPD. *Chest.* 1980;77:311–314.

10. Bebout DE, Hodgkin JE, Zorn EG, et al. Clinical and physiological outcomes of a university-hospital pulmonary rehabilitation program. *Respir Care.* 1983;28:1468.

11. Ries AL. The scientific basis for pulmonary rehabilitation. *J Cardiovasc Pulm Rehab 10*: 418–441.

12. Casaburi R, Patessio A, Ioli F, Zanaboni S, Donner CF, Wasserman K. Reductions in lactic acidosis and ventilation as a result of exercise training in patient with obstructive lung disease. *Am Rev Respir Dis.* 1991;143:9–18.

13. Maltais F, Simard AA, Simard C, Jobin J, Desgagnés P, LeBlanc P. Oxidative capacity of the skeletal muscle and lactic acid kinetics during exercise in normal subjects and in patients with COPD. *Am J Respir Crit Care Med.* 1996;153:288–293.

14. Maltais F, LeBlanc P, Simard C, et al. Skeletal muscle adaptation to endurance training in patients with chronic obstructive pulmonary disease. *Am J Respir Crit Care Med.* 1996;154:442–447.

15. Porszasz J, Emtner M, Goto S, Somfay A, Whipp BJ, Casaburi R. Exercise training decreases ventilatory requirements and exercise-induced hyperinflation at submaximal intensities in patients with COPD. *Chest.* 2005;128:2025–2034.

16. Reardon J, Awad E, Normandin E, Vale F, Clark B, ZuWallack RL. The effect of comprehensive outpatient pulmonary rehabilitation on dyspnea. *Chest.* 1994;105:1046–1052.

17. O'Donnell DE, McGuire M, Samis L, Webb KA. General exercise training improves ventilatory and peripheral muscle strength and endurance in chronic airflow limitation. *Am J Respir Crit Care Med.* 1998;157:1489–1497.

18. Goldstein RS, Gort EH, Stubbing D, Avendano MA, Guyatt GH. Randomised controlled trial of respiratory rehabilitation. *Lancet.* 1994;344:1394–1397.

19. Ries AL, Kaplan RM, Limberg TM, Prewitt LM. Effects of pulmonary rehabilitation on physiologic and psychosocial outcomes in patients with chronic obstructive pulmonary disease. *Ann Intern Med.* 1995;122:823–832.

20. National Emphysema Treatment Trial Research Group. A randomized trial comparing lung-volume–reduction surgery with medical therapy for severe emphysema. *New Engl J Med.* 2003;348:2059–2073.

21. Ries AL, Make BJ, Shing ML, et al. The effects of pulmonary rehabilitation in the National Emphysema Treatment Trial. *Chest.* 2005;128:3799–3809.

22. ACCP/AACVPR Pulmonary Rehabilitation Guidelines Panel. Pulmonary rehabilitation: joint ACCP/AACVPR evidence-based guidelines. *Chest.* 1997;112:1363–1396.

23. Griffiths TL, Burr ML, Campbell IA, et al. Results at 1 year of outpatient multidisciplinary pulmonary rehabilitation: a randomised controlled trial. *Lancet.* 2000;29:362–369.

24. California Pulmonary Rehabilitation Collaborative Group. Effects of pulmonary rehabilitation on dyspnea, quality of life and health care costs in California. *J Cardiopulm Rehabil.* 2004;24:52–62.

25. Raskin J, Spiegler P, McCusker C, et al. The effect of pulmonary rehabilitation on healthcare utilization in chronic obstructive pulmonary disease: the Northeast Pulmonary Rehabilitation Consortium. *J Cardiopulm Rehabil.* 2006;26:231–236.

26. Bourbeau J, Julien M, Maltais F, et al. Reduction of hospital utilization in patients with chronic obstructive pulmonary disease: a disease-specific self-management intervention. *Arch Intern Med.* 2003;163:585–591.

27. Medicare program: changes to the hospital outpatient prospective payment system and CY 2010 payment rates. *Fed Regist.* 2009;74(223):60566–60574. 42 CFR §§410, 416, 419. 13.

28. Camp PG, Hernandez P, Bourbeau J, Kirkham A, Debigare R, Stickland MK, Goodridge D, Marciniuk DD, Road JD, Bhutani M, Dechman G. Pulmonary rehabilitation in Canada: a report from the Canadian Thoracic Society COPD Clinical Assembly. *Can Respir J.* 2015;22(3):147–152.

29. Alison JA, McKeough ZJ, Johnston K, McNamara RJ, Spencer LM, Jenkins SC, Hill CJ, McDonald VM, Frith P, Cafarella P, Brooke M, Cameron-Tucker HL, Candy S, Cecins N, Chan ASL, Dale M, Dowman LM, Granger C, Halloran S, Jung P, Lee A, Leung R, Matulik T, Osadnik C, Roberts M, Walsh J, Wootton S, Holland AE. On behalf of the Lung Foundation Australia and the Thoracic Society of Australia and New Zealand. Australian and New Zealand Pulmonary Rehabilitation Guidelines. *Respirology.* 2017;22:800–819.

30. Nishi SP, Zhang W, Kuo YF, Sharma G. Pulmonary rehabilitation utilization in older adults with chronic obstructive pulmonary disease, 2003 to 2012. *J Cardiopulm Rehab Prev.* 2016;36(5):375–382.

31. Camp PG, et al. Pulmonary rehabilitation in Canada.

32. Marciniuk DD, Brooks D, Butcher S, Debigare R, et al. Optimizing pulmonary rehabilitation in chronic obstructive pulmonary disease-practical issues: A Canadian Thoracic Society Clinical Practice Guideline. *Can Respir J.* July/August 2010;17(4):159-168.

33. Nakazawa A, Cox NS, Holland AE. Current best practice in rehabilitation in interstitial lung disease. *Ther Adv Respir Dis.* 2017;11(2):115–128

34. Guell MR, Cejudo P, Ortego F, Puy MC, et al. Benefits of a long-term maintenance pulmonary rehabilitation program for patients with COPD. *Ann Am Thorac Soc.* 2017;195:622–629.

## Chapter 2

1. Spruit MA, Singh SJ, Garvey C, et al. An official American Thoracic Society/European Respiratory Society statement: Key concepts and advances in pulmonary rehabilitation. *Am J Respir Crit Care Med.* 2013;188(8):e13-e64.

2. Rochester CL, Fairburn C, Crouch RH. Pulmonary rehabilitation for respiratory disorders other than chronic obstructive pulmonary disease. *Clin Chest Med.* 2014;35(2):369–389.

3. McCarthy B, Casey D, Devane D, Murphy K, Murphy E, Lacasse Y. Pulmonary rehabilitation for chronic obstructive pulmonary disease. *Cochrane DB Syst Rev.* 2015;(2):CD003793.

4. Global Initiative for Chronic Obstructive Lung Disease. *Global Strategy for the Diagnosis, Management, and Prevention of Chronic Obstructive Pulmonary Disease 2017 Report.* https://goldcopd.org/gold-2017-global-strategy-diagnosis-management-prevention-copd/\

5. Fried L, Tangen C, Walston J, Newman A, Hirsch C, Gottdiener J, Seeman T, Tracy R, Kop W, Burke G, McBurnie M. Frailty in older adults: evidence for a phenotype. *J Gerontol.* 2001;56(3):M146-M157.

6. Maddocks M, Kon SSC, Canavan JL, et al. Physical frailty and pulmonary rehabilitation in COPD: a prospective cohort study. *Thorax.* 2016;71(11):988–995.

7. Sahin H, Naz I, Varol Y, Aksel N, Tuksavul F, Ozsoz A. Is a pulmonary rehabilitation program effective in COPD patients with chronic hypercapnic failure? *Expert Rev Respir Med.* 2016;10(5):593–598.

8. Wedzicha JA, Miravitlles M, Hurst JR, et al. Management of COPD exacerbations: a European Respiratory Society/American Thoracic Society guideline. *Eur Respir J.* 2017;49(3):1600791.

9. *CDC 033 Asthma surveillance data.* www.cdc.gov/asthma/asthmadata.htm.

10. Carson KV, Chandratilleke MG, Picot J, Brinn MP, Esterman AJ, Smith BJ. Physical training for asthma. *Cochrane DB Syst Rev.* 2013;(9):CD001116.

11. Alexander BM, Petren EK, Rizvi S, et al. *Annual Data Report 2015. Cyst Fibrosis Foundation Patient Registry.* 2016:1–94. www.cff.org/Our-Research/CF-Patient-Registry/2015-Patient-Registry-Annual-Data-Report.pdf.

12  Yankaskas JR, Marshall BC, Sufian B, Simon RH, Rodman D. Cystic fibrosis adult care: consensus conference report. *Chest.* 2004;125(1 Suppl.).

13  Radtke T, Nolan SJ, Hebestreit H, Kriemler S. Physical exercise training for cystic fibrosis. *Cochrane DB Syst Rev.* 2015;(6):CD002768.

14  Newall C, Stockley RA, Hill SL. Exercise training and inspiratory muscle training in patients with bronchiectasis. *Thorax.* 2005;60:943–948.

15  Huppmann P, Sczepanski B, Boensch M, et al. Effects of inpatient pulmonary rehabilitation in patients with interstitial lung disease. *Eur Respir J.* 2013;42(2):444–453.

16  Dowman L, Hill CJ, Holland AE. Pulmonary rehabilitation for interstitial lung disease (review). *Cochrane DB Syst Rev Pulm.* 2014;(10):1–53.

17  Raghu G, Collard HR, Egan JJ, et al. An official ATS/ERS/JRS/ALAT statement: Idiopathic pulmonary fibrosis: evidence-based guidelines for diagnosis and management. *Am J Respir Crit Care Med.* 2011;183(6):788–824.

18  Morisset J, Bube BP, Garvey C, et al. The unmet educational needs of patients with interstitial lung disease. Setting the stage for tailored pulmonary rehabilitation. *Ann Am Thorac Soc.* 2016;13(7):1026–1033.

19  Morris NR, Kermeen FD, Holland AE. Exercise-based rehabilitation programmes for pulmonary hypertension. *Cochrane DB Syst Rev.* 2017;2017(1).

20  Galie N, Corris PA, Frost A, et al. Updated treatment algorithm of pulmonary arterial hypertension. *J Am Coll Cardiol.* 2013;62:D60–D72.

21  Li M, Mathur S, Chowdhury NA, et al. Pulmonary rehabilitation in lung transplant candidates. *J Heart Lung Transplant.* 2013;32.

22  Dierich M, Tecklenburg A, Fuehner T, et al. The influence of clinical course after lung transplantation on rehabilitation success. *Transpl Int.* 2013;26:322–330.

23  Rochester CL. Pulmonary rehabilitation for patients who undergo lung-volume-reduction surgery or lung transplantation. *Respir Care.* 2008;53(9):1196–1202.

24  Jones LW, Peddle CJ, Eves ND, et al. Effects of presurgical exercise training on cardiorespiratory fitness among patients undergoing thoracic surgery for malignant lung lesions. *Cancer.* 2007;110(3):590–598.

25  Franssen FME, Rochester CL. Comorbidities in patients with COPD and pulmonary rehabilitation: do they matter? *Eur Respir Rev.* 2014;23(131):131–141.

26  King CS, Nathan SD. Idiopathic pulmonary fibrosis: effects and optimal management of comorbidities. *Lancet Respir Med.* 2017;5(1):72–84.

27  Tashkin DP, Murray RP. Smoking cessation in chronic obstructive pulmonary disease. *Respir Med.* 2009;103(7):963–974.

28  Siu AL. U.S. Preventive Services Task Force. Behavioral and pharmacotherapy interventions for tobacco smoking cessation in adults, including pregnant women: U.S. Preventive Services Task Force recommendation statement. *Ann Intern Med.* 2015;163:622–634.

29  Van Eerd EAM, Van der Meer RM, Van Schayck OCP, et al. Smoking cessation for people with chronic obstructive pulmonary disease. *Cochrane DB Syst Rev.* 2016;8:1–76.

30  Pires-Yfantouda R, Absalom G, Clemens F. Smoking cessation interventions for COPD: a review of the Literature. *Respir Care.* 2013;58(11);1955–1962.

31  World Health Organization. Adherence to long-term therapies: evidence for action. 2003. http://apps.who.int/iris/bitstream/handle/10665/42682/9241545992.pdf.

32  Blackstock FC, ZuWallack R, Nici L, Lareau S. Why don't our patients with chronic obstructive pulmonary disease listen to us? The enigma of nonadherence. *Ann Am Thorac Soc.* 2016;13(3):317–323.

33  Spruit MA, Vercoulen JH, Sprangers MA, Wouters EF. Fatigue in COPD: an important yet ignored symptom. *Lancet Resp Med.* 2017;5(7):542–544.

34  Atkins CP, Gilbert D, Brockwell GD, Wilson RS. Fatigue in sarcoidosis and idiopathic pulmonary fibrosis: differences in character and severity between disease. *Sarcoidosis Vasc Diffuse Lung Dis.* 2016;33(2):130–138.

35  Sasaki H, Kasagi F, et al. Grip strength predicts cause-specific mortality in middle-aged and elderly persons. *Am J Medicine.* 2007;120:337–342.

36  Cortopassi F, Celli B, et al. Longitudinal changes in handgrip strength, hyperinflation, and 6-minute walk distance in patients with COPD and a control group. *Chest.* 2015;148(4):986–994.

37  Soler X, Gaio E, Powell FL, et al. High prevalence of obstructive sleep apnea in patients with moderate to severe chronic obstructive pulmonary disease. *Ann Am Thorac Soc.* 2015;12(8):1219–1225.

38  Schiza S, Mermigkis C, Margaritopoulos GA, et al. Idiopathic pulmonary fibrosis and sleep disorders: no longer strangers in the night. *Eur Respir Rev.* 2015;24(136):327–339.

39  Collins EG, Bauldoff G, Carlin B, et al. Clinical competency guidelines for pulmonary rehabilitation professionals: position statement of the American Association of Cardiovascular and Pulmonary Rehabilitation. *J Cardiopulm Rehabil Prev.* 2014;34(5):291–302.

40  Villa A, Lui A, Limberg T, Larsen C, Baylon M, Mohney A, Soler X, Ries A. Pulmonary rehabilita-

tion corrects oxygen prescriptions in chronic lung disease patients. Abstract 1148485. *Resp Care.* 2011;1692.

41. eCFR Code of Federal Regulations Title 42: Public 410.47 Pulmonary rehabilitation program: conditions for coverage. www.gpo.gov/fdsys/granule /CFR-2010-title42-vol2/CFR-2010-title42-vol2 -sec410-47.

42. Popa-Velea O. Psychological intervention—a critical element of rehabilitation in chronic pulmonary disease. *J Med Life.* 2014;7(2):274–281.

43. Celli BR, Cote CG, Marin JM, et al. The body-mass index, airflow obstruction, dyspnea, and exercise capacity index in chronic obstructive pulmonary disease. *N Engl J Med.* 2004;350(10):1005–1012.

44. Cote CG, Celli BR. Pulmonary rehabilitation and the BODE index in COPD. *Eur Respir J.* 2005;26(4):630–636.

45. Jones PW, Harding G, Berry P, et al. Development and first validation of the COPD Assessment Test. *Eur Respir J.* 2009;34:648e54.

46. Hurst JR, Vestbo J, Anzueto A, et al. Susceptibility to exacerbation in chronic obstructive pulmonary disease. *N Engl J Med.* 2010;363(12):1128–1138.

## Chapter 3

1. Spruit MA, Singh SJ, Garvey C, et al. An official American Thoracic Society/European Respiratory Society statement: key concepts and advances in pulmonary rehabilitation. *Am J Respir Crit Care Med.* 2013;188:13–64.

2. Nici L, Donner C, Wouters E, et al. American Thoracic Society/European Respiratory Society statement on pulmonary rehabilitation. *Am J Respir Crit Care Med.* 2006;173:1390–1413.

3. Casaburi R, Porszasz J, Burns MR, Carithers ER, Chang RS, Cooper CB. Physiologic benefits of exercise training in rehabilitation of patients with severe chronic obstructive pulmonary disease. *Am J Respir Crit Care Med.* 1997;5:1541–1551.

4. O'Shea SD, Taylor NF, Paratz J. Peripheral muscle strength training in COPD—a systematic review. *Chest.* 2004;126:903–914.

5. Kongsgaard M, Backer V, Jorgensen K, Kjaer M, Beyer N. Heavy resistance training increases muscle size, strength and physical function in elderly male COPD patients. *Respir Med.* 2004;98:1000–1007.

6. Kofod LM, Dossing M, Steentoft J, Kristensen MT. Resistance training with ankle weight cuffs is feasible in patients with acute exacerbation of COPD. *J Cardiopulm Rehabil Prev.* 2017;37:49–56.

7. Phillips WT, Benton MJ, Wagner CL, Riley C. The effect of a single set resistance training on strength and functional fitness in pulmonary rehabilitation patients. *J Cardiopulm Rehabil.* 2006;26: 330–337.

8. Spruit MA, Gosselink R, Troosters T, De Paepe K, Decramer M. Resistance versus endurance training in patients with COPD and peripheral muscle weakness. *Eur Respir J.* 2002;19:1072–1078.

9. Zambom-Ferraresi F, Cebollero P, Gorostiaga EM, et al. Effects of combined resistance and endurance training versus resistance training alone on strength, exercise capacity, and quality of life in patients with COPD. *J Cardiopulm Rehabil Prev.* 2015;35:446–453.

10. Iepsen UW, Jorgensen KJ, Ringbaek T, Hansen H, Skrubbeltrang C, Lange P. A systematic review of resistance training versus endurance training in COPD. *J Cardiopulm Rehabil Prev.* 2015;35:163–172.

11. Mador MJ, Bozkanat E, Aggarwal A, Shaffer NP, Kufel TJ. Endurance and strength training in patients with COPD. *Chest.* 2004;125:2036–2045.

12. Kenn K, Gloeckl R, Behr J. Pulmonary rehabilitation in patients with idiopathic pulmonary fibrosis—a review. *Respiration.* 2013;86(2):89–99.

13. Holland A, Hill C. Physical training for interstitial lung disease. *Cochrane DB Syst Rev.* 2008;4:CD006322.

14. Dowman L, Hill CJ, Holland AE. Pulmonary rehabilitation for interstitial lung disease. *Cochrane DB Syst Rev.* 2014;10:CD006322.

15. Huppmann P, Sczepanski B, Boensch M, et al. Effects of inpatient pulmonary rehabilitation in patients with interstitial lung disease. *Eur Respir J.* 2013;42(2):444–453.

16. American College of Sports Medicine. *ACSM's Guidelines for Exercise Testing and Prescription.* 10th ed. Philadelphia: Wolters Kluwer/Lippincott Williams & Wilkins; 2018:118, 123, 125, 251–261.

17. Bolton CE, Bevan-Smith EF, Blakey JD, et al. British Thoracic Society guideline on pulmonary rehabilitation in adults. *Thorax.* 2013;68:ii1-ii30.

18. Maltais F, Decramer M, Casaburi R, et al. An official American Thoracic Society/European Respiratory Society statement: update on limb muscle dysfunction in chronic obstructive pulmonary disease. *Am J Respir Crit Care Med.* 2014;189(9):e15-e62.

19. Singer J, Yelin EH, Katz PP, et al. Respiratory and skeletal muscle strength in chronic obstructive pulmonary disease: impact on exercise capacity and lower extremity function. *J Cardiopulm Rehab Prev.* 2011;31:111–119.

20. Gea J, Pascual S, Casadevall C, Orozco-Levi M, Barreiro E. Muscle dysfunction in chronic obstructive pulmonary disease: update on causes and biological findings. *Thorac Dis.* 2015;7(10):e418-e438.

21. Casaburi R. Skeletal muscle dysfunction in chronic obstructive pulmonary disease. *Med Sci Sports Exerc.* 2001;33:S662-S670.

22. Gosselink R, Troosters T, Decramer M. Peripheral muscle weakness contributes to exercise limitation in COPD. *Am J Respir Crit Care Med.* 1996;153:976–980.

23. Crouch R. Physical and respiratory therapy for the medical and surgical patient. In: Hodgkin JE, Celli BR, Connors GL, eds. *Pulmonary Rehabilitation: Guidelines to Success.* 4th ed. St. Louis: Mosby/Elsevier; 2009:154–179.

24. Dean E. Optimizing outcomes: relating interventions to an individual's needs. In: Frownfelter D, Dean E, eds. *Cardiovascular and Pulmonary Physical Therapy: Evidence and Practice.* 4th ed. St. Louis: Mosby/Elsevier; 2006:247–261.

25. Gibbons RJ, Balady GJ, Bricker JT, et al. ACC/AHA 2002 guideline update for exercise testing: summary article. A report of the American College of Cardiology/American Heart Association Task Force on Practice Guidelines Committee to update the 1997 exercise testing guidelines. *J Am Coll Cardiol.* 2002;40(8):1531–1540.

26. American Thoracic Society/American College of Chest Physicians. ATS/ACCP statement on cardiopulmonary exercise testing. *Am J Respir Crit Care Med.* 2003;167:211–277.

27. Mezzani A. Cardiopulmonary exercise testing: basics of methodology and measurements. *Ann Am Thorac Soc.* 2017;14:S3-S11.

28. ZuWallack RL, Haggerty MC. Clinically meaningful outcomes in patients with chronic obstructive pulmonary disease. *Am J Med.* 2004;117(12A):49S-59S

29. American Association of Cardiovascular and Pulmonary Rehabilitation. *Guidelines for Pulmonary Rehabilitation Programs.* 4th ed. Champaign, IL: Human Kinetics; 2011.

30. Chatterjee AB, Rissmiller RW, Meade K, Paladenech C, Confort J, Adair NE, Haponik EF, Chin R. Reproducibility of the 6-minute walk test for ambulatory oxygen prescription. *Respiration.* 2010;79:121–127.

31. Ringbaek TJ, Broendum E, Hemmingsen L, Lybeck K, Nielsen D, Andersen C, Lange P. Rehabilitation of patients with chronic obstructive pulmonary disease: exercise twice a week is not sufficient! *Respir Med.* 2000;94:150–154.

32. Cahalin LP. Pulmonary evaluation. In: DeTurk WE, Cahalin LP, eds. *Cardiovascular and Pulmonary Physical Therapy: An Evidence-Based Approach.* New York: McGraw-Hill; 2004:221–272.

33. American Thoracic Society Committee on Pulmonary Function Standards. Guidelines for methacholine and exercise challenge testing, 1999. *Am J Respir Crit Care Med.* 2000;161:309–329.

34. Australian Lung Foundation and Australian Physiotherapy Association. Six-minute walk test. Pulmonary Rehabilitation Toolkit. www .pulmonaryrehab.com.au.

35. Holland AE, Spruit MA, Troosters T, Puhan MA, Pepin V, Saey D, McCormack MC, Carlin BW, Sciurba FC, Pitta F, et al. An official European Respiratory Society/American Thoracic Society technical standard: field walking tests in chronic respiratory disease. *Eur Respir J.* 2014;44:1428–1446.

36. Singh SJ, Puhan MA, Andrianopoulos V, et al. An official systematic review of the European Respiratory Society/American Thoracic Society: measurement properties of field walking tests in chronic respiratory disease. *Eur Respir J.* 2014;44:1447–1478.

37. Garvey C, Bauldoff, G. Teneback C, Collins E, Donesky D, Eichenauer K, Buckley M. AACVPR Pulmonary Rehabilitation Outcome Toolkit. www .aacvpr.org/Member-Center/Pulmonary-Rehab-Outcomes-Resource-Guide 2017.

38. Crisafulli E, Beneventi C, Bortolotti V, Kidonias N, Fabbri LM, Chetta A, et al. Energy expenditure at rest and during walking in patients with chronic respiratory failure: a prospective two-phase case-control study. *PLoS ONE.* 2011;6(8):e23770.

39. Enright PL. The six-minute walk test. *Respir Care.* 2003;48(8):783–785.

40. Sciurba F, Criner GJ, Lee SM, Mohsenifar Z, Shade D, Slivka W, Wise RA. Six-minute walk distance in chronic obstructive pulmonary disease: reproducibility and effect of walking course layout and length. *Am J Respir Crit Care Med.* 2003;167:1522–1527.

41. Puhan MA, Mador MJ, Held U, Goldstein R, Guyatt GH, et al. Interpretation of treatment changes in 6-minute walk distance in patients with COPD. *Eur Respir J.* 2008;32:637–643.

42. Singh SJ, Morgan MDL, Scott S, et al., Development of a shuttle walking test of disability in patients with chronic airways obstruction. *Thorax.* 1992;47:1019–1024.

43. Hill K, Dolmage T, Woon L, Counts D, Goldstein, Brook D. A simple method to derive speed for the endurance shuttle walk test. *Respir Med.* 2012;12:1665–1670.

44. Fletcher GF, Ades PA, Kligfield P, et al. Exercise standards for testing and training: a scientific statement from the American Heart Association. *Circulation.* 2013;128(8):873–934.

45. Arena R, Guazzi M, Myeers J, Grinnen D, Forman DE, Lavie CJ. Cardiopulmonary exercise testing

in the assessment of pulmonary hypertension. *Expert Rev Respir Med.* 2011;2:281–293.

46. Myers J, Forman DE, Balady GJ, et al. Supervision of exercise testing by nonphysicians—a scientific statement from the American heart Association. *Circulation.* 2014;130:1014–1027.

47. Smith G, Reyes JT, Russell JL, Humpi T. Safety of maximal cardiopulmonary exercise testing in pediatric patients with pulmonary hypertension. *Chest.* 2009;135(5):1209–1214.

48. Arena R, Lavie CJ, Milani RV, Myers J, Guazzi M. Cardiopulmonary exercise testing in patients with pulmonary arterial hypertension: an evidence-based review. *J Heart Lung Transplant.* 2102;2:159–173.

49. Collins EG, Bauldoff G, Carlin B, et al. Clinical competency guidelines for pulmonary rehabilitation professionals. *J Cardiopulm Rehabil.* 2014;34:291–302.

50. Kortianou EA, Nasis IG, Spetsioti ST, Daskalakis AM, Vogiatzis I. Effectiveness of interval exercise training in patients with COPD. *Cardiopulm Phys Ther J.* 2010;3:12–19.

51. Langer D, Hendricks E, Burtin C, et al. A clinical practice guideline for physiotherapists treating patients with chronic obstructive lung disease based on a systematic review of available evidence. *Clin Rehabil.* 2009;23(5):445–462.

52. Ries AL, Bauldoff GS, Carlin BW, et al. Pulmonary rehabilitation: joint ACCP/AACVPR evidence-based clinical practice guidelines. *Chest.* 2007;131:4S-42S.

53. Carson KV, Chandratilleke MG, Picot J, Brinn MP, Esterman AJ, Smith BJ. Physical training for asthma. *Cochrane DB Syst Rev.* 2013:CD001116.

54. Morton AR, Fitch KD. Australian association for exercise and sports science position statement on exercise and asthma. *J Sci Med Sport.* 2011;14:312–316.

55. Gimenez M, Servera E, Vergara P, Bach JR, Polu JM. Endurance training in patients with chronic obstructive pulmonary disease: a comparison of high versus moderate intensity. *Arch Phys Med Rehabil.* 2000;81:102–109.

56. Vogiatzis I, Terzis G, Nanas S, Stratakos G, Simoes DCM, Georgiadou O, Zakynthinos S, Roussos C. Skeletal muscle adaptations to interval training in patients with advanced COPD. *Chest.* 2005;128:3838–3845.

57. Maltais F, LeBlanc P, Jobin J, et al. Intensity of training and physiologic adaptation in patient with chronic obstructive pulmonary disease. *Am J Respir Crit Care Med.* 1997;155:555–561.

58. Casaburi R, Patessio A, Ioli F, et al. Reductions in exercise lactic acidosis and ventilation as a result of exercise training in patients with obstructive lung disease. *Am Rev Respir Dis.* 1991;143:9–18.

59. Coppoolse R, Schols AM, Baarends EM, Mostert R, Akkermans MA, Janssen PP, Wouters EF. Interval versus continuous training in patients with severe COPD: a randomized clinical trial. *Eur Respir J.* 1999;14:258–263.

60. Ries AL, Kaplan RM, Limberg TM, Prewitt LM. Effects of pulmonary rehabilitation on physiologic and psychosocial outcomes in patients with chronic obstructive pulmonary disease. *Ann Intern Med.* 1995;122(11):823–832.

61. Datta D, ZuWallack R. High versus low intensity exercise training in pulmonary rehabilitation: is more better? *Chron Respir Dis.* 2004;1:143–149.

62. Ries AL, Make BJ, Lee SM, Krasna MJ, Bartels M, Crouch R, Fishman AP. The effects of pulmonary rehabilitation in the National Emphysema Treatment Trial. *Chest.* 2005;128(6):3799–3809.

63. Puente-Maestu L, Sanz ML, Sanz P, Cubillo JM, Mayol J, Casaburi R. Comparison of effects of supervised versus self-monitored training programs in patients with chronic obstructive pulmonary disease. *Eur Respir J.* 2000;15:517–525.

64. Lacasse Y, Martin S, Lasserson TJ, Goldstein RS. Meta-analysis of respiratory rehabilitation in chronic obstructive pulmonary disease: a Cochrane systematic review. *Eura Medicophys.* 2007;43:475–485.

65. Plankeel JF, McMullen B, MacIntyre NR. Exercise outcomes after pulmonary rehabilitation depend on the initial mechanism of exercise limitation among non-oxygen-dependent COPD patients. *Chest.* 2005;127:110–116.

66. Bailey SP, Brown L, Bailey EK. Lack of relationship between functional and perceived quality of life outcomes following pulmonary rehabilitation. *Cardiopulm Phys Ther J.* 2008;19(1):3–10.

67. Hassanein SE, Narsavage GL. The dose effect of pulmonary rehabilitation on physical activity, perceived exertion, and quality of life. *J Cardiopulm Rehabil Prev.* 2009;29:255–260.

68. Guell M-R, Cejudo P, Ortega F, et al. Benefits of long-term pulmonary rehabilitation maintenance program in severe COPD patients: 3 year follow-up. *Amer J Respir Crit Care Med.* 2017;5:622–629.

69. Strijbos JH, Postma DS, Van Altena R, et al. A comparison between an outpatient hospital-based pulmonary rehabilitation program and a home-care pulmonary rehabilitation program in patients with COPD: a follow-up of 18 months. *Chest.* 1996;109:366–372.

70. Wijkstra PJ, Van der Mark TW, Kraan J, et al. Long-term effects of home rehabilitation on physical performance in chronic obstructive

pulmonary disease. *Am J Respir Crit Care Med.* 1996;153:1234–1241.

71. Griffiths TL, Burr ML, Campbell IA, et al. Results at 1 year of outpatient multidisciplinary pulmonary rehabilitation: a randomised controlled trial. *Lancet.* 2000;355:362–368.

72. Neunhauserer D, Steidle-Kloc E, Weiss G, et al. Supplemental oxygen during high-intensity exercise training in nonhypoxemic chronic obstructive pulmonary disease. *Am J Med.* 2016;11:1185–1193.

73. Guell R, Casan P, Belda J, et al. Long-term effects of outpatient rehabilitation of COPD: a randomized trial. *Chest.* 2000;117:976–983.

74. Centers for Disease Control and Prevention. Falls among older adults: an overview. www.cdc.gov /HomeandRecreationalSafety/Falls/adultfalls .html.

75. Verrill D, Barton C, Beasley W, Lippard WM. The effects of short- and long-term pulmonary rehabilitation on functional capacity, perceived dyspnea, and quality of life. *Chest.* 2005;128:673–683.

76. Berry MJ, Rejeski WJ, Adair NE, et al. A randomized, controlled trial comparing long-term and short-term exercise in patients with chronic obstructive pulmonary disease. *J Cardiopulm Rehabil.* 2003;23:60–68.

77. Ochmann U, Jorres RA, Nowak D. Long-term efficacy of pulmonary rehabilitation—a state of the art review. *J Cardiopulm Rehabil Prev.* 2012;32:117–126.

78. Pitta F, Troosters T, Probst VS, Langer D, Decramer M, Gosselink R. Are patients with COPD more active after pulmonary rehabilitation? *Chest.* 2008;134:273–280.

79. Troosters T, Casaburi R, Gosselink R, Decramer M. Pulmonary rehabilitation in chronic obstructive pulmonary disease. *Am J Respir Crit Care Med.* 2005;172:19–38.

80. Punzal PA, Ries AL, Kaplan RM, Prewitt LM. Maximum intensity exercise training in patients with chronic obstructive pulmonary disease. *Chest.* 1991;100:618–623.

81. Troosters T, Gosselink R, Langer D, Decramer M. Pulmonary rehabilitation in chronic obstructive pulmonary disease. *Respir Med: COPD Update.* 2007;3:57–64.

82. Beauchamp MK, Janaudis-Ferreira T, Goldstein RS, Brooks D. Optimal duration of pulmonary rehabilitation for individuals with chronic obstructive lung disease—a systematic review. *Chron Respir Dis.* 2011;8:129–140.

83. Rossi G, Florini F, Romagnoli M, Bellantone T, Lucic S, Lugli D, Clini E. Length and clinical effectiveness of pulmonary rehabilitation in outpatients with chronic airway obstruction. *Chest.* 2005;127:105–109.

84. Dowman L, Hill CJ, Holland AE. Pulmonary rehabilitation for interstitial lung disease. *Cochrane DB Syst Rev.* 2014;10:CD006322.

85. Protas EJ. The aging patient. In: Frownfelter D, Dean EJ, eds. *Cardiovascular and Pulmonary Physical Therapy: Evidence and Practice.* 4th ed. St. Louis: Mosby/Elsevier; 2006:685–693.

86. Lotters F, Van Tol B, Kwakkel G, et al. Effects of controlled inspiratory muscle training in patients with COPD: a meta-analysis. *Eur Respir J.* 2002;20:570–576.

87. Rodrigues J, Watchie J. Cardiovascular and pulmonary physical therapy treatment. In: Watchie J, ed. *Cardiovascular and Pulmonary Physical Therapy: A Clinical Manual.* 2nd ed. St. Louis: Saunders/ Elsevier; 2010:298–341.

88. Porto EF, Castro AA, Velloso M, Nascimento O, Dal Maso F, Jardim JR. Exercises using the upper limbs hyperinflate COPD patients more than exercises using the lower limbs at the same metabolic demand. *Monaldi Arch Chest Dis.* 2009;71:21–26.

89. Costi S, Crisafulli E, Antoni FD, Beneventi C, Fabbri LM, Clini EM. Effects of unsupported upper extremity exercise training in patients with COPD: a randomized clinical trial. *Chest.* 2009;136:387–395.

90. Biskobing DM. COPD and osteoporosis. *Chest.* 2002;12:609–620.

91. Borg G. Perceived exertion as an indicator of somatic stress. *Scand J Rehab Med.* 1970;2:92–98.

92. Borg G. Psychophysical bases of perceived exertion. *Med Sci Sports Exerc.* 1982;14:377–381.

93. Borg G. Psychophysical scaling with applications in physical work and the perception of exertion. *Scand J Work Environ Health.* 1990;(Suppl 1):55–58.

94. Gift AG, Narsavage G. Validity of the numerical rating scale as a measure of dyspnea. *Am J Crit Care.* 1998;3:200–204

95. Zanini A, Aiello M, Adamo D, et al. Estimation of minimal clinically important difference in EQ-5D visual analog scale score after pulmonary rehabilitation in subjects with COPD. *Respir Care.* 2015;60:88–95.

96. Crisafuli E, Clini EM. Measures of dyspnea in pulmonary rehabilitation. *Multidiscip Respir Med.* 2010;5:202–210.

97. Ries AL, Farrow JT, Clausen JL. Pulmonary function tests cannot predict exercise-induced hypoxemia in chronic obstructive pulmonary disease. *Chest.* 1988;93:454–459.

98. Nocturnal Oxygen Therapy Trial Group. Continuous or nocturnal oxygen therapy in hypoxemic

chronic obstructive lung disease: a clinical trial. *Ann Intern Med.* 1980;93:391–398.

99. American Thoracic Society and European Respiratory Society Task Force, Standards for the Diagnosis and Management of Patients with COPD. *Eur Respir J.* 2004:23:932–946.

100. Emtner M, Porszasz J, Burns M, et al. Benefits of supplemental oxygen in exercise training in non-hypoxemic COPD patients. *Am J Respir Crit Care Med.* 2003;168:1034–1042.

101. Puhan MA, Schunemann HJ, Frey M, et al. Value of supplemental interventions to enhance the effectiveness of physical exercise during respiratory rehabilitation in COPD: a systematic review. *Respir Res.* 2004;5:25.

102. Jarosch I, Gloeckl R, Damm E, Schwedhelm AL, Buhrow D, Jerrentrup A, Spruit MA, Kenn K. Short-term effects of supplemental oxygen on 6-minute walk test outcomes in COPD patients: a randomized, placebo-controlled, single-blind, crossover trial. *Chest.* 2017;151:795–803.

103. Roig M, Eng JJ, MacIntyre DL, Road JD, Reid WD. Deficits in muscle strength, mass, quality, and mobility in people with chronic obstructive pulmonary disease. *J Cardiopulm Rehabil.* 2011;31:120–124.

104. Robertson RJ, Goss FL, Dube J, et al. Validation of the adult OMNI scale of perceived exertion for cycle ergometer exercise. *Med Sci Sports Exerc.* 2004;36(1):102–108.

105. Utter AC, Robertson RJ, Green JM, Suminski RR, McAnulty SR, Nieman DC. Validation of the adult OMNI scale of perceived exertion for walking/running exercise. *Med Sci Sports Exerc.* 2004;36(10):1776–1780.

106. Garvey C, Bayles MP, Hamm LF. Pulmonary rehabilitation exercise prescription in chronic obstructive pulmonary disease: review of selected guidelines. *J Cardiopulm Rehabil.* 2016;36:75–83.

107. Kaelin ME, Swank A, Adams KJ, Barnard KL, Berning J, Green A. Cardiopulmonary responses, muscle soreness responses, muscle soreness, and injury during the one repetition maximum assessment in pulmonary rehabilitation patients. *J Cardiopulm Rehabil.* 1999;6:366–372.

108. American College of Sports Medicine. Progression models in resistance training for healthy adults—position stand. *Med Sci Sports Exerc.* 2009;41:687–708.

109. Williams MA, Haskell WL, Ades PA, et al. Resistance exercise in individuals with and without cardiovascular disease: 2007 update: a scientific statement from the American Heart Association Council on Clinical Cardiology and Council on Nutrition, Physical Activity, and Metabolism. *Circulation.* 2007;116:572–584.

110. Bellet RN, Francis RL, Jacob JS, et al. Timed up and go tests in cardiac rehabilitation. *J Cardiopulm Rehabil Prev.* 2013;33:99–105.

111. Jones CJ, Rikli RE. Measuring functional fitness of older adults. *J Act Aging.* 2002:2:24–30.

112. Miotto JM, Chodzko-Zaijko WJ, Reich JL, Supler MM. Reliability and validity of the Fullerton Functional Fitness Test: an independent replication study. *J Aging Phys Activ.* 1999;7:339–353.

113. Smith WN, Gianluca DR, Adams JB, et al. Simple equations to predict concentric lower-body muscular power in older adults using the 30-second chair-rise test: a pilot study. *Clin Interven Aging.* 2010;5:173–180.

114. Takeda K, Kawasaki Y, Yoshida K, et al. The 6-minute pegboard and ring test is correlated with upper extremity activity of daily living in chronic obstructive pulmonary disease. *Intern J COPD.* 2013;8:347–351.

115. Gee MA, Redfern MS, Furman JM, Whitney SL, Wrisley DM, Marchetti GF. Clinical measurement of sit-to-stand performance in people with balance disorders: validity of data for the five-times-sit-to-stand test. *Phys Ther.* 2005;85:1034–1045.

116. Rikli RE, Jones CJ. Functional fitness normative scores for community-residing older adults, ages 60–94. *J Aging Phys Activ.* 1999;7:162–181.

117. Bohannon RW. Reference values for extremity muscle strength obtained by hand-held dynamometry from adults aged 20 to 79 years. *Arch Phys Med Rehabil.* 1997;78:26–32.

118. Mroszczyk-McDonald A, Savage PD, Ades PA. Handgrip strength in cardiac rehabilitation. *J Cardiopulm Rehabil Prev.* 2007;27:298–302.

119. Shechtman O, Mann WC, Justiss MD, Tomita M. Grip strength in the frail elderly. *Am J Phys Med Rehabil.* 2004;83:819–826.

120. Rantanen T, Guralnik JM, Foley D, et al. Midlife handgrip strength as a predictor of old age disability. *JAMA.* 1999;281:558–560.

121. Rantanen T, Volpato S, Ferrucci L, Heikkinen E, Fried LP, Guralnik JM. Handgrip strength and cause-specific and total mortality in older disabled women: exploring the mechanism. *J Am Geriatr Soc.* 2003;51:636–641.

122. Harris C, Wattles AP, DeBeliso M, Sevene-Adams PG, Berning JM, and Adams KJ. The seated medicine ball throw as a test of upper body power in older adults. *J Strength Cond Res.* 2011;25:2344–2348.

123. Signorile JF, Sandler DJ, Ma F, et al. The gallon jug shelf transfer test: an instrument to evaluate deteriorating function in older adults. *J Aging Phys Act.* 2007;15:56–74.

124. Raub JA. Psychophysiologic effects of hatha yoga on musculoskeletal and cardiopulmonary func-

tion: a literature review. *J Altern Complement Med.* 2002;8(6):797–812.

125. Zafrir B. Exercise training and rehabilitation in pulmonary arterial hypertension. *J Cardiopulm Rehabil Prev.* 2013;33:263–273.

126. Robles P, Araujo T, Brooks D, et al. Cardiorespiratory responses to short bouts of resistance training exercises in individuals with chronic obstructive pulmonary disease—a comparison of exercise intensities. *J Cardiopulm Rehabil Prev.* 2017;37:356–362.

127. Probst VS, Troosters T, Pitta F, Decramer M, Gosselink R. Cardiopulmonary stress during exercise training in patients with COPD. *Eur Respir J.* 2006;27:1110–1118.

128. Kuehne T, Yilmaz S, Steendijk P. Magnetic resonance imaging analysis of right ventricular pressure-volume loops: in vivo validation and clinical application in patients with pulmonary hypertension. *Circulation.* 2004;110:2010–2016.

129. Sun XG, Hansen JE, Oudiz RJ, Wasserman K. Exercise pathophysiology in patients with primary pulmonary hypertension. *Circulation.* 2001;104:429–435.

130. Naeije R, Vanderpool R, Dhakal BP, Saggar R, Saggar R, Vachiéry J-L, Lewis GD. Exercise-induced pulmonary hypertension: physiological basis and methodological concerns. *Am J Respir Crit Care Med.* 2013;187:576–583.

131. Galiè N, Corris P, Frost F, Girgis R, Granton J, et al. Updated treatment algorithm of pulmonary arterial hypertension. *J Am Col Card.* 2013;62:25.

132. Mereles D, Ehlken N, Kreuscher S, Ghofrani S, Hoeper M, et al. Exercise and respiratory training improve exercise capacity and quality of life in patients with severe chronic pulmonary hypertension. *Circulation.* 2006;114:1482–1489.

133. Weinstein AA, Chin LMK, Keyser RE, et al. Effect of aerobic exercise training on fatigue and physical activity in patients with pulmonary arterial hypertension. *Respir Med.* 2013;107:778–784.

134. Chan L, Chin LM, Kennedy M, et al. Benefits of intensive treadmill exercise training on cardiorespiratory function and quality of life in patients with pulmonary hypertension. *Chest.* 2013;143: 333-343.

135. Morris NR, Kermeen FD, Holland AE. Exercise-based rehabilitation programmes for pulmonary hypertension. *Cochrane DB Syst Rev.* 2017;1: CD011285.

136. Pandey A, Garg S, Khunger M, Garg S, Kumbhani DJ, Chin KM, Berry JD. Efficacy and safety of exercise training in chronic pulmonary hypertension: systematic review and meta-analysis. *Circ Heart Fail.* 2015;8:1032–1043.

137. Desai SA, Channick RN. Exercise in patients with pulmonary arterial hypertension. *J Cardiopulm Rehabil Prev.* 2008;28:12–16.

138. Astrand PO, Rodahl K. *Textbook of Work Physiology: Physiological Bases of Exercise.* New York: McGraw Hill; 1977:456.

139. Garvey C, Tiep B, Carter R, et al. Severe exercise-induced hypoxemia. *Respir Care.* 2012;7:1154–1160.

140. Aubier M, Murciano D, Fournier M, Milic-Emili J, Pariente R, Derenne JP. Central respiratory drive in acute respiratory failure of patients with chronic obstructive pulmonary disease. *Am Rev Respir Dis.* 1980;122:191–199.

141. Sassoon CSH, Hassell KT, Mahutte CK. Hyperoxic-induced hypercapnia in stable chronic obstructive pulmonary disease. *Am Rev Respir Dis.* 1987;135: 907–911.

142. Austin MA, Wills KE, Blizzard L, Walters EH, Wood-Baker R. Effect of high flow oxygen on mortality in chronic obstructive pulmonary disease patients in prehospital setting: randomised controlled trial. *BMJ.* 2010;341:C562.

143. Wagner PD, Dantzker DR, Dueck R, Clausen JL, West JB. Ventilation-perfusion inequality in chronic obstructive pulmonary disease. *J Clin Invest.* 1977;59(2):203–226.

144. Hopkins SR. Exercise induced arterial hypoxemia: the role of ventilation-perfusion inequality and pulmonary diffusion limitation. *Adv Exp Med Biol.* 2006;588:17–30.

145. Wang T, Kernstine K, Tiep B, Venkataraman K, Horak D, Barnett M. Intrapulmonary shunting through tumor causing refractory hypoxemia. ATS Clinical Cases 2007. www.thoracic.org/professionals/clinical-resources/clinical-cases/intrapulmonary-shunting-through-tumor-causing-refractory-hypoxemia.php.

146. Chetty KG, Dick C, McGovern J, Conroy RM, Mahutte CK. Refractory hypoxemia due to intrapulmonary shunting associated with bronchioloalveolar carcinoma. *Chest.* 1997;111:1120–1121.

147. Carter R. The physiologic principles of oxygen delivery. In: Tiep BL, ed. *Portable Oxygen Therapy: Including Oxygen Conserving Methodology.* Mount Kisco, NY: Futura; 1991:81–124.

148. Maltais F, Bourbeau J, Shapiro S, et al. Chronic Obstructive Pulmonary Disease Axis of Respiratory Health Network; Fonds de Recherche en Santé du Québec. Effects of home-based pulmonary rehabilitation in patients with chronic obstructive pulmonary disease: a randomized trial. *Ann Intern Med.* 2008;149:869–878.

149. Güell M, de Lucas P, Gáldiz J, et al. Home vs. hospital-based pulmonary rehabilitation for

patients with chronic obstructive pulmonary disease: a Spanish multicenter trial. *Arch Bronconeumol.* 2008;44:512–518.

150. Fernández A, Pascual J, Ferrando C, et al. Home-based pulmonary rehabilitation in very severe COPD: is it safe and useful? *J Cardiopulm Rehabil Prev.* 2009;29:325–331.

151. Smith A. Older adults and technology use. Pew Research Center. www.pewinternet.org/2014/04/03/older-adults-and-technology-use/.

152. Burkow T, Vognild L, Johnsen E, Risberg M, Bratvold A, Breivik E, et al. Comprehensive pulmonary rehabilitation in home-based online groups: a mixed method pilot study in COPD. *BMC Res Notes.* 2015;10(8):766.

153. Vorrink SN, Kort HS, Troosters T, Zanen P, Lammers JJ. Efficacy of an mHealth intervention to stimulate physical activity in COPD patients after pulmonary rehabilitation. *Eur Respir J.* 2016;48(4):1019–1029.

154. Smith A. Older adults and technology use. Pew Research Center. www.pewinternet.org/2014/04/03/older-adults-and-technology-use/.

155. Probst V, Troosters T, Coosemans I, et al. Mechanisms of improvement in exercise capacity using a rollator in patients with COPD. *Chest.* 2004;126:1102–110.

156. Breyer M, Breyer-Kohansal R, Funk G, Dornhofer N, Spruit M, Wouters E, et al. Nordic walking improves daily physical activities in COPD: a randomised controlled trial. *Respir Res.* 2010;11:112.

157. Pierson DJ. Thomas L Petty's lessons for the respiratory care clinician of today. *Respir Care 59.* 2014 (8):1287–1301.

158. O'Donnell D. Hyperinflation, dyspnea, and exercise intolerance in chronic obstructive pulmonary disease. *Proc Am Thorac Soc.* 2006;3:180–184.

159. Garvey C, Singer JP, Bruun AM, Soong A, Rigler J, Hays S. Moving pulmonary rehabilitation into the home. *J Cardiopulm Rehabil Prev.* 2018;38(1):8–16.

160. Mazzuca S. Does patient education in chronic disease have therapeutic value? *J Chronic Dis* 1982;35:521–529.

161. Bischoff E, Hamd D, Sedeno M, et al. Effects of written action plan adherence on COPD exacerbation recovery. *Thorax.* 2011;66:26–31.

162. Rice K, Dewan N, Bloomfield H, et al. Disease management program for chronic obstructive pulmonary disease: a randomized controlled trial. *Am J Respir Crit Care Med* 2010;182:890–896.

163. Effing T, Monninkhof E, Van der Valk P, et al. Self management education for patients with chronic obstructive pulmonary disease. *Cochrane DB Syst Rev.* 2007;4:CD002990.

164. Trappenburg J, Monninkhof E, Bourbeau J, et al. Effect of an action plan with ongoing support by a case manager on exacerbation-related outcome in patients with COPD: a multicentre randomised controlled trial. *Thorax.* 2011;66:977–984.

165. Effing T, Kerstjens H, Van der Valk P, Zielhuis G, et al. (Cost)-effectiveness of self-treatment of exacerbations on the severity of exacerbations in patients with COPD: the COPE II Study. *Thorax.* 2009;64:956–962.

166. Camillo CA, Osadnik CR, Van Remoortel H, Burtin C, Janssens W, Troosters T. Effect of "add-on" interventions on exercise training in individuals with COPD: a systematic review. *ERJ Open Res.* 2016;2:1. www.ncbi.nlm.nih.gov/pubmed/27730178.

## Chapter 4

1. McCarthy B, Casey D, Devane D, et al. Pulmonary rehabilitation for chronic obstructive pulmonary disease. *Cochrane DB Syst Rev.* 2015;2(Art):CD003793.

2. Bourbeau J, Lavoie KL, Sedeno M. Comprehensive self-management strategies. *Semin Respir Crit Care Med.* 2015;36:630–638.

3. Zwerink M, Brusse-Keizer M, Van der Valk PD, Zielhuis GA, Monninkhof EM, Van der Palen J, Frith PA, Effing T. Self management for patients with chronic obstructive pulmonary disease. *Cochrane DB Syst Rev.* 2014;3(Art):CD002990.

4. Global Initiative for Chronic Obstructive Lung Disease. Global strategy for the diagnosis, management, and prevention of chronic obstructive pulmonary disease. 2017 Report. http://goldcopd.org.

5. Jolly K, Majothi S, Sitch AJ, et al. Self-management of health care behaviors for COPD: a systematic review and meta-analysis. *Int J COPD.* 2016;11:305–326.

6. Blackmore C, Johnson-Warrington VL, Williams JEA, et al. Development of a training program to support health care professionals to deliver the SPACE for COPD self-management program. *Int J COPD.* 2017;12:1669–1681.

7. Dritsaki M, Johnson-Warrington V, Mitchell K, et al. An economic evaluation of a self-management programme of activity, coping and education for patients with chronic obstructive pulmonary disease. Chron Respir Dis. 2016;13(1):48–56.

8. Blackstock FC, ZuWallack R, Nici L, Lareau SC. Why don't our patients with chronic obstructive pulmonary disease listen to us? The enigma of non-adherence. *Ann Am Thorac Soc.* 2016;13(3):317–323.

9. Benzo RP, Abascal-Bolado B, Dulohery MM. Self-management and quality of life in chronic

obstructive pulmonary disease (COPD): the mediating effects of positive affect. *Patient Educ Couns.* 2016;99(4);617–623.

10. Cabral LF, D'Elia T, Marins D, et al. Pursed lip breathing improves exercise tolerance in COPD: a randomized crossover study. *Euro J Phys Rehabil Med.* 2015;51(1):79–88.

11. Spruit MA, Singh SJ, Garvey C, et al. An official American Thoracic Society/European Respiratory Society statement: key concepts and advances in pulmonary rehabilitation. *Am J Respir Crit Care Med.* 2013;188(8):e13-e64.

12. Kon SS, Canavan CK, Man WD. Pulmonary rehabilitation and acute exacerbations of COPD. *Expert Rev Respir Med.* 2012;6(5):523–531.

13. Heffner JE, Fahy B, Hilling L, et al. Attitudes regarding advance directives among patients in pulmonary rehabilitation. *Am J Respir Crit Care Med.* 1996;154:1735–1740.

## Chapter 5

1. Collins EG, Bauldoff G, Carlin B, Crouch R, Emery CF, Garvey C, et al. Clinical competency guidelines for pulmonary rehabilitation professionals: position statement of the American Association of Cardiovascular and Pulmonary Rehabilitation. *J Cardiopulm Rehabil Prev.* 2014;34(5):291–302.

2. CFR 42 CFR §410.47 Pulmonary rehabilitation program: conditions for coverage.

3. Stage KB, Middelboe T, Stage TB, Sørensen CH. Depression in COPD—management and quality of life considerations. *Int J Chron Obstruct Pulmon Dis.* 2006;1(3):315–320.

4. Spruit M, Sing S, Garvey C, ZuWallack R, Nici L, Rochester C, Hill K, Holland A, Lareau S, Man D, et al. An official American Thoracic Society/European Respiratory Society statement: key concepts and advances in pulmonary rehabilitation. *Am J Respir Crit Care Med.* 2013;188:e13-e64.

5. Yohannes A, Willgoss T, Baldwin R, Connolly M. Depression and anxiety in chronic heart failure and chronic obstructive disease: prevalence, relevance, clinical implications and management principles. *Int J Geriatr Psychiatry.* 2010;25:1209–1221.

6. Kunik M, Roundy K, Veazey C, et al. Surprisingly high prevalence of anxiety and depression in chronic breathing disorders. *Chest.* 2005;127:1205–1211.

7. Ouellette DR, Lavoie KL. Recognition, diagnosis, and treatment of cognitive and psychiatric disorders in patients with COPD. *Int J Chron Obstruct Pulmon Dis.* 2017;12:639–650.

8. Holland AE, Fiore JF, Bell EC, Goh N, Westall G, Symons, K, et al. Dyspnoea and comorbidity contribute to anxiety and depression in interstitial lung disease. *Respirology.* 2014;19(8):1215–1221.

9. Harzheim D, Klose H, Pinado FP, Ehlken N, Nagel C, Fischer C, et al. Anxiety and depression disorders in patients with pulmonary arterial hypertension and chronic thromboembolic pulmonary hypertension. *Resp Res.* 2013;14(1):104.

10. Olveira C, Olveira G, Gaspar I, Dorado A, Cruz I, Soriguer F, et al. Depression and anxiety symptoms in bronchiectasis: associations with health-related quality of life. *Qual Life Res.* 2013;22(3):597–605.

11. American Psychiatric Association. *Diagnostic and statistical manual of mental disorders: DSM-5.* Washington, DC: American Psychiatric Association; 2013.

12. Spruit MA, Watkins ML, Edwards LD, Vestbo J, Calverley PMA, et al. Determinants of poor 6-min walking distance in patients with COPD: the ECLIPSE cohort. *Respir Med.* 2010;104:849–857.

13. Dimatteo M, Lepper H, Croghan T. Depression is a risk factor for noncompliance with medical treatment: meta-analysis of the effects of anxiety and depression and adherence. *Arch Intern Med.* 2000;160:2101–2107.

14. Kim HF, Kunik ME, Molinari VA, et al. Functional impairment in COPD patients: the impact of anxiety and depression. *Psychosomatics.* 2000;41:461–465.

15. Keating A, Lee A, Holland A. What prevents people with chronic obstructive pulmonary disease from attending pulmonary rehabilitation? A systematic review. *Chr Respir Dis.* 2011;8:89–99.

16. Busch AM, Scott-Sheldon LA, Pierce J, Chattillion EA, Cunningham K, Buckley ML, et al. Depressed mood predicts pulmonary rehabilitation completion among women, but not men. *Resp Med.* 2014;108(7):1007–1013.

17. Ng TP, Niti M, Tan WC, Cao Z, Ong KC, Eng P. Depressive symptoms and chronic obstructive pulmonary disease: effect on mortality, hospital readmission, symptom burden, functional status, and quality of life. *Arch Intern Med.* 2007;167(1):60–67.

18. Fan VS, Ramsey SD, Giardino ND, et al. Sex, depression, and risk of hospitalization and mortality in chronic obstructive pulmonary disease. *Arch Intern Med.* 2007;(21):2345–2253.

19. Beck A, Steer R, Brown G. *Manual for the Beck Depression Inventory-II: A Comprehensive Review.* San Antonio, TX: Psychological Corporation; 1996.

20. Kroenke K, Spitzer R. The PHQ-9: a new diagnostic and severity measure. *Psychc Annals.* 2002;32:509–521.

21. Zigmond AS, Snaith RP. The hospital anxiety and depression scale. *Acta Psychiatr Scand.* 1983;67(6):361–370.

22. Eichenauer K, Feltz G, Wilson J, Brookings J. Measuring psychosocial risk factors in cardiac rehabilitation: validation of the psychosocial risk factor survey. *J Cardiopulm Rehabil Prev.* 2010;30:309–318.

23. Smarr, K, Keefer, A. Measures of depression and depressive symptoms: Beck Depression Inventory II (BDI-II), Center for Epidemiological Studies Depression Scale (CES-D), Geriatric Depression Scale (GDS), Hospital Anxiety and Depression Scale (HADS), and Patient Health Questionnaire (PHQ-9). *Arthrit Care Res.* 2011;63:S454-S466.

24. American Association of Cardiovascular and Pulmonary Rehabilitation. Outcomes Resource Guide. Available at www.aacvpr.org/Member-Center/Pulmonary-Rehab-Outcomes-Resource-Guide.

25. Posner K, Brown GK, Stanley B, Brent DA, Yershova KV, Oquendo MA, et al. The Columbia–Suicide Severity Rating Scale: initial validity and internal consistency findings from three multisite studies with adolescents and adults. *Am J Psych.* 2011;168(12):1266–1277. www.cssrs.columbia.edu.

26. Department of Veterans Affairs. *VA Suicide Risk Assessment Guide.* 2017. www.mentalhealth.va.gov/docs/VA029AssessmentGuide.pdf.

27. Joint Commission. *Joint Commission Sentinel Event Alert.* 2016;56. www.jointcommission.org/assets/1/18/SEA_56_Suicide.pdf.

28. Janssen DJ, Spruit MA, Leue C, Gijsen C, Hameleers H, Schols JM, Ciro Network, et al. Symptoms of anxiety and depression in COPD patients entering pulmonary rehabilitation. *Chr Respir Dis.* 2010;7(3):147–157.

29. Livermore N, Sharpe L, McKenzie D. Panic attacks and panic disorder in chronic obstructive pulmonary disease: a cognitive behavioral perspective. *Resp Med.* 2010;104:1246–1253.

30. Giardino ND, Curtis JL, Andrei AC, Fan VS, Benditt JO, Lyubkin M, et al. Anxiety is associated with diminished exercise performance and quality of life in severe emphysema: a cross-sectional study. *Resp Res.* 2010;11(1):29.

31. Gudmundsson G, Gislason T, Janson C, Lindberg E, Hallin R, Ulrik CS, et al. Risk factors for rehospitalisation in COPD: role of health status, anxiety and depression. *Eur Respir J.* 2005;26(3):414–419.

32. Ries AL. Position paper of the American Association of Cardiovascular and Pulmonary Rehabilitation: scientific basis of pulmonary rehabilitation. *J Cardiopulm Rehabil.* 1990;10:418–441.

33. Beck A, Epstein N, Brown G, Steer R. An inventory for measuring clinical anxiety: psychometric properties. *J Consult Clin Psychol.* 1988;56:893–897.

34. Spitzer R, Kroenke K, Williams J, Lowe B. A brief measure for assessing generalized anxiety disorder: the GAD-7. *Arch Intern Med.* 2006;166:1092–1097.

35. Jackson B, Kubzansky LD, Cohen S, Jacobs DR Jr, Wright RJ; CARDIA study investigators. Does harboring hostility hurt? Associations between hostility and pulmonary function in the Coronary Artery Risk Development in (Young) Adults (CARDIA) study. *Health Psychol.* 2007;26(3):333–340.

36. Kubzansky LD, Sparrow D, Jackson B, Cohen S, Weiss ST, Wright RJ. Angry breathing: a prospective study of hostility and lung function in the Normative Aging Study. *Thorax.* 2006;61(10):863–868.

37. Spielberger, CD. *Manual for the State-Trait Anger Expression Inventory-II (STAXI-2).* Odessa, FL: Psychological Assessment Resources; 1999.

38. Marino P, Sirey JA, Raue PJ, Alexopoulos GS. Impact of social support and self-efficacy on functioning in depressed older adults with chronic obstructive pulmonary disease. *Int J Chr Obstr Pulm Dis.* 2008;3(4):713–718.

39. Grodner S, Prewitt LM, Jaworsk BA, Myers R, Kaplan RM, Ries AL. The impact of social support in pulmonary rehabilitation of patients with chronic obstructive pulmonary disease. *Ann Behav Med.* 1996;18(3):139–145.

40. RAND Corporation. Social support survey instrument. 2017. www.rand.org/health/surveys_tools/mos/social-support/survey-instrument.html.

41. Berkman LF, Enhancing Recovery in Coronary Heart Disease Patients investigators (ENRICHD). Effects of treating depression and low perceived social support on clinical events after myocardial infarction: the Enhancing Recovery in Coronary Heart Disease Patients (ENRICHD) randomized trial. *JAMA.* 2003;289:3106–3116.

42. Köseoğlu N, Köseoğlu H, Ceylan E, Cimrin HA, Özalevli S, Esen A. Erectile dysfunction prevalence and sexual function status in patients with chronic obstructive pulmonary disease. *J Urology.* 2005;174(1):249–252.

43. Dias M, Oliveira MJ, Oliveira P, Ladeira I, Lima R, Guimarães M. Does any association exist between chronic obstructive pulmonary disease and erectile dysfunction? The DECODED study. *Revista Portuguesa de Pneumologia* (English ed.). 2017.

44. Kaptein AA, Van Klink RC, De Kok F, Scharloo M, Snoei L, Broadbent E, et al. Sexuality in patients with asthma and COPD. *Resp Med.* 2008;102(2):198–204.

45. Vincent EE, Singh SJ. Addressing the sexual health of patients with COPD: the needs of the patient and implications for health care professionals. *Chr Resp Dis.* 2007;4(2):111–115.

46. Nici L, Donner C, Wouters E, Zuwallack R, Ambrosino N, Bourbeau J, et al. American Thoracic Society/European Respiratory Society statement on pulmonary rehabilitation. *Am J Respir Crit Care Med.* 2006;173(12):1390–1413.

47. Eekhof J, Van Selm J, Tombrock CG, Hoogslag G, Kaptein A. De seksualiteitsbeleving van oudere patiënten met COPD [Sexual experiences of elderly patients with COPD]. *Huisarts Wet.* 1991;34:527–530

48. Vennix P. NISSO-schalen: Vragenlijsten voor de man en voor de vrouw [NISSO-scales: questionnaires for the man and for the woman]. NISSO, Netherlands Institute for Social Sexuality Research, Zeist, the Netherlands (1985).

49. Traphagen N, Tian Z, Allen-Gipson D. Chronic ethanol exposure: pathogenesis of pulmonary disease and dysfunction. *Biomolecules.* 2015;5(4):2840–2853

50. Singh G, Zhang W, Kuo YF, Sharma G. Association of psychological disorders with 30-day readmission rates in patients with COPD. *Chest.* 2016;149(4):905–915.

51. Hijjawi SB, Abu Minshar M, Sharma G. Chronic obstructive pulmonary disease exacerbation: a single-center perspective on hospital readmissions. *Postgrad Med.* 2015;127(4):343–348.

52. Yadavilli R, Collins A, Ding WY, Garner N, Williams J, Burhan H. Hospital readmissions with exacerbation of obstructive pulmonary disease in illicit drug smokers. *Lung.* 2014;192(5):669–673.

53. Safa M, Boroujerdi FG, Talischi F, Masjedi MR. Relationship of coping styles with suicidal behavior in hospitalized asthma and chronic obstructive pulmonary disease patients: substance abusers versus non- substance abusers. *Tanaffos.* 2014;13(3):23–30.

54. Rapsey CM, Lim CC, Al-Hamzawi A, Alonso J, Bruffaerts R, Caldas-de-Almeida JM, Florescu S, De Girolamo G, Hu C, Kessler RC, Kovess-Masfety V, Levinson D, Medina-Mora ME, Murphy S, Ono Y, Piazza M, Posada-Villa J, ten Have M, Wojtyniak B, Scott KM. Associations between DSM-IV mental disorders and subsequent COPD diagnosis. *J Psychosom Res.* 2015;79(5):333–339.

55. Vetrano DL, Bianchini E, Onder G, Cricelli I, Cricelli C, Bernabei R, Bettoncelli G, Lapi F. Poor adherence to chronic obstructive pulmonary disease medications in primary care: role of age, disease burden and polypharmacy. *Geriatr Gerontol Int.* 2017;17(12):2500–2506.

56. Ewing JA. Detecting alcoholism: the CAGE questionnaire. *JAMA.* 1984;252(14):1905–1907.

57. Brown RL, Rounds LA. Conjoint screening questionnaires for alcohol and other drug abuse: criterion validity in a primary care practice. *Wisc Med J.* 1995;94(3):135–140.

58. Saunders JB, Aasland OG, Babor TF, De la Fuente JR, Grant M. Development of the alcohol use disorders identification test (AUDIT): WHO collaborative project on early detection of persons with harmful alcohol consumption-II. *Addiction.* 1993;88(6):791–804.

59. Incalzi AR, Gemma A, et al. Chronic obstructive pulmonary disease: an original model of cognitive decline. *Am Rev Respir Dis.* 1993;148:418–424.

60. Kozora E, Filley CM, et al. Cognitive functioning in patients with chronic obstructive pulmonary disease and mild hypoxemia compared with patients with mild Alzheimer disease and normal controls. *Neuropsych Neuropsychol Behav Neurol.* 1999;12:178–183.

61. Dodd JW, Getov SV, Jones PW. Cognitive function in COPD. *EurResp J.* 2010;35(4):913–922.

62. Hung WW, Wisnivesky JP, Siu AL, Ross JS. Cognitive decline among patients with chronic obstructive pulmonary disease. *Am J Respir Crit Care Med.* 2009;180(2):134–137.

63. Incalzi RA, Corsonello A, Trojano L, et al. Cognitive training is ineffective in hypoxemic COPD: a six-month randomized controlled trial. *Rejuvenation Res.* 2008;11:239–250.

64. Roberts R, Knopman DS. Classification and epidemiology of MCI. *ClinGeri Med.* 2013;29(4).

65. Grant I, Heaton RK, McSweeny AJ, Adams KM, Timms RM. Neuropsychologic findings in hypoxemic chronic obstructive pulmonary disease. *Arch Int Med.* 1982;142(8):1470–1476.

66. Kizilbash A, Venderploeg R, Curtiss G. The effects of depression and anxiety on memory performance. *Arch Clin Neuropsychol.* 2002;17:57–67.

67. Bremner J, Narayan M, Anderson E, Staib L, Miller H, Charney D. Hippocampal volume reduction in major depression. *Am J Psychiatry.* 2000;157:115–117.

68. Kozora E, Tran ZV, Make B. Neurobehavioral improvement after brief rehabilitation in patients with chronic obstructive pulmonary disease. *J Cardio Pulm Rehabil.* 2002;22:426–430.

69. Khatri P, Blumenthal J, Babyak M, Craighead W, Herman S, Baldewisz, T. Effects of exercise training on cognitive functioning among depressed older men and women. *J Aging Phys Act.* 2001;9:43–57.

70. Kramer A, Hanh S, Cohen N, McAuley E, Scalf P, Erickson, K. Aging, fitness and neurocognitive function. *Nature.* 1999;40006743:418–419.

71. Schou L, Østergaard B, Rasmussen LS, Rydahl-Hansen S, Phanareth K. Cognitive dysfunc-

tion in patients with chronic obstructive pulmonary disease—a systematic review. *Resp Med.* 2012;106(8):1071–1081.

72. Cleutjens F, Spruit MA, Ponds R, et al. Cognitive functioning in obstructive lung disease: results from the United Kingdom biobank. *J Am Med Dir Assoc.* 2014;15:214–219.

73. Nasreddine Z, Phillips N, Bédirian V, et al. The Montreal Cognitive Assessment, MoCA: a brief screening tool for mild cognitive impairment. *J Am Geriat Soc.* 2005;53:695–699.

74. Folstein M, Folstein S, McHugh P. Mini-mental state: A practical method for grading the cognitive state of patients for the clinician. *J Psychiatr Res.* 1975;12:189–198.

75. Blackstock FC, ZuWallack R, Nici L, Lareau SC. Why don't our patients with chronic obstructive pulmonary disease listen to us? The enigma of nonadherence. *Ann Am Thorac Soc.* 2016;13(3):317–323.

76. George J, Kong D, Thoman R, Stewart K. Factors associated with medication nonadherence in patients with COPD. *Chest.* 2005;128:3198–3204.

77. Young P, Dewse M, Fergusson W, Kolbe J. Respiratory rehabilitation in chronic obstructive pulmonary disease: predictors of nonadherence. *Eur Respir J.* 1999;13:855–859.

78. Oates GR, Hamby BW, Stepanikova I, Knight SJ, Bhatt SP, Hitchcock J, et al. Social determinants of adherence to pulmonary rehabilitation for chronic obstructive pulmonary disease. *COPD: J Chr Obstr Pulm Dis.* 2017;11:1–8.

79. Vogelmeier CF, Criner GJ, Martinez FJ, Anzueto A, Barnes PJ, Bourbeau J, et al. Global Strategy for the diagnosis, management and prevention of chronic obstructive lung disease 2017 report. *Respirology.* 2017;22(3):575–601.

80. Schuch FB, Vancampfort D, Richards J, Rosenbaum S, Ward PB, Stubbs B. Exercise as a treatment for depression: a meta-analysis adjusting for publication bias. *J Psychiatr Res.* 2016;77:42–51.

81. Emery C. Neuropsychiatric function in chronic lung disease: the role of pulmonary rehabilitation. *Resp Care.* 2008;53:1208–1216.

82. Bornstein DA, Borkovec TD. *Progressive Muscle Relaxation: A Manual for the Helping Professions.* Champaign, IL: Research Press; 1973.

83. Farver-Vestergaard I, Jacobsen D, Zachariae R. Efficacy of psychosocial interventions on psychological and physical health outcomes in chronic obstructive pulmonary disease: a systematic review and meta-analysis. *Psychother Psychomat.* 2015;84:37–50.

84. von Leupoldt A, Fritzsche A, Trueba AF, Meuret AE, Ritz, T. Behavioral medicine approaches to chronic obstructive pulmonary disease. *Ann Behavi Med.* 2012;44(1):52–65.

85. Beck AT, Rush AJ, Shaw BF, Emery G. *Cognitive Therapy of Depression.* New York: Guilford; 1979.

86. Abramowitz JS, Deacon BJ, Whiteside SPH. *Exposure Therapy for Anxiety: Principles and Practice.* New York: Guilford; 2011.

87. Vozoris NT, Fischer HD, Wang X, Anderson GM, Bell CM, Gershon AS, Stephenson AL, Gill SS, Rochon PA. Benzodiazepine use among older adults with chronic obstructive pulmonary disease: a population-based cohort study. *Drugs Aging.* 2013;30(3):183–192.

88. Griffin CE, Kaye AM, Bueno FR, Kaye AD. Benzodiazepine pharmacology and central nervous system–mediated effects. *Ochsner J.* 2013;13(2):214–223.

89. George CF, Bayliff CD. Management of insomnia in patients with chronic obstructive pulmonary disease. *Drugs.* 2003;63:379.

90. Ensrud KE, Blackwell TL, Mangione CM, Bowman PJ, Whooley MA, Bauer DC, Schwartz AV, Hanlon JT, Nevitt MC, for the Study of Osteoporotic Fractures Research Group. Central nervous system–active medications and risk for falls in older women. *J Am Geriat Soc.* 2002;50:1629–1637.

91. Miller WR, Rollnick S. *Motivational Interviewing: Preparing People for Change.* New York: Guilford; 2002.

92. Rubak S, Sandbæk A, Lauritzen T, Christensen B. Motivational interviewing: a systematic review and meta-analysis. *Br J Gen Pract.* 2005;55(513):305–312.

93. O'Halloran P, Blackstock F, Shields N, Holland A, Iles R, Kingsley M, Bernhardt J, Lanin N, Morris M, Taylor N. Motivational interviewing to increase physical activity in people with chronic health conditions: a systematic review and meta-analysis. *Clin Rehabil.* 2014;28:1159–1171.

94. Benzo R, Vickers K, Ernst D, Tucker S, McEvoy C, Lorig K. Development and feasibility of a self-management intervention for chronic obstructive pulmonary disease delivered with motivational interviewing strategies. *Journal of Cardiopulmonary Rehabilitation and Prevention.* 2013;33:113–122.

95. Miller WR, Rollnick S. Ten things that motivational interviewing is not. *Behav Cogn Psychoth.* 2009;37(2):129–140.

96. McGinnis JM, Foege WH. Actual causes of death in the United States. *JAMA.* 1993;270:2207–2212.

97. US Department of Health and Human Services. *The Health Consequences of Smoking—50 Years of Progress: A Report of the Surgeon General.* 2014.

98. Centers for Disease Control and Prevention. Annual smoking-attributable mortality, years of potential

life lost, and productivity losses—United States, 1997–2001. *MMWR*. 2005;54:625–628.

99. Quickstats: Percentage of adults who ever used an e-cigarette and percentage who currently use e-cigarettes, by age. National Health Interview Survey, United States, 2016.

100. Patnode CP, Henderson JT, Thompson JH, Senger CA, Fortmann SP, Whitlock EP. *Behavioral Counseling and Pharmacotherapy Interventions for Tobacco Cessation in Adults, Including Pregnant Women: A Review of Reviews for the U.S. Preventive Services Task Force*. Evidence Synthesis No. 134. AHRQ Publication No. 14-05200-EF-1. Rockville, MD: Agency for Healthcare Research and Quality; 2015.

101. Doll R, Peto R, Boreham J, Sutherland I. Mortality in relation to smoking: 50 years' observations on male British doctors. *BMJ*. 2004;328:1519.

102. Garcia-Rodrigueza O, et al. Probability and predictors of relapse to smoking: results of the National Epidemiologic Survey on Alcohol and Related Conditions (NESARC). *Drug Alcohol Depen*. 2013;132:470–485

103. National Institute of Drug Abuse. Fagerstrom test for nicotine dependence. https://cde.drugabuse.gov/instrument/d7c0b0f5-b865-e4de-e040-bb89ad43202b. 2017.

104. Niaura R, Abrams DB. Smoking cessation: progress, priorities, and prospectus. *J Consult Clin Psychol*. 2002;70(3):494.

105. Fiore MC, Jaen CR, Baker T, Bailey WC, Benowitz NL, Curry S, et al. Treating tobacco use and dependence: 2008 update. Rockville, MD: US Department of Health and Human Services.

## Chapter 6

1. Schols AM, Ferreira IM, Franssen FM, et al. Nutritional assessment and therapy in COPD: a European Respiratory Society statement. *Eur Respir J*, 2014;44:1504–1520.

2. Maltais F, Decramer M, Casaburi R, et al. An official American Thoracic Society/European Respiratory Society statement: update on limb muscle dysfunction in chronic obstructive pulmonary disease. *Am J Respir Crit Care Med*. 2014;189:e15-e62.

3. Schols AM, Soeters PB, Dingemans AM, Mostert R, Frantzen PJ, Wouters EF. Prevalence and characteristics of nutritional depletion in patients with stable COPD eligible for pulmonary rehabilitation. *Am Rev Respir Dis*. 1993;147:1151–1156.

4. Filley GF, Beckwitt HJ, Reeves JT, et al. Chronic obstructive bronchopulmonary disease. II. Oxygen transport in two clinical types. *Am J Med*. 1968;44:26–38.

5. Goris AH, Vermeeren MA, Wouters EF, Schols AM, Westerterp KR. Energy balance in depleted ambulatory patients with chronic obstructive pulmonary disease: the effect of physical activity and oral nutritional supplementation. *Br J Nutr*. 2003;89(5):725–731.

6. Schols AM, Soeters PB, Mostert R, Saris WH, Wouters EF. Energy balance in chronic obstructive pulmonary disease. *Am Rev Respir Dis*. 1991;143(6):1248–1252.

7. Kao CC, Hsu JW, Bandi V, Hanania NA, Kheradmand F, Jahoor F. Resting energy expenditure and protein turnover are increased in patients with severe chronic obstructive pulmonary disease. *Metabolism*. 2011;60(10):1449–1455.

8. Engelen MP, Deutz NE, Wouters EF, Schols AM. Enhanced levels of whole-body protein turnover in patients with chronic obstructive pulmonary disease. *Am J Respir Crit Care Med*. 2000;162(4 part 1):1488–1492.

9. Baarends EM, Schols AM, Akkermans MA, et al. Decreased mechanical efficiency in clinically stable patients with COPD. *Thorax*. 1997;52:981–986.

10. Baarends EM, Schols AM, Pannemans DL, et al. Total free living energy expenditure in patients with severe chronic obstructive pulmonary disease. *Am J Respir Crit Care Med*. 1997;155:549–554.

11. Kim V, Kretschman DM, Sternberg AL, et al. Weight gain after lung reduction surgery is related to improved lung function and ventilatory efficiency. *Am J Respir Crit Care Med*. 2012;186:1109–1116.

12. Wouters EFM. Chronic obstructive pulmonary disease: systemic effects of COPD. *Thorax*. 2002;57:1067–1070.

13. Landbo C, Prescott E, Lange P, et al. Prognostic value of nutritional status in chronic obstructive pulmonary disease. *Am J Respir Crit Care Med*. 1999;160:1856–1861.

14. Lainscak M, von Haehling S, Doehner W, et al. Body mass index and prognosis in patients hospitalized with acute exacerbation of chronic obstructive pulmonary disease. *J Cachexia Sarcopenia Muscle*. 2011;2:81–86.

15. Van den Borst B, Gosker HR, Koster A, et al. The influence of abdominal visceral fat on inflammatory pathways and mortality risk in obstructive lung disease. *Am J Clin Nutr*. 2012;96:516–526.

16. Schols AM, Broekhuizen R, Weling-Scheepers CW, Wouters EF. Body composition and mortality in chronic obstructive pulmonary disease. *Am J Clin Nutr*. 2005;82:53–59.

17. Kao CC, Hsu JW, Bandi V, Hanania NA, Kheradmand F, Jahoor F. Resting energy expenditure and

protein turnover are increased in patients with severe chronic obstructive pulmonary disease. *Metabolism.* 2011;60(10):1449–1455.

18. Engelen MP, Deutz NE, Wouters EF, Schols AM. Enhanced levels of whole-body protein turnover in patients with chronic obstructive pulmonary disease. *Am J Respir Crit Care Med.* 2000;162(4 part 1):1488–1492.

19. Rutten EP, Franssen FM, Engelen MP, Wouters EF, Deutz NE, Schols AM. Greater whole-body myofibrillar protein breakdown in cachectic patients with chronic obstructive pulmonary disease. *Am J Clin Nutr.* 2006;83(4):829–834.

20. Remels AH, Schrauwen P, Broekhuizen R, et al. Peroxisome proliferator-activated receptor expression is reduced in skeletal muscle in COPD. *Eur Respir J.* 2007;30(2):245–252.

21. Engelen MP, Wouters EF, Deutz NE, Menheere PP, Schols AM. Factors contributing to alterations in skeletal muscle and plasma amino acid profiles in patients with COPD. *Am J Clin Nutr.* 2000;72(6):1480–1487.

22. Haegens A, Schols AM, Van Essen AL, Van Loon LJ, Langen RC. Leucine induces myofibrillar protein accretion in cultured skeletal muscle through mTOR dependent and independent control of myosin heavy chain mRNA levels. *Mol Nutr Food Res.* 2012;56(5):741–752.

23. Engelen MP, De Castro CL, Rutten EP, Wouters EF, Schols AM, Deutz NE. Enhanced anabolic response to milk protein sip feeding in elderly subjects with COPD is associated with a reduced splanchnic extraction of multiple amino acids. *Clin Nutr.* 2012;31(5):616–624.

24. Rutten, E. Issues related to obesity in COPD. Nutritional Support in Pulmonary Disease Module 38.2. Online publication of Life Long Learning (LLL) Programme in Clinical Nutrition and Metabolism; 2017. ESPEN. http://lllnutrition.com /mod_lll/TOPIC38/m382.pdf.

25. Sin DD, Jones RL, Man SF. Obesity is a risk factor for dyspnea but not for airflow obstruction. *Arch Int Med.* 2002;162(13):1477–1481.

26. Cecere LM, Littman AJ, Slatore CG, et al. Obesity and COPD: associated symptoms, health-related quality of life, and medication use. *COPD.* 2011;8(4):275–284.

27. Ramachandran K, McCusker C, Connors M, ZuWallack R, Lahiri B. The influence of obesity on pulmonary rehabilitation outcomes in patients with COPD. *Chron Respir Dis.* 2008;5(4):205–209.

28. Leone N, Courbon D, Thomas F, et al. Lung function impairment and metabolic syndrome: the critical role of abdominal obesity. *Am J Respir Crit Care Med.* 2009;179(6):509–516.

29. Chailleux E, Laaban JP, Veale D. Prognostic value of nutritional depletion in patients with COPD treated by long-term oxygen therapy: data from the ANTADIR observatory. *Chest.* 2003;123(5):1460–1466.

30. Ora J, Laveneziana P, Ofir D, Deesomchok A, Webb KA, O'Donnell DE. Combined effects of obesity and COPD on dyspnea and exercise tolerance. *Am J Respir Crit Care Med.* 2009;180(10):964–971.

31. Kalantar-Zadeh K, Horwich TB, Oreopoulos A, et al. Risk factor paradox in wasting diseases. *Curr Opin Clin Nutr Metab Care.* 2007;10(4):433–442.

32. Hanson C, Rutten EP, Woutes EF, and Rennard S. Diet and vitamin D as risk factors for lung impairment and COPD. *Translat Res.* 2013;162(4):219–236.

33. McKeever TM, Lewis SA, Smit HA, Burney P, Cassano PA, Britton J. A multivariate analysis of serum nutrient levels and lung function. *Respir Res.* 2008;9:67.

34. Schunemann HJ, Grant BJ, Freudenheim JL, et al. The relation of serum levels of antioxidant vitamins C and E, retinol and carotenoids with pulmonary function in the general population. *Am J Respir Crit Care Med.* 2001;163(5):1246–1255.

35. Rautalahti M, Virtamo J, Haukka J, et al. The effect of alphatocopherol and beta-carotene supplementation on COPD symptoms. *Am J Respir Crit Care Med.* 1997;156:1447–1452.

36. Shaheen SO, Jameson KA, Robinson SM, et al. Relationship of vitamin D status to adult lung function and COPD. *Thorax.* 2011;66:692–698.

37. Kukuljan S, Nowson CA, Sanders K, Daly RM. Effects of resistance exercise and fortified milk on skeletal muscle mass, muscle size, and functional performance in middle-aged and older men: an 18-mo randomized controlled trial. *J Appl Physiol.* 2009;107:1864–1873.

38. Janssens W, Bouillon R, Claes B, Carremans C, Lehouck A, Buysschaert I, Coolen J, Mathieu C, Decramer M, Lambrechts D. Vitamin D deficiency is highly prevalent in COPD and correlates with variants in the vitamin D–binding gene. *Thorax.* 2010;65:215–220.

39. Romme EA, Rutten EP, Smeenk FW, Spruit MA, Menheere PP, Wouters EF. Vitamin D status is associated with bone mineral density and functional exercise capacity in patients with chronic obstructive pulmonary disease. *Ann Med.* 2012;45(1):91–96.

40. Lange NE, Sparrow D, Vokonas P, Litonjua AA. Vitamin D deficiency, smoking, and lung function in the normative aging study. *Am J Respir Crit Care Med.* 2012;186(7):616–621.

41. Kasper DL. *Harrison's Principles of Internal Medicine.* 19th ed. New York: McGraw-Hill; 2015.

42. Silverberg DS, Mor R, Weu MT, et al. Anemia and iron deficiency in COPD patients: prevalence and the effects of correction of the anemia with erythropoiesis stimulating agents and intravenous iron. *BMC Pulm Med.* 2014;14:24.

43. Van de Bool C, Mattijssen-Verdonschot C, Van Melick PPMJ, Spruit MA, Franssen FME, Wouters EFM, Schols A, Rutten EP. Quality of dietary intake in relation to body composition in patients with chronic obstructive pulmonary disease eligible for pulmonary rehabilitation. *Eur J Clin Nutr.* 2014;68(2):159–165.

44. Keranis E, Makris D, Rodopoulou P, et al. Impact of dietary shift to higher-antioxidant foods in COPD: a randomised trial. *Eur Respir J.* 2010;36(4):774–780.

45. Shaheen SO, Jameson KA, Syddall HE, et al. The relationship of dietary patterns with adult lung function and COPD. *Eur Respir J.* 2010;36:277–284.

46. Varraso R, Fung TT, Hu FB, et al. Prospective study of dietary patterns and chronic obstructive pulmonary disease among US men. *Thorax.* 2007;62:786–791.

47. Varraso R, Fung TT, Barr RG, et al. Prospective study of dietary patterns and chronic obstructive pulmonary disease among US women. *Am J Clin Nutr.* 2007;86:488–495.

48. Kaluza J, Larsson SC, Orsini N, Linden A, Wolk A. Fruit and vegetable consumption and risk of COPD: a prospective cohort study of men. *Thorax.* 2017;72(6):500–509.

49. Shalit N, Tierney A, Holland A, Miller B, Norris N, King S. Factors that influence dietary intake in adults with stable COPD. *Nutr Diet.* 2016;73:455–462.

50. Hronek M, Kovarik M, Aimova P, Koblizek V, Pavlikova L, Salajka F, Zadak Z. Skinfold anthropometry—the accurate method for fat free mass measurement in COPD. *COPD.* 2013;10:597–603.

51. Holley E, Thompson D. *Fitness Professionals Handbook.* 7th ed. Champaign, IL: Human Kinetics; 2016.

52. Heber D, Ingles S, Ashley JM, Maxwell MH, Lyons RF, Elashoff RM. Clinical detection of sarcopenic obesity by bioelectrical impedance analysis. *Am J Clin Nutr.* 1996;64:472S-477S.

53. Schutz Y, Kyle UU, Prichard C. Fat-free mass index and fat mass index percentiles in Caucasians aged 18–98 years. *Int J Obesity.* 2002;26(7):953–960.

54. Durnin JV, Womersley J. Body fat assessed from total body density and its estimation from skinfold thickness: measurements on 481 men and women aged from 16 to 72 years. *Br J Nutr.* 1974;32(1):77–97.

55. Jackson AS, Pollock ML. Generalized equations for predicting body density of men. *Br J Nutr.* 1978;40:497–504.

56. Jackson AS, Pollock ML, Ward A. Generalized equations for predicting body density of women. *Med Sci Sports Exerc.* 1980;12:175–181.

57. Nevill AN, Metsios GS, Jackson AS, Wang J, Thornton J, Gallagher D. Can we use the Jackson and Pollock equations to predict body density/fat of obese individuals in the 21st century? *Int J Body Compos Res.* 2008;6(3):114–121.

58. Cruz-Jentoft AJ, Baeyens JP, Bauer JM, et al. Sarcopenia: European consensus on definition and diagnosis: report of the European Working Group on Sarcopenia in Older People. *Age Ageing.* 2010;39(4):412–423.

59. Grodner M, Long S, DeYoung S. Nutrition in patient care. In: DeYoung S. *Foundations and Clinical Applications of Nutrition: A Nursing Approach.* 3rd ed. St. Louis, MO: Elsevier Health Sciences; 2004:406–407.

60. Kasper DL. *Harrison's Principles of Internal Medicine.* 19th ed. New York: McGraw-Hill; 2015.

61. Kim KM, Jang HC, Lim S. Differences among skeletal muscle mass indices derived from height-, weight-, and body mass index–adjusted models in assessing sarcopenia. *Korean J of Int Med.* 2016;31(4):643–650.

62. Calder, P, Laniano A, Lonnqvist F, Muscaritoll M, Ohlander M, Schols A. Targeted medical nutrition for cachexia in chronic obstructive pulmonary disease: a randomized, controlled trial. *J Cachexia Sarcopen.* 2018;9(1):28–40.

63. Atkins JL, Whincup PH, Morris RW, Lennon LT, Papacosta O, Wannamethee SG. Sarcopenic obesity and risk of cardiovascular disease and mortality: a population-based cohort study of older men. *J Am Geriatr Soc.* 2014;62:253-260.

64. Schols, AM. Nutritional advances in patients with respiratory diseases. *Eur Respir Rev.* 2015;24:17–22.

65. Thompson FE, Subar AF. Dietary assessment methodology. In: Coulston AM, Boushey C. *Nutrition in Prevention and Treatment of Disease.* San Diego: Academic Press; 2008:5–41.

66. Root M, Housera SM, Anderson JB, Dawson R. Healthy Eating Index 2005 and selected macronutrients are correlated with improved lung function in humans. *Nutr Res.* 2014;34(4):277–284.

67. Schwingshackl L, Hoffman G. Diet quality as assessed by the Healthy Eating Index, the Alternate Healthy Eating Index, the Dietary Approaches to Stop Hypertension Score, and health outcomes: a systematic review and meta-analysis of cohort studies. *J Acad Nutr Diet.* 2015;115:780–800.

68. Ferreira IM, Brooks D, White J, et al. Nutritional supplementation for stable chronic obstruc-

tive pulmonary disease. *Cochrane DB Syst Rev.* 2012;(12);CD000998.

69. Schols AM. The 2014 ESPEN Arvid Wretlind lecture: metabolism and nutrition: shifting paradigms in COPD management. *Clin Nutr.* 2015;34(6):1074–1079.

70. Vermeeren MA, Wouters EF, Nelissen LH, Van Lier A, Hofman Z, Schols AM. Acute effects of different nutritional supplements on symptoms and functional capacity in patients with chronic obstructive pulmonary disease. *Am J Clin Nutr.* 2001;73(2):295–301.

71. Talpers SS, Romberger D, et al. Nutritionally associated increased carbon dioxide production-excess total calories vs. high proportion of carbohydrate calories. *Chest.* 1992;102:551–555.

72. Schols AM. Nutrition as a metabolic modulator in COPD. *Chest.* 2013;144(4):1340–1345.

73. Steiner MC, Barton RL, Singh SJ, et al. Nutritional enhancement of exercise performance in chronic obstructive pulmonary disease: a randomised controlled trial. *Thorax.* 2003;58(9):745–751.

74. Varraso R, Chiuve SE, Fung TT, Barr RG, Hu F, Willett WC, Camargo CA. Alternate Healthy Eating Index 2010 and risk of chronic obstructive pulmonary disease among US women and men: prospective study. *BMJ.* 2015;350:h286.

75. Kan H, Stevens J, Heiss G, et al. Dietary fiber, lung function, and chronic obstructive pulmonary disease in the atherosclerosis risk in communities study. *Am J Epidemiol.* 2008;167:570–578.

76. Varraso R, Willett WC, Camargo CA Jr. Prospective study of dietary fiber and risk of chronic obstructive pulmonary disease among US women and men. *Am J Epidemiol.* 2010;171:776–784.

77. Agler AH, Kurth T, Gaziano JM, et al. Randomised vitamin E supplementation and risk of chronic lung disease in the Women's Health Study. *Thorax.* 2011;66:320–325.

78. Sinha A, Hollingsworth KG, Ball S, Cheetham T. Improving the vitamin D status of vitamin D deficient adults is associated with improved mitochondrial oxidative function in skeletal muscle. *J Clin Endocrinol Metab.* 2013;98(3):E509-E513.

79. Malinovschi A, Masoero M, Bellocchia M, Ciuffreda A, Solidoro P, Mattei A, et al. Severe vitamin D deficiency is associated with frequent exacerbations and hospitalization in COPD patients. *Respir Res.* 2014;15:131.

80. Hornikx M, Van Remoortel H, Lehouck A, et al. Vitamin D supplementation during rehabilitation in COPD: a secondary analysis of a randomized trial. *Resp Res.* 2012;13:84.

81. Bjerk SM, Edgington BD, Rector TS, Kunisaki, KM. Supplemental vitamin D and physical performance in COPD: a pilot randomization trial. *Int J Chron Obstruc Pulmon Dis.* 2013;8:97–104.

82. Brug J, Schols A, Mesters I. Dietary change, nutrition education and chronic obstructive pulmonary disease. *Patient Educ Counsel.* 2004;52(3):249–257.

## Chapter 7

1. Munro BH, ed. *Statistical Methods for Health Care Research.* 5th ed. Philadelphia: Lippincott Williams & Wilkins; 2005.

2. Troosters T, Gosselink R, Decramer M. Short- and long-term effects of outpatient rehabilitation in patients with chronic obstructive pulmonary disease: a randomized trial. *Am J Med.* 2000;109:207–212.

3. Pitta F, Troosters T, Probst VS, et al. Are patients with COPD more active after pulmonary rehabilitation? *Chest.* 2008;134:273–280.

4. Holland AE, Spruit MA, et al. Official ERS/ATS technical standard: field walking tests in chronic respiratory disease. *Eur Respir J.* 2014;44:1428–1446.

5. Singh SJ, Puhan MA, Andrianopoulos V, et al. An official systematic review of the ERS/ATS: measurement properties of field walking tests in chronic respiratory disease. *ERJ J.* 2014;44:1447–1478.

6. Dyer CAE, Singh SJ, Stockley RA, et al. The incremental shuttle walking test in elderly people with chronic airflow limitation. *Thorax.* 2002;57:34–38.

7. Revill SM, Morgan MDL, Singh SJ, et al. The endurance shuttle walk: a new field test for the assessment of endurance capacity in chronic obstructive pulmonary disease. *Thorax.* 1999;54:213–222.

8. Singh SJ, Morgan MD, Scott S, et al. Development of a shuttle walking test of disability in patients with chronic airways obstruction. *Thorax.* 1992;47:1019–1024.

9. Borg G. Perceived exertion as an indicator of somatic stress. *Scand J Rehab Med.* 1970;2:92–98.

10. Meek PM, Lareau SC. Critical outcomes in pulmonary rehabilitation: assessment and evaluation of dyspnea and fatigue. *J Rehab Res Dev.* 2003;40:13–24.

11. Aitken RCB. Measurement of feelings using visual analogue scales. *Proc R Soc Med.* 1969;62:989–993.

12. Fletcher CM. The clinical diagnosis of pulmonary emphysema: an experimental study. *Proc R Soc Med.* 1952;45:577–584.

13. Archibald CJ, Guidotti TL. Degree of objectively measured impairment and perceived shortness of breath with activities of daily living in patients with chronic obstructive pulmonary disease. *Can J Rehab.* 1987;1:45–54.

14. Eakin EG, Resnikoff PM, Prewitt LM, et al. Validation of a new dyspnea measure: the UCSD shortness of breath questionnaire. *Chest.* 1998;113:619–624.

15. Mahler D, Weinberg D, Wells C, et al. The measurement of dyspnea: contents, interobserver agreement and physiologic correlates of two new clinical indexes. *Chest.* 1984;85:751–758.

16. Guyatt GH, Berman LB, Townsend M, et al. A measure of quality of life for clinical trials in chronic lung disease. *Thorax.* 1987;42:773–778.

17. Yorke J, et al. Dyspnea-12 is a valid and reliable measure of breathlessness in patients with interstitial lung disease. *Chest.* 2011;139(1):159–164.

18. Norweg A, et al. A multidimensional computer adaptive test approach to dyspnea assessment. *Arch Phys Med Rehabil.* 2011;92(10):1561–1569.

19. FACIT-Dyspnea available at www.facit.org/facitorg/questionnaires.

20. Partridge MR, et al. Development and validation of the Capacity of Daily Living during the Morning questionnaire and the Global Chest Symptoms Questionnaire in COPD. *Eur Respir J.* 2010;36:96–104.

21. Meek PM, Banzett R, Parshall MB, Gracely RH, Schwartzstein RM, Lansing R. Reliability and validity of the multidimensional dyspnea profile. *Chest.* 2012;141(6):1546–1553.

22. Lareau SC, Carrieri-Kohlman V, Janson-Bjerklie S, et al. Development and testing of the Pulmonary Functional Status and Dyspnea Questionnaire (PFSDQ). *Heart Lung.* 1994;23:242–250.

23. Lareau SC, Meek PM, Roos PJ. Development and testing of a modified version of the Pulmonary Functional Status and Dyspnea Questionnaire (PFSDQ-M). *Heart Lung.* 1998;27:159–168.

24. Dodd JW, Mars PL, Clark AL, Ingram KA, Fowler RP, Canavan JL, et al. The COPD Assessment Test (CAT): short- and medium-term response to pulmonary rehabilitation. *COPD.* 2012;9(4):390–394.

25. Jones PW, Quirk FH, Baveystock CM, et al. A self-complete measure of health status for chronic airflow limitation: the St. George's Respiratory Questionnaire. *Am Rev Respir Dis.* 1992;145:1321–1327.

26. Ware JE, Sherbourne CD. The MOS 36-item short-form health survey (SF-36). I. Conceptual framework and item selection. *Med Care.* 1992;30:473–481.

27. Ferrans C, Powers M. Psychometric assessment of the Quality of Life Index. *Res Nurs Health.* 1992;15:29–38.

28. Stavem K, Jodalen H. Reliability and validity of the COOP/WONCA health status measure in patients with chronic obstructive pulmonarydisease. *Qual Life Res.* 2002;11(6):527–33.

29. Weaver TE, Narsavage GL, Guilfoyle MJ. The development and psychometric evaluation of the pulmonary functional status scale: an instrument to assess functional status in pulmonary disease. *J Cardiopulm Rehabil.* 1998;18:105–111.

30. Tu S-P, McDonell MB, Spertus JA, et al. Ambulatory Care Quality Improvement Project Investigators. A new self-administered questionnaire to monitor health-related quality of life in patients with COPD. *Chest.* 1997;112:614–622.

31. Guyatt GH, Berman LB, Townsend M, Pugsley SO, Chambers LW. A measure of quality of life for clinical trials in chronic lung disease. *Thorax.* 1987;42:773–778.

32. Williams JE, Singh SJ, Sewell L, Guyatt GH, Morgan MD. Development of a self-reported Chronic Respiratory Questionnaire (CRQ-SR). *Thorax.* 2001;56(12):954–959.

33. Schünemann HJ, Puhan M, Goldstein R, Jaeschke R, Guyatt GH. Measurement properties and interpretability of the chronic respiratory disease questionnaire (CRQ). *COPD.* 2005;2:81–89.

34. Wigal JK, Creer TL, Kotses H. The COPD self-efficacy scale. *Chest.* 1991;99:1193–1196.

35. Frei A, Svarin A, Steurer-Stey C, et al. Self-efficacy instruments for patients with chronic diseases suffer from methodological limitations—a systematic review. *Health Qual Life Outcomes.* 2009: 7:86–95.

36. Nishimura K, Izumi T, Tsukino M, et al. Dyspnea is a better predictor of 5-year survival than airway obstruction in patients with COPD. *Chest.* 2002;121:1434–1440.

37. Gerardi DA, Lovett L, Benoit-Connors ML, et al. Variables related to increased mortality following out-patient pulmonary rehabilitation. *Eur Respir J.* 1996;9:431–435.

38. Domingo-Salvany A, Lamarca R, Ferrer M, et al. Health-related quality of life and mortality in male patients with chronic obstructive pulmonary disease. *Am J Respir Crit Care Med.* 2002;166:680–685.

39. Bowen JB, Votto JJ, Thrall RS, et al. Functional status and survival following pulmonary rehabilitation. *Chest.* 2000;118:697–703.

40. Camillo CA, Langer D, Osadnik CR, Pancini L, Demeyer H, Burtin C, Gosselink R, Decramer M, Janssens W, Troosters T. Survival after pulmonary rehabilitation in patients with COPD: impact of functional exercise capacity and its changes. *Int J Chron Obstruct Pulmon Dis.* 2016;11:2671–2679.

41. Hakamy A, Bolton CE, McKeever TM. The effect of pulmonary rehabilitation on mortality, balance, and risk of fall in stable patients with chronic obstructive pulmonary disease: a systematic review. *Chr Resp Dis.* 2017;14(1):54–62.

42. Griffiths TL, Burr ML, Campbell IA, et al. Results at 1 year of outpatient multidisciplinary pulmonary rehabilitation: a randomised controlled trial. *Lancet.* 2000;355(9201):362–368.

43. Ries AL, Kaplan RM, Limberg TM, et al. Effects of pulmonary rehabilitation on physiologic and psycho-social outcomes in patients with chronic obstructive pulmonary disease. *Ann Intern Med.* 1995;122(11):823–832.

## Chapter 8

1. Ries AL. ACCP/AACVPR evidence-based guidelines for pulmonary rehabilitation. Round 3: another step forward. *J Cardiopulm Rehabil Prev.* 2007;27(4): 233–236.

2. Spruit MA, Singh SJ, Garvey C, et al. An official American Thoracic Society/European Respiratory Society statement: key concepts and advances in pulmonary rehabilitation. *Am J Respir Crit Care Med.* 2013;188(8):e13–e64.

3. Kitsantas A, Zimmerman BJ. Self-efficacy, activity participation, and physical fitness of asthmatic and nonasthmatic adolescent girls. *J Asthma.* 2000;37(2):163–174.

4. Folgering H, Van Herwaarden C. Pulmonary rehabilitation in asthma and COPD, physiological basics. *Respir Med.* 1993;87(Suppl B):41–44.

5. Kapadia SG, Wei C, Bartlett SJ, et al. Obesity and symptoms of depression contribute independently to the poor asthma control of obesity. *Respir Med.* 2014;108(8):1100–1107.

6. Carson KV, Chandratilleke MG, Picot J, Brinn MP, Esterman AJ, Smith BJ. Physical training for asthma. *Cochrane DB Syst Rev.* 2013;30(9):CD001116.

7. Mendes FA, Goncalves RC, Nunes MP, et al. Effects of aerobic training on psychosocial morbidity and symptoms in patients with asthma: a randomized clinical trial. *Chest.* 2010;138(2):331–337.

8. Rochester CL, Fairburn C, Crouch RH. Pulmonary rehabilitation for respiratory disorders other than chronic obstructive pulmonary disease. *Clin Chest Med.* 2014;35(2):369–389.

9. Harnett CM, Hunt EB, Bowen BR, et al. A study to assess inhaler technique and its potential impact on asthma control in patients attending an asthma clinic. *J Asthma.* 2014;51(4):440–445.

10. Clark NM, Gotsch A, Rosenstock IR. Patient, professional, and public education on behavioral aspects of asthma: a review of strategies for change and needed research. *J Asthma.* 1993;30(4):241–255.

11. Freitas DA, Holloway EA, Bruno SS, Chaves GS, Fregonezi GA, Mendonca KP. Breathing exercises for adults with asthma. *Cochrane DB Syst Rev.* 2013(10):Cd001277.

12. Carlin BW. Outcome measurement in pulmonary rehabilitation. *Respir Care Clin N Am.* 1998;4(1):113–127.

13. Basaran S, Guler-Uysal F, Ergen N, Seydaoglu G, Bingol-Karakoc G, Ufuk Altintas D. Effects of physical exercise on quality of life, exercise capacity and pulmonary function in children with asthma. *J Rehabil Med.* 2006;38(2):130–135.

14. Dyer CA, Hill SL, Stockley RA, Sinclair AJ. Quality of life in elderly subjects with a diagnostic label of asthma from general practice registers. *Eur Respir J.* 1999;14(1):39–45.

15. MacKenzie T, Gifford AH, Sabadosa KA, et al. Longevity of patients with cystic fibrosis in 2000 to 2010 and beyond: survival analysis of the Cystic Fibrosis Foundation patient registry. *Ann Intern Med.* 2014;161(4):233–241.

16. Moorcroft AJ, Dodd ME, Morris J, Webb AK. Individualised unsupervised exercise training in adults with cystic fibrosis: a 1 year randomised controlled trial. *Thorax.* 2004;59(12):1074–1080.

17. Boas SR. Exercise recommendations for individuals with cystic fibrosis. *Sports Med.* 1997;24(1): 17–37.

18. Selvadurai HC, Blimkie CJ, Meyers N, Mellis CM, Cooper PJ, Van Asperen PP. Randomized controlled study of in-hospital exercise training programs in children with cystic fibrosis. *Pediatr Pulmonol.* 2002;33(3):194–200.

19. McKone EF, Barry SC, FitzGerald MX, Gallagher CG. The role of supplemental oxygen during submaximal exercise in patients with cystic fibrosis. *Eur Respir J.* 2002;20(1):134–142.

20. Stevens D, Stephenson A, Faughnan ME, Leek E, Tullis E. Prognostic relevance of dynamic hyperinflation during cardiopulmonary exercise testing in adult patients with cystic fibrosis. *J Cyst Fibros.* 2013;12(6):655–661.

21. Dekerlegand RL, Hadjiliadis D, Swisher AK, Parrott JS, Heuer AJ, Myslinski MJ. Inspiratory muscle strength relative to disease severity in adults with stable cystic fibrosis. *J Cyst Fibros.* 2015;14(5):639–645.

22. Schneiderman JE, Wilkes DL, Atenafu EG, et al. Longitudinal relationship between physical activity and lung health in patients with cystic fibrosis. *Eur Respir J.* 2014;43(3):817–823.

23. Nixon PA, Orenstein DM, Kelsey SF, Doershuk CF. The prognostic value of exercise testing in patients with cystic fibrosis. *N Engl J Med.* 1992;327(25):1785–1788.

24. Hebestreit H, Kieser S, Junge S, et al. Long-term effects of a partially supervised conditioning programme in cystic fibrosis. *Eur Respir J.* 2010;35(3): 578–583.

25. Klijn PH, Oudshoorn A, Van der Ent CK, Van der Net J, Kimpen JL, Helders PJ. Effects of anaerobic training in children with cystic fibrosis: a randomized controlled study. *Chest.* 2004;125(4): 1299–1305.

26. Kriemler S, Kieser S, Junge S, et al. Effect of supervised training on FEV₁ in cystic fibrosis: a randomised controlled trial. *J Cyst Fibros.* 2013;12(6): 714–720.

27. Cerny FJ. Relative effects of bronchial drainage and exercise for in-hospital care of patients with cystic fibrosis. *Phys Ther.* 1989;69(8):633–639.

28. Flume PA, Robinson KA, O'Sullivan B, et al. Cystic fibrosis pulmonary guidelines: airway clearance therapies. *Respiratory Care.* 2009;54(4):15.

29. Frangolias DD, Holloway CL, Vedal S, Wilcox PG. Role of exercise and lung function in predicting work status in cystic fibrosis. *Am J Respir Crit Care Med.* 2003;167(2):150–157.

30. Moorcroft AJ, Dodd ME, Webb AK. Exercise limitations and training for patients with cystic fibrosis. *Disabil Rehabil.* 1998;20(6–7):247–253.

31. Enright S, Chatham K, Ionescu AA, Unnithan VB, Shale DJ. Inspiratory muscle training improves lung function and exercise capacity in adults with cystic fibrosis. *Chest.* 2004;126(2):405–411.

32. Sawyer EH, Clanton TL. Improved pulmonary function and exercise tolerance with inspiratory muscle conditioning in children with cystic fibrosis. *Chest.* 1993;104(5):1490–1497.

33. Dasenbrook EC, Merlo CA, Diener-West M, Lechtzin N, Boyle MP. Persistent methicillin-resistant Staphylococcus aureus and rate of FEV₁ decline in cystic fibrosis. *Am J Respir Crit Care Med.* 2008;178(8): 814–821.

34. Snell G, Reed A, Stern M, Hadjiliadis D. The evolution of lung transplantation for cystic fibrosis: a 2017 update. *J Cyst Fibros.* 2017;16(5):553–564.

35. Saiman L, Siegel JD, LiPuma JJ, et al. Infection prevention and control guideline for cystic fibrosis: 2013 update. *Infect Control Hosp Epidemiol.* 2014;35(Suppl 1):S1-S67.

36. Stallings VA, Stark LJ, Robinson KA, et al. Evidence-based practice recommendations for nutrition-related management of children and adults with cystic fibrosis and pancreatic insufficiency: results of a systematic review. *J Am Diet Assoc.* 2008;108(5):832–839.

37. Orenstein DM, Nixon PA, Ross EA, Kaplan RM. The quality of well-being in cystic fibrosis. *Chest.* 1989;95(2):344–347.

38. Quittner AL, Sweeny S, Watrous M, et al. Translation and linguistic validation of a disease-specific quality of life measure for cystic fibrosis. *J Pediatr Psychol.* 2000;25(6):403–414.

39. Gee L, Abbott J, Conway SP, Etherington C, Webb AK. Development of a disease specific health related quality of life measure for adults and adolescents with cystic fibrosis. *Thorax.* 2000;55(11): 946–954.

40. Pasteur MC, Bilton D, Hill AT, British Thoracic Society Non CFBGG. British Thoracic Society guideline for non-CF bronchiectasis. *Thorax.* 2010;65(7):577.

41. Newall C, Stockley RA, Hill SL. Exercise training and inspiratory muscle training in patients with bronchiectasis. *Thorax.* 2005;60(11):943–948.

42. Mandal P, Sidhu MK, Kope L, et al. A pilot study of pulmonary rehabilitation and chest physiotherapy versus chest physiotherapy alone in bronchiectasis. *Respir Med.* 2012;106(12):1647–1654.

43. Lee AL, Hill CJ, Cecins N, et al. The short and long term effects of exercise training in non-cystic fibrosis bronchiectasis—a randomised controlled trial. *Respir Res.* 2014;15:44.

44. Ryerson CJ, Abbritti M, Ley B, Elicker BM, Jones KD, Collard HR. Cough predicts prognosis in idiopathic pulmonary fibrosis. *Respirology.* 2011;16(6): 969–975.

45. Markovitz GH, Cooper CB. Exercise and interstitial lung disease. *Curr Opin Pulm Med.* 1998;4(5):272–280.

46. Marciniuk DD, Gallagher CG. Clinical exercise testing in interstitial lung disease. *Clin Chest Med.* 1994;15(2):287–303.

47. O'Donnell DE, Chau LK, Webb KA. Qualitative aspects of exertional dyspnea in patients with interstitial lung disease. *J Appl Physiol* 1998;84(6): 2000–2009.

48. Hsia CC. Cardiopulmonary limitations to exercise in restrictive lung disease. *Med Sci Sports Exerc.* 1999;31(1 Suppl):S28–32.

49. Khanna D, Clements PJ, Furst DE, et al. Correlation of the degree of dyspnea with health-related quality of life, functional abilities, and diffusing capacity for carbon monoxide in patients with systemic sclerosis and active alveolitis: results from the Scleroderma Lung Study. *Arthritis Rheum.* 2005;52(2):592–600.

50. Foster S, Thomas HM 3rd. Pulmonary rehabilitation in lung disease other than chronic obstructive pulmonary disease. *Am Rev Respir Dis.* 1990;141(3):601–604.

51. Nonn RA, Garrity ER Jr. Lung transplantation for fibrotic lung diseases. *Am J Med Sci.* 1998;315(3): 146–154.

52. Johnson-Warrington V, Mitchell KE, Singh SJ. Is a practice incremental shuttle walk test needed for patients with chronic obstructive pulmonary disease admitted to hospital for an acute exacerbation? *Respiration.* 2015;90(3):206–210.

53. Nishiyama O, Kondoh Y, Kimura T, et al. Effects of pulmonary rehabilitation in patients with idiopathic pulmonary fibrosis. *Respirology.* 2008;13(3):394–399.

54. Ferreira A, Garvey C, Connors GL, et al. Pulmonary rehabilitation in interstitial lung disease: benefits and predictors of response. *Chest.* 2009;135(2): 442–447.

55. Bajwah S, Ross JR, Peacock JL, et al. Interventions to improve symptoms and quality of life of patients with fibrotic interstitial lung disease: a systematic review of the literature. *Thorax.* 2013;68(9): 867–879.

56. Dowman L, Hill CJ, Holland AE. Pulmonary rehabilitation for interstitial lung disease. *Cochrane DB Syst Rev.* 2014;6(10):CD006322.

57. Ryerson CJ, Cayou C, Topp F, et al. Pulmonary rehabilitation improves long-term outcomes in interstitial lung disease: a prospective cohort study. *Respir Med.* 2014;108(1):203–210.

58. Dowman LM, McDonald CF, Hill CJ, et al. The evidence of benefits of exercise training in interstitial lung disease: a randomised controlled trial. *Thorax.* 2017;72(7):610–619.

59. Nagata K, Tomii K, Otsuka K, et al. Evaluation of the chronic obstructive pulmonary disease assessment test for measurement of health-related quality of life in patients with interstitial lung disease. *Respirology.* 2012;17(3):506–512.

60. Aboussouan LS. Mechanisms of exercise limitation and pulmonary rehabilitation for patients with neuromuscular disease. *Chron Respir Dis.* 2009;6(4):231–249.

61. Kilmer DD. Response to aerobic exercise training in humans with neuromuscular disease. *Am J Phys Med Rehabil.* 2002;81(11 Suppl):S148–150.

62. Bach JR. A historical perspective on the use of noninvasive ventilatory support alternatives. *Respir Care Clin N Am.* 1996;2(2):161–181.

63. Cup EH, Pieterse AJ, Ten Broek-Pastoor JM, et al. Exercise therapy and other types of physical therapy for patients with neuromuscular diseases: a systematic review. *Arch Phys Med Rehabil.* 2007;88(11):1452–1464.

64. Morrow B, Zampoli M, Van Aswegen H, Argent A. Mechanical insufflation-exsufflation for people with neuromuscular disorders. *Cochrane DB Syst Rev.* 2013;12:CD010044.

65. Morris NR, Kermeen FD, Holland AE. Exercise-based rehabilitation programmes for pulmonary hypertension. *Cochrane DB Syst Rev.* 2017;1: CD011285.

66. Mainguy V, Maltais F, Saey D, et al. Peripheral muscle dysfunction in idiopathic pulmonary arterial hypertension. *Thorax.* 2010;65(2):113–117.

67. Thabut G, Dauriat G, Stern JB, et al. Pulmonary hemodynamics in advanced COPD candidates for lung volume reduction surgery or lung transplantation. *Chest.* 2005;127(5):1531–1536.

68. Benza RL, Miller DP, Gomberg-Maitland M, et al. Predicting survival in pulmonary arterial hypertension: insights from the Registry to Evaluate Early and Long-Term Pulmonary Arterial Hypertension Disease Management (REVEAL). *Circulation.* 2010;122(2):164–172.

69. Matthay RA, Niederman MS, Wiedemann HP. Cardiovascular-pulmonary interaction in chronic obstructive pulmonary disease with special reference to the pathogenesis and management of cor pulmonale. *Med Clin North Am.* 1990;74(3):571–618.

70. Miyamoto S, Nagaya N, Satoh T, et al. Clinical correlates and prognostic significance of six-minute walk test in patients with primary pulmonary hypertension. Comparison with cardiopulmonary exercise testing. *Am J Respir Crit Care Med.* 2000;161(2 Pt 1):487–492.

71. Puente-Maestu L, Palange P, Casaburi R, et al. Use of exercise testing in the evaluation of interventional efficacy: an official ERS statement. *Eur Respir J.* 2016;47(2):429–460.

72. Stiebellehner L, Quittan M, End A, et al. Aerobic endurance training program improves exercise performance in lung transplant recipients. *Chest.* 1998;113(4):906–912.

73. Troosters T, Gosselink R, Decramer M. Chronic obstructive pulmonary disease and chronic heart failure: two muscle diseases? *J Cardiopulm Rehabil.* 2004;24(3):13.

74. Troosters T, Van Remoortel H. Pulmonary rehabilitation and cardiovascular disease. *Semin Respir Crit Care Med.* 2009;30(6):675–683.

75. Buys R, Avila A, Cornelissen VA. Exercise training improves physical fitness in patients with pulmonary arterial hypertension: a systematic review and meta-analysis of controlled trials. *BMC Pulm Med.* 2015;15:40.

76. Raskin J, Qua D, Marks T, Sulica R. A retrospective study on the effects of pulmonary rehabilitation in patients with pulmonary hypertension. *Chron Respir Dis.* 2014;11(3):153–162.

77. Crouch R, MacIntyre NR. Pulmonary rehabilitation of the patient with nonobstructive lung disease. *Respir Care Clin N Am.* 1998;4(1):59–70.

78. Desai SA, Channick RN. Exercise in patients with pulmonary arterial hypertension. *J Cardiopulm Rehabil Prev.* 2008;28(1):12–16.

79. Jemal A, Thomas A, Murray T, et al. Cancer statistics. *Cancer J Clin.* 2002;52:23–47.

80. Maione P, Perrone F, Gallo C, et al. Pretreatment quality of life and functional status assessment

significantly predict survival of elderly patients with advanced non-small-cell lung cancer receiving chemotherapy: a prognostic analysis of the multicenter Italian lung cancer in the elderly study. *J Clin Oncol.* 2005;23(28):6865–6872.

81. MacDonald N. Cancer cachexia and targeting chronic inflammation: a unified approach to cancer treatment and palliative/supportive care. *J Support Oncol.* 2007;5(4):157–162.

82. Dimeo F, Schwartz S, Wesel N, et al. Effects of an endurance and resistance exercise program on persistent cancer-related fatigue after treatment. *Ann Oncol.* 2008;19:1495–1499.

83. Benzo RP. Pulmonary rehabilitation in lung cancer: a scientific opportunity. *J Cardiopulm Rehabil Prev.* 2007;27:61–64.

84. Bobbio A, Chetta A, Ampollini L, Primomo L, Internullo I, Carbognani P, Rusca M, Olivieri D. Preoperative pulmonary rehabilitation in patients undergoing lung resection for non-small cell lung cancer. *Eur J Card Thorac Surg.* 2008;33(1):95–98.

85. Benzo R, Wigle D, Novotny P, Wetzstein M, Nichols F, Shen RK, Cassivi S, Deschamps C. Preoperative pulmonary rehabilitation before lung cancer resection: results from two randomized studies. *Lung Cancer.* 2011;74(3):441–445.

86. Shannon VR. Role of pulmonary rehabilitation in the management of patients with lung cancer. *Curr Opin Pulm Med.* 2010;16(4):334–339.

87. Jones LW, Peddle CJ, Eves ND, et al. Effects of pre-surgical exercise training on cardiorespiratory fitness among patients undergoing thoracic surgery for malignant lung lesions. *Cancer.* 2007;110:590–598.

88. Bobbio A, Chetta A, Ampollini L, et al. Preoperative pulmonary rehabilitation in patients undergoing lung resection for non-small cell lung cancer. *Eur J Cardiothorac Surg.* 2008;33:95–98.

89. Warner MA, Offord KP, Warner ME, et al. Role of preoperative cessation of smoking and other factors in postoperative pulmonary complications: a blinded prospective study of coronary artery bypass patients. *Mayo Clin Proc.* 1989;64:609.

90. Wilson DJ. Pulmonary rehabilitation exercise program for high risk thoracic surgical patients. *Chest Surg Clin N Am.* 1997;7(4):697–706.

91. Bartels MN, Kim H, Whiteson JH, et al. Pulmonary rehabilitation in patients undergoing lung-volume reduction surgery. *Arch Phys Med Rehabil.* 2006;87(3 Suppl 1):S84–90.

92. Morano T, Araujo AS, Nascimento FB, DaSilva F, Mewquita R, Pinto JS, de Moraes Fiho MO, Pereira D. Preoperative pulmonary rehabilitation versus chest physical therapy in patients under-

going lung cancer resection: a pilot randomized controlled trial. *Arch Phys Med and Rehabil.* 2013;94(1):53–58.

93. Kaneda H, Saito Y, Okamoto M, et al. Early postoperative mobilization with walking at 4 hours after lobectomy in lung cancer patients. *Gen Thorac Cardiovasc Surg.* 2007;55(12):493–498.

94. Cesario A, Ferri L, Galetta D, et al. Post-operative respiratory rehabilitation after lung resection for non-small cell lung cancer. *Lung Cancer.* 2007;57:175–180.

95. Spruit MA, Janssen PP, Willemsen SCP, et al. Exercise capacity before and after an 8-week multidisciplinary inpatient pulmonary rehabilitation program in lung cancer patients: a pilot study. *Lung Cancer.* 2006;52:257–260.

96. Granger CL, McDonald CF, Berney S, Chao C, Denehy L. Exercise intervention to improve exercise capacity and health related quality of life for patients with non-small cell lung cancer: a systematic review. *Lung Cancer.* 2011;72(2):139–153.

97. Flaherty KR, Martinez FJ. Lung volume reduction surgery for emphysema. *Clin Chest Med.* 2000;21:819–848.

98. Cordova FC, Criner GJ. Surgery for chronic obstructive pulmonary disease: the place for lung volume reduction and transplantation. *Curr Opin Pulm Med.* 2001;7(2):93–104.

99. National Emphysema Treatment Trial Research Group. Rationale and design of the National Emphysema Treatment Trial: a prospective randomized trial of lung volume reduction surgery. *J Cardiopulm Rehabil.* 2000;20(1):24–36.

100. National Emphysema Treatment Trial Research Group. A randomized controlled trial comparing lung volume reduction surgery with medical therapy for severe emphysema. *N Engl J Med.* 2003;348(21):2059–2073.

101. Ries AL, Make BJ, Lee SM, et al. The effects of pulmonary rehabilitation in the National Emphysema Treatment Trial. *Chest.* 2005;128(6):3799–3809.

102. Debigare R, Maltais F, Whittom F, et al. Feasibility and efficacy of home exercise training before lung volume reduction. *J Cardiopulm Rehabil.* 1999;19(4):235–241.

103. Rochester CL. Pulmonary rehabilitation for patients who undergo lung-volume-reduction surgery or lung transplantation. *Respir Care.* 2008;53(9):1–7.

104. Arcasoy SM, Wild J. Medical complications after lung transplantation. *Semin Respir Crit Care Med.* 2006;27(5):508–520.

105. Hoffman M, Chaves G, Ribeiro-Samora GA, Britto RR, Parreira VF. Effects of pulmonary rehabilita-

tion in lung transplant candidates: a systematic review. *BMJ Open*. 2017;7:e013445.

106. Maury G, Langer D, Verleden G, et al. Skeletal muscle force and functional exercise tolerance before and after lung transplantation: a cohort study. *Am J Transplant*. 2008;8(6):1275–1281.

107. Reinsma GD, Ten Hacken NH, Grevnik RG, et al. Limiting factors of exercise performance 1 year after lung transplantation. *J Heart Lung Transplant*. 2006;25(11):1310–1316.

108. Van Der Woude BT, Kropmans TJ, Douma KW, et al. Peripheral muscle force and exercise capacity in lung transplant candidates. *Int J Rehabil Res*. 2002;25(4):351–355.

109. American Association of Cardiovascular and Pulmonary Rehabilitation (AACVPR). *Guidelines for Cardiac Rehabilitation and Secondary Prevention Programs*. 5th ed. Champaign, IL: Human Kinetics; 2013.

## Chapter 10

1. Committee on Quality Health Care in America, Institute of Medicine. *Crossing the Quality Chasm: A New Health System for the 21st Century*. Washington, DC: National Academy Press; 2001.

2. AACVPR Clinical Competency Guidelines for Pulmonary Rehabilitation Professionals. *J Cardiopulm Rehabil Prev*. 2014;34:291–302.

# Index

*Note:* The italicized *f* and *t* following page numbers refer to figures and tables, respectively.

# About the AACVPR

The **American Association of Cardiovascular and Pulmonary Rehabilitation (AACVPR)** is dedicated to improving the quality of life for patients and their families by reducing morbidity, mortality, and disability from cardiovascular and pulmonary disease through education, prevention, rehabilitation, research, and disease management. AACVPR is a multidisciplinary professional association composed of health professionals who serve in the field of cardiac and pulmonary rehabilitation. AACVPR also provides educational and professional development opportunities to its members, which include cardiovascular and pulmonary physicians, nurses, exercise physiologists, physical therapists, behavioral scientists, respiratory therapists, and nutritionists.